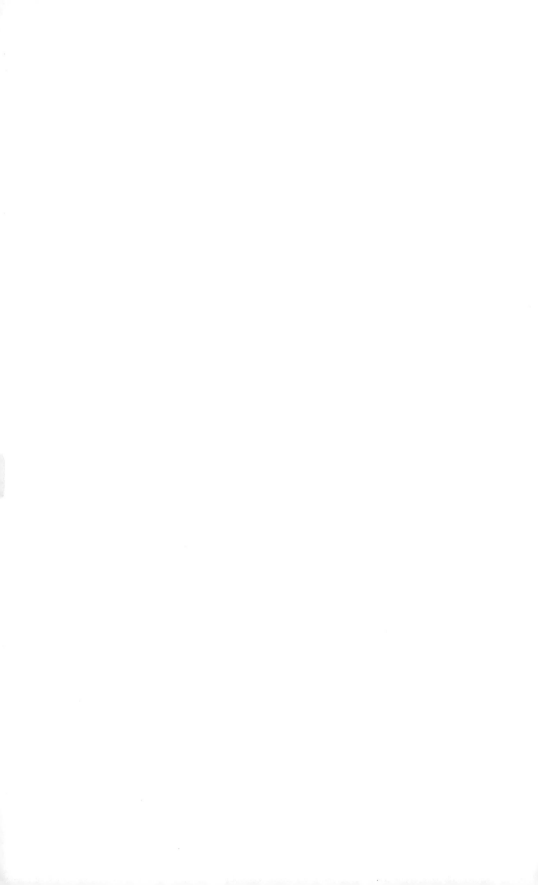

HEALTHY FOODS

HEALTHY FOODS

Fact versus Fiction

Myrna Chandler Goldstein
and Mark A. Goldstein, MD

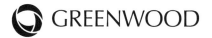 GREENWOOD

AN IMPRINT OF ABC-CLIO, LLC
Santa Barbara, California • Denver, Colorado • Oxford, England

Library of Congress Cataloging-in-Publication Data
Goldstein, Myrna Chandler, 1948–
   Healthy foods : fact versus fiction / Myrna Chandler Goldstein
and Mark A. Goldstein.
      p. cm.
   Includes bibliographical references and index.
   ISBN 978-0-313-38096-9 (hard copy : alk. paper)—ISBN 978-0-313-38097-6
(ebook) 1. Food. 2. Nutrition. I. Goldstein, Mark A. (Mark Allan), 1947– II. Title.
   TX355.G67 2010
   641.3—dc22   2010013684

ISBN: 978-0-313-38096-9
EISBN: 978-0-313-38097-6

14   13   12   11   2   3   4   5

This book is also available on the World Wide Web as an eBook.
Visit www.abc-clio.com for details.

Greenwood Press
An Imprint of ABC-CLIO, LLC

ABC-CLIO, LLC
130 Cremona Drive, P.O. Box 1911
Santa Barbara, California 93116-1911

This book is printed on acid-free paper ∞

Manufactured in the United States of America

Copyright Acknowledgments

All photographs are courtesy of Mark A. Goldstein, MD.

CONTENTS

INTRODUCTION

Every day, consumers are bombarded with information about food. Wherever they go and whatever they do, consumers are confronted with a never-ending commentary on the topic. And, all too often, the material that is presented may be heralded one day and denounced the next. Dietitians and nutritionists may sing endless praises for certain foods; later, consumers may be advised to eliminate these same foods from their diets. For example, for years, all fats were lumped together in one giant pot. People were told to reduce or eliminate fat from their diets. It is now recognized that some fats, such as olive oil, may play an integral role in a healthful diet.

The goal of this book is to investigate the research behind some 50 supposedly healthful foods. In many cases, that is relatively easy. There are a number of foods that have been extensively studied. But, that is not true for some supposedly healthful foods. In numerous instances, we were unable to locate a sufficient amount of research to write an entry. Moreover, there are about a dozen healthier foods that are grown with large amounts of pesticides. It is our belief that the benefits obtained from eating those foods may well be compromised by the pesticides. (Those consumers who wish to reduce their intake of pesticides should purchase the organically grown versions of those foods.)

It is also important to realize that even truly beneficial foods should be eaten as part of an overall wholesome and nourishing diet. Thus, though blueberries are a superb addition to the diet, no one would advise people to eat them three times a day. It is especially important not to eat large amounts of dried fruit, with their concentrations of sugar. And, while the consumption of organic apples strongly supports good health, they will do very little to assist a daily lunch of pizza and a bag of chips.

For most people, their diet should consist primarily of fruits, vegetables, beans, legumes, nuts, seeds, and whole grains. However, their diet should also include lean protein obtained from lean poultry, cold-water fish (such as sardines, halibut, and wild salmon), and tofu, and healthier fatty foods, such as olive oil, sesame seeds, and avocados. Foods with saturated fat, such as red meat, should be consumed sparingly. Sometimes, it is advantageous to eliminate them from the diet. In fact, many vegans, people who eat no animal products, report improvements in their health and well-being and a greater ease in maintaining a healthful weight.

At present, about two-thirds of Americans are overweight or obese. These conditions are associated with other medical problems such as diabetes, cancer, and cardiovascular disease. If more Americans could find ways to include greater amounts of healthier foods in their diets, the prevalence of these illnesses could be reduced. We hope that this book plays a role in that undertaking.

ALMONDS

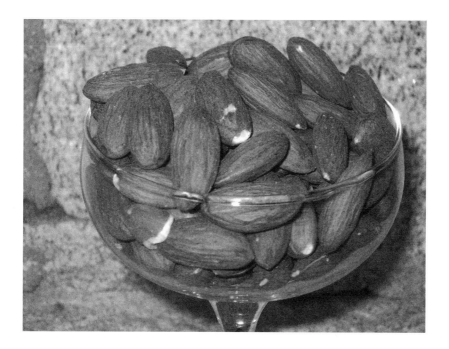

Although the vast majority of people view almonds as a type of nut, technically, they are not. In fact, almonds are actually the seeds of the fruit of the almond tree, a mid-sized tree that has aromatic pink and white flowers. There are two types of almonds: sweet and bitter. Only the sweet are eaten; bitter almonds are used to make almond oil.

Believed to have originated in North Africa and western Asia, almonds have been grown for thousands of years. They are even mentioned in the Bible. Today, almonds flourish in countries that border the Mediterranean Sea, such as Spain and Italy. In the United States, they are grown in California.[1]

Known to be high in fat, almonds have been shunned by some people concerned about weight gain. Is that a wise choice?

CARDIOVASCULAR HEALTH

Led by Canadian David J. A. Jenkins, MD, a group of researchers have conducted a number of studies on almonds and other foods that tend to lower bad (low-density lipoprotein, or LDL) cholesterol. One study that is frequently noted was published in 2002 in *Circulation*. The three-month study included 15 men and 12 postmenopausal women (average age 64) who had elevated levels of cholesterol. Their mean total cholesterol level was 260 milligrams per deciliter (mg/dl). During the first month, the participants consumed an average of 74 grams of almonds each day. That meant that almonds comprised almost 25 percent of their diets. During the second month, they ate about 37 grams of almonds each day. In the last month, they ate a low-saturated-fat whole-wheat muffin. The results were truly stunning. When the participants ate the half-portion of almonds, their levels of LDL cholesterol dropped an average of 4.4 percent; when they ate the full portion, their LDL levels dropped an average of 9.4 percent. The whole-wheat muffins did not appear to have any significant effects on cholesterol levels. The researchers concluded that, "almonds used as snacks in the diets of hyperlipidemic subjects significantly reduce coronary heart disease risk factors, probably in part because of the nonfat (protein and fiber) and monounsaturated fatty acid components of the nuts."[2]

Another study led by Dr. Jenkins was published in 2006 in *The American Journal of Clinical Nutrition*. In the study, people followed a dietary plan known as the Portfolio Eating Plan (which includes lipid-lowering foods such as plant sterols, viscous fiber, soy protein, and almonds) for a year. Of the 55 people who completed the study, almost one-third reduced their LDL (bad) cholesterol by more than 20 percent. That's the same reduction seen by people who take the first generation of statin drugs, such as Pravachol.[3]

Dr. Jenkins was also interested in the role that the Portfolio diet could play in helping to control blood pressure. When he and his associates studied the association between cholesterol-lowering foods and blood pressure, they found that these foods had a strong impact. In fact, in an article published in June 2008 in the *European Journal of Clinical Nutrition*, the researchers noted that, "A dietary portfolio of plant-based cholesterol-lowering foods reduced blood pressure significantly, related to almond intake. The dietary portfolio of combining a range of cholesterol-lowering foods may benefit cardiovascular disease risk both by reducing serum lipids and also blood pressure."[4]

WEIGHT MANAGEMENT

Could eating almonds actually help people lose weight? A study published in 2003 in the *International Journal of Obesity* placed 65 overweight or obese people on either an almond-enriched low-calorie diet or a low-calorie diet high in complex carbohydrates. While both diets contained the same amount of calories and equivalent amounts of protein, the people eating the almond enriched diet consumed 39 percent of their calories from fat, 25 percent from monounsaturated fat; the people on the high-complex-carbohydrates diet consumed only 18 percent of their calories from fat, of which 5 percent was monounsaturated fat. Fifty-three percent of their calories came from carbohydrates. At the end of 24 weeks, the almond-eating people lost more weight, more body fat, and had greater reductions in their waistlines. They also had reductions in total body water and systolic blood pressure. The almond diet even appeared to be more beneficial for those subjects with type 1 diabetes. Ninety-six percent of the subjects with type 1 diabetes who ate the almond diet were able to reduce their medication; only 50 percent of those on the complex carbohydrate diet could do that. The researchers concluded that, "Almond supplementation of a formula-based LCD [low-calorie diet] is a novel alternative to self-selected complex carbohydrates and has a potential role in reducing the public health implications of obesity."[5]

Another almond weight study was conducted by two Purdue University researchers and published in 2007 in the *British Journal of Nutrition*. In a 23-week crossover study, which included 20 women with a mean age of 24 and a mean body mass index (BMI) of 25, participants were randomized to either eat a diet with almonds or eat their usual diet. The almond group added about two ounces per day of almonds to their regular diet. That's a whopping 344 calories! The control group ate their regular diet and no almonds. After ten weeks, everyone had a three-week washout period. Then, the control group ate daily almonds for ten weeks, and the original almond group ate no almonds. The researchers found that participants who ate the almonds did not gain weight. How could that be? Apparently, since the participants felt satisfied, they reduced their consumption of other foods. The researchers also observed that the subjects who ate almonds tended to eat smaller amounts of carbohydrates. So, the almonds replaced carbohydrate-rich foods.[6]

OVERALL HEALTH AND WELL-BEING

In a study published in 2004 in the *British Journal of Nutrition*, researchers from California's Loma Linda University studied some of the benefits of adding almonds to the diet of 81 men and women between the ages of 25 and 70. During the first six months of the study, the participants ate their usual diet; during the second six months of the study, everyone added an average of 52 grams of almonds to their daily diet (about two ounces). The researchers found that by including almonds in their diets, the subjects increased their intake of monounsaturated and polyunsaturated fats, dietary fiber, vegetable protein, alpha-tocopherol vitamin E, magnesium, and copper. At the same time, the subjects reduced their intake of trans fats, sodium, cholesterol, and sugars. The researchers noted that, "These spontaneous nutrient changes closely match the dietary recommendations to prevent cardiovascular and other chronic diseases."[7]

In a study conducted at the Jean Mayer U.S. Department of Agriculture (USDA) Human Nutrition Research Center on Aging at Tufts University in Boston and published in 2005 in *The Journal of Nutrition*, researchers determined that the antioxidants in the skin of almonds and the vitamin E contained within almonds are a strong antioxidant team. Thus, while the flavonoids in almond skins enhanced LDL's resistance to oxidation by 18 percent (thereby making them less sticky and therefore less likely to clog arteries), when combined with the vitamin E from inside almonds, LDL's resistance to oxidation soared. The researchers also identified 20 powerful antioxidants in almond skins. People who eat almonds with skins significantly increase the amount of flavonoids and vitamin E in their bodies.[8]

ONE CAVEAT

Those who have kidney or gallbladder problems are often told not to eat foods with oxalates. Since almonds contain oxalates, people with kidney or gallbladder problems should discuss this issue with their health providers before consuming almonds. Should almonds be a regular part of the diet? Absolutely.

NOTES

1. The George Mateljan Foundation Website. http://whfoods.com.

2. Jenkins, David J. A., Cyril W. C. Kendall, Augustine Marchie, et al. 2002. "Dose Response of Almonds on Coronary Heart Disease Risk Factors: Blood Lipids, Oxidized Low-Density Lipoproteins, Lipoprotein(a), Homocysteine, and Pulmonary Nitric Oxide." *Circulation* 106: 1327–1332.

3. Jenkins, David J. A., Cyril W. C. Kendall, Dorothea A. Faulkner, et al. March 2006. "Assessment of the Longer-Term Effects of a Dietary Portfolio of Cholesterol-Lowering Foods in Hypercholesterolemia." *The American Journal of Clinical Nutrition* 83(3): 582–591.

4. Jenkins, D. J. A., C. W. C. Kendall, D. A. Faulkner, et al. June 2008. "Long-Term Effects of a Plant-Based Dietary Portfolio of Cholesterol-Lowering Foods on Blood Pressure." *European Journal of Clinical Nutrition* 62: 781–788.

5. Wien, M. A., J. M. Sabaté, D. N. Iklé, et al. 2003. "Almonds vs Complex Carbohydrates in a Weight Reduction Program. *International Journal of Obesity* 27: 1365–1372.

6. Hollis, James and Richard Mattes. September 2007. "Effect of Chronic Consumption of Almonds on Body Weight in Healthy Humans." *British Journal of Nutrition* 98(3): 651–656.

7. Jaceldo-Siegl, Karen, Joan Sabaté, Sujatha Rajaram, and Gary E. Fraser. 2004. "Long-Term Almond Supplementation Without Advice on Food Replacement Induces Favourable Nutrient Modifications to the Habitual Diets of Free-Living Individuals." *British Journal of Nutrition* 92(3): 533–540.

8. Chen, Chung-Yen, Paul E. Milbury, Karen Lapsley, and Jeffrey B. Blumberg. June 2005. "Flavonoids from Almond Skins Are Bioavailable and Act Synergistically

with Vitamins C and E to Enhance Hamster and Human LDL Resistance to Oxidation." *The Journal of Nutrition* 135: 1366–1373.

REFERENCES AND RESOURCES
Magazines, Journals, and Newspapers

Chen, Chung-Yen, Paul E. Milbury, Karen Lapsley, and Jeffrey B. Blumberg. June 2005. "Flavonoids from Almond Skins Are Bioavailable and Act Synergistically with Vitamins C and E to Enhance Hamster and Human LDL Resistance to Oxidation." *The Journal of Nutrition* 135: 1366–1373.

Hollis, James, and Richard Mattes. September 2007. "Effects of Chronic Consumption of Almonds on Body Weight in Healthy Humans." *British Journal of Nutrition* 98(3): 651–656.

Jaceldo-Siegl, Karen, Joan Sabaté, Sujatha Rajaram, and Gary E. Fraser. September p2004. "Long-Term Almond Supplementation Without Advice on Food Replacement Induces Favourable Nutrient Modifications to the Habitual Diets of Free-Living Individuals." *British Journal of Nutrition* 92(3): 533–540.

Jenkins, D. J. A., C. W. C. Kendall, D. A. Faulkner, et al. June 2008. "Long-Term Effects of a Plant-Based Dietary Portfolio of Cholesterol-Lowering Foods on Blood Pressure." *European Journal of Clinical Nutrition* 62: 781–788.

Jenkins, David J. A., Cyril W. C. Kendall, Dorothea A. Faulkner, et al. March 2006. "Assessment of the Longer-Term Effects of a Dietary Portfolio of Cholesterol-Lowering Foods in Hypercholesterolemia." *The American Journal of Clinical Nutrition* 83(3): 582–591.

Jenkins, David J. A., Cyril W. C. Kendall, Augustine Marchie, et al. 2002. "Dose Response of Almonds on Coronary Heart Disease Risk Factors: Blood Lipids, Oxidized Low-Density Lipoproteins, Lipoprotein(a), Homocysteine, and Pulmonary Nitric Oxide." *Circulation* 106: 1327–1332.

Wien, M. A., J. M. Sabaté, D. N. Iklé, et al. 2003. "Almonds vs Complex Carbohydrates in a Weight Reduction Program." *International Journal of Obesity* 27: 1365–1372.

Website

The George Mateljan Foundation. http://whfoods.com.

APPLES

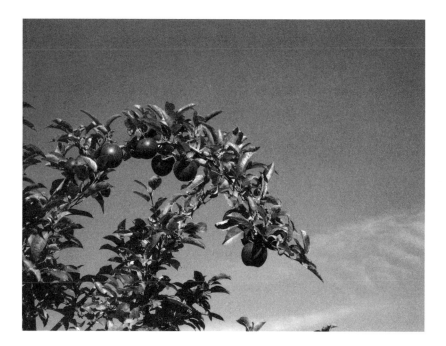

Apples, which originated in eastern Europe and southwestern Asia, have long been considered a healthful food that is readily available in most temperate climates. There are a seemingly endless number of varieties. In fact, it has been estimated that throughout the world there are now about 7,000 different types of apples.

Apples have good amounts of soluble and insoluble dietary fiber as well as vitamin C. They contain many phytonutrients, such as quercetin, catechin, phloridzin, and chlorogenic acid that act as antioxidants. So, they support cardiovascular health. Most of these benefits are found in the skins.

The pulp and skin of apples also contain flavonoids. Flavonoids have been found to be useful for inflammation, clot prevention, reducing blood pressure, and lowering the production of fat in liver cells.

Moreover, apples have been associated with reducing the risk of cancer and protection against asthma.[1] But, what have researchers learned?

CARDIOVASCULAR HEALTH

In a study published in 2007 in *The Journal of Nutrition*, researchers at the University of Utah studied the use of 730 mg of quercetin supplementation in 19 men and women with prehypertension and 22 men and women with stage 1 hypertension. While no changes were seen in the subjects with prehypertension, quercetin supplementation was associated with a reduction in systolic, diastolic, and mean arterial pressure in subjects with stage 1 hypertension. The researchers believe that quercetin lowers blood pressure because it blocks the effects of a chemical that causes the constriction of blood vessels. In effect, it causes blood vessels to dilate.[2]

METABOLIC SYNDROME PREVENTION

In a study published in 2008 in *The FASEB Journal*, researchers used data from the National Health and Nutrition Examination Survey (1999–2004) to review the association between apples and apple products (apple juice and applesauce) and metabolic syndrome in adults. Their results were noteworthy. Adults who regularly ate apples and apple products–the equivalent of about one medium apple per day—reduced their risk for metabolic syndrome by 27 percent. Metabolic syndrome is a cluster of medical problems that include insulin resistance, abnormal blood fat, and borderline or elevated blood pressure. These problems have been linked to chronic illnesses such as cardiovascular disease and diabetes. Regular consumers of apples and apple products tended to have lower blood pressure readings, lower C-reactive protein levels, and smaller waistlines than the people who were not regular consumers of apples and apple products.[3]

Commenting on the study, a 2008 article in *Psychology Today* noted that apples contain the soluble fiber pectin, which lowers fats in the body, including cholesterol. Apples also have an "array of phytochemical antioxidants" which helps to prevent blood fats from hardening. Most of the antioxidants and insoluble fibers are found in the peel, but pectin is found in the flesh. "Neither the pectin alone nor the phytochemicals alone–or any one phytochemical–is as effective as the combination of fiber and antioxidants." Or, as the lead author of the study is quoted, "It seems to be one of those situations where the whole is greater than the sum of its parts."[4]

CANCER

In a study published in 2009 in *The FASEB Journal*, British researchers from the Institute of Food Research in Norwich determined that in laboratory research, pectin binds to and may inhibit a protein that fosters the spread of cancer throughout the body. Specifically, some sugars in pectin attach to a protein known as galectin-3, which is on the surface of tumor cells. Galectin-3 helps the tumor cells grow and spread. When pectin binds to galectin-3, it inhibits the growth and may, possibly, reverse the spread of cancer cells.[5]

In a study published in 2009 in the *Journal of Agricultural and Food Chemistry*, Cornell University researchers explained that fresh apple extract inhibited the size of mammary tumors in rats. Furthermore, as the amount of extract increased so did the amount of inhibition. Only 23 percent of the rats fed the largest amount of apple extract, the equivalent of humans eating six apples per day, developed mammary tumors. That stands in sharp contrast to the 81 percent of rats who developed tumors in the control group. Not only did the treated animals have fewer tumors, their tumors were smaller, slower growing, and they contained fewer malignant cells. The researchers noted that, the "results demonstrate the potent capacity of fresh apples to suppress . . . mammary cancers in rats."[6]

LOWERS SUSCEPTIBILITY TO INFLUENZA

In a study published in 2008 in the *American Journal of Physiology: Regulatory, Integrative and Comparative Physiology*, researchers from South Carolina investigated the effects of quercetin on the influenza status of mice. Mice were randomly assigned to one of four groups. On three consecutive days, two of the groups exercised on a treadmill for about 140 minutes. Only one group of runners received quercetin. The other two groups of mice did not exercise. Only one group of non-exercise mice received quercetin. All of the mice were intranasally (within the nose) inoculated with the common and well-known influenza virus H1N1.

The study yielded the following findings:

- Excessive exercising increases the susceptibility to flu. The mice that exercised until they were fatigued were far more likely to become ill with the flu.
- The mice that exercised became ill with the flu sooner than those who did not exercise.
- The mice that exercised and took quercetin become ill at about the same rate as the mice that did not exercise.
- The mice that did not exercise and the mice that exercised and took quercetin had about the same severity of symptoms.

The researchers concluded that the data indicate, "that short-term quercetin feedings may prove to be an effective strategy to lessen the impact of stressful exercise on susceptibility to respiratory infection."[7]

PROTECT STOMACH FROM ASPIRIN THERAPY

In a laboratory rat study published in 2008 in the *British Journal of Nutrition*, Italian researchers attempted to determine if polyphenol extracts from apples could protect the stomach from ulcers and other complications that are associated with aspirin therapy. The rats were divided into two groups. One received apple polyphenol extract—the equivalent of about two apples per day for a human—before aspirin therapy; the other group received no pretreatment. The researchers found that both macroscopic and microscopic stomach injuries were dramatically reduced when rats ate apple polyphenols before aspirin therapy. They concluded that apple polyphenol extract "might be of therapeutic use in the prophylaxis of aspirin-related gastropathy."[8]

IMPROVED STRENGTH

In a study published in 2007 in *Medicine & Science in Sports & Exercise*, researchers divided sixteen 11-week-old male rats into two groups. One group was fed a diet that included apple polyphenols; the other group, the control, had no apple polyphenols. The study continued for three weeks. In truly striking findings, when compared to the control rats, the rats that ate the apple polyphenols had almost a 100 percent increase in muscle strength in their gastrocnemius muscles. (The gastrocnemius muscles are found in the back of the legs, and they make up the greater part of the calf.) In addition, they dropped body fat and experienced less muscle fatigue.[9]

ONE CAVEAT

Apples tend to be grown with lots of pesticides. Some of these may be avoided by washing the apples and peeling the skin. However, since the skin contains so many valuable properties, such as the fiber, the majority of the quercetin, and flavonoids, important nutrients are lost when it is discarded. To avoid the pesticides, it is best to eat apples that have been organically grown. And, eat lots of them as part of the diet.

NOTES

1. The George Mateljan Foundation Website. www.whfoods.com.

2. Edwards, Randi L., Tiffany Lyon, Sheldon E. Litwin, et al. November 2007. "Quercetin Reduces Blood Pressure in Hypertensive Subjects." *The Journal of Nutrition* 137: 2405–2411.

3. Fulgoni, Victor L., Sally A. Fulgoni, Stacie Haaga, and Andrew Ebert. 2008. "Apple Consumption Is Associated with Increased Nutrient Intakes and Reduced Risk of Metabolic Syndrome in Adults from the National Health and Nutrition Examination Survey (1999–2004)." *The FASEB Journal* 22: 1081.7.

4. Mickenberg, Kimberly. September–October 2008. "The Apple of Your Eyes (and Heart and Brain): There are Dozens of New Reasons an Apple a Day Keeps the Doctor Away." *Psychology Today* 41(5): 63.

5. Gunning, A. Patrick, Roy J. M. Bongaerts, and Victor J. Morris. 2009. "Recognition of Galactan Components of Pectin by Galectin-3." *The FASEB Journal* 23: 415–424.

6. Liu, Jia-Ren, Hong-Wei, Bing-Qing Chen, et al. 2009. "Fresh Apples Suppress Mammary Carcinogenesis and Proliferative Activity and Induce Apoptosis in

Mammary Tumors of the Sprague-Dawley Rat." *Journal of Agricultural and Food Chemistry* 57(1): 297–304.

7. Davis, J. M., E. A. Murphy, J. L. McClellan, et al. 2008. "Quercetin Reduces Susceptibility to Influenza Infection Following Stressful Exercise." *American Journal of Physiology: Regulatory, Integrative and Comparative Physiology* 295: R505–R509.

8. D'Argenio, Giuseppe, Giovanna Mazzone, Concetta Tuccillo, et al. 2008. "Apple Polyphenol Extracts Prevent Aspirin-Induced Damage to the Rat Gastric Mucosa." *British Journal of Nutrition* 100: 1228–1236.

9. Nakazato, Koichi, Hongsun Song, and Toshiaki Waga. June 2007. "Dietary Apple Polyphenols Enhance Gastrocnemius Function in Wistar Rats." *Medicine & Science in Sports & Exercise* 39(6): 934–940.

REFERENCES AND RESOURCES
Magazines, Journals, and Newspapers

D'Argenio, Giuseppe, Giovanna Muzzone, Concetta Tuccillo, et al. 2008. "Apple Polyphenol Extracts Prevent Aspirin-Induced Damage to the Rat Gastric Mucosa." *British Journal of Nutrition* 100: 1228–1236.

Davis, J. M., E. A. Murphy, J. L. McClellan, et al. 2008. "Quercetin Reduces Susceptibility to Influenza Infection Following Stressful Exercise." *American Journal of Physiology: Regulatory, Integrative and Comparative Physiology* 295: R505–R509.

Edwards, Randi L., Tiffany Lyon, Sheldon E. Litwin, et al. November 2007. "Quercetin Reduces Blood Pressure in Hypertensive Subjects." *The Journal of Nutrition* 137: 2405–2411.

Fulgoni, Victor L., Sally A. Fulgoni, Stacie Haaga, and Andrew Ebert. 2008. "Apple Consumption Is Associated with Increased Nutrient Intakes and Reduced Risk of Metabolic Syndrome in Adults from the National Health and Nutrition Examination Survey (1999–2004)." *The FASEB Journal* 22: 1081.7.

Gunning, A. Patrick, Roy J. M. Bongaerts, and Victor J. Morris. 2009. "Recognition of Galactan Components of Pectin by Galectin-3." *The FASEB Journal* 23: 415–424.

Liu, Jia-Ren, Hong-Wei Dong, Bing-Qing Chen, et al. 2009. "Fresh Apples Suppress Mammary Carcinogenesis and Proliferative Activity and Induce Apoptosis in Mammary Tumors of the Sprague-Dawley Rat." *Journal of Agricultural and Food Chemistry* 57(1): 297–304.

Mickenberg, Kimberly. September–October 2008. "The Apple of Your Eyes (and Heart and Brain): There Are Dozens of New Reasons an Apple a Day Keeps the Doctor Away." *Psychology Today* 41(5): 63.

Nakazato, Koichi, Hongsun Song, and Toshiaki Waga. June 2007. "Dietary Apple Polyphenols Enhance Gastrocnemius Function in Wistar Rats." *Medicine & Science in Sports & Exercise* 39(6): 934–940.

Website

The George Mateljan Foundation. www.whfoods.com.

AVOCADOS

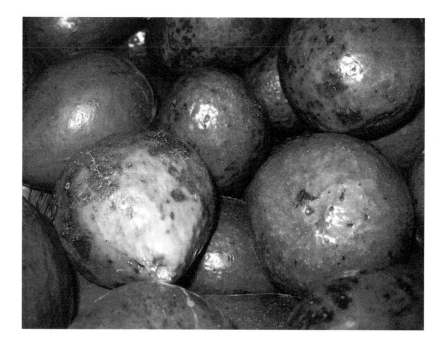

It is true. Avocados contain lots of fat. Approximately three-quarters of each avocado is fat. And, for a relatively small fruit with a rather large seed, it has a whopping 290 calories.

So, it should surprise no one that many people have avoided eating any avocados. Perhaps it is time for them to reconsider. A 2007 article in *Better Nutrition* explains that the fat in avocados is almost entirely "the health-protective monounsaturated variety, primarily oleic acid."[1] In addition, avocados are hosts to more than 20 nutrients such as potassium, folate, copper, and vitamins C, B_3 (niacin), B_6, E, and K. They have fiber, phytosterols, and the eye-protective lutein and zeaxanthin. Moreover, avocados have only modest amounts of carbohydrates and protein.[2] Paul A. Lachance, PhD, the director of the Nutraceuticals Institute at Rutgers University, has noted that avocados should be considered one of the ten most nutrient-dense foods.[3] But what does the research say?

LOWERS LEVELS OF CHOLESTEROL

A study conducted in Australia in the 1990s and reported in the *American Journal of Clinical Nutrition* placed middle-aged women on either diets high in monounsaturated fatty acids and enriched with avocado or high in complex carbohydrates. After three weeks, each group switched to the other diet. While both diets improved the subjects' blood cholesterol levels, the high monounsaturated diet that was enriched with avocados saw greater improvement. Of even more significance, the monounsaturated/avocado diet did not lower the levels of high-density lipoprotein (HDL) or "good cholesterol," but the high-complex-carbohydrate diet did. High levels of HDL are important for the prevention of cardiovascular disease.[4]

In a letter to the editors of the *Journal of the American Dietetic Association*, which was published in 2001, Karen C. Duester, MS, RD, explains that studies have shown that avocados are a "significant source of dietary phytosterols," which are "anticholesterolemic agents." They reduce the creation of new cholesterol and lower the intestinal absorption of existing cholesterol. Beta-sitosterol is a phytosterol that is found in abundance in avocados.[5]

CANCER

A study published in 2007 in *Seminars in Cancer Biology* reports that Ohio State University researchers used extracts taken from Hass avocados (the most common type of avocado grown in the United States) to kill or stop the growth of precancerous oral cancer cells. At the same time, the extracts did not harm normal cells. The researchers believe that the anti-cancer activity is a result of the high levels of phytochemicals (plant compounds) found in avocados. "These studies suggest that individual and combinations of phytochemicals from avocado fruit may offer an advantageous dietary strategy in cancer prevention."[6] When interviewed about the research, Steven D'Ambrosio, PhD, one of the researchers, noted that the study focused on oral cancer, "but the findings might have implications for other types of cancer. These are preliminary findings, and more research is needed."[7]

An article published in 2005 in *The Journal of Nutritional Biochemistry* indicates that avocados, which contain lutein, may also be useful in the fight against prostate cancer. Researchers at the UCLA Center for Human Nutrition exposed prostate cancer cells to pure lutein as well as an extract of whole avocado. Although there was no change in the cancer cells when exposed to pure lutein, when exposed to avocado extract cell growth was inhibited by up to 60 percent. "In common with other colorful fruits and vegetables, the avocado contains numerous bioactive carotenoids. Because the avocado also contains a significant amount of monounsaturated fat, these bioactive carotenoids are likely to be absorbed into the bloodstream, where, in combination with other diet-derived phytochemicals, they may contribute to the significant cancer risk reduction associated with a diet of fruits and vegetables."[8]

WEIGHT LOSS

Considering that avocados contain so much fat, it is truly remarkable that some research has associated them with weight loss. Yet an Israeli study published in 2002 in *The Journal of Nutrition* describes research in which rats were fed either avocado pulp or cellulose as dietary fiber. The rats that ate the avocado pulp consumed lower amounts of food and gained less weight than the rats that ate cellulose. The researchers believe that there is some form of "appetite depressant" in avocados.[9]

Six years later, research may have revealed the identity of that "appetite depressant." A study published in 2008 in *Cell Metabolism* explained that oleic acid, which is found in abundance in avocados, is transformed into oleoylethanolamide (OEA) in the top portion of the small intestine. There, it connects to the nerve-endings that send hunger-curbing messages—telling the brain to stop eating.[10] In essence, according to this research, people who eat avocados will eat less food than they might otherwise consume.

NUTRIENT BOOSTER

In 2005, *The Journal of Nutrition* published research findings that found that avocados enabled the body to absorb more healthy nutrients. In the study, men and women ate salads and salsa with and without fresh avocados. The subjects who ate the salads with 2.5 tablespoons of avocado absorbed far more alpha-carotene and beta-carotene than those who ate the salads without avocados. Furthermore, the subjects who ate salsa with five tablespoons of avocado took in far more lycopene and beta-carotene than those who ate salsa without avocado. The researchers believe that the higher levels of absorption are the direct result of the avocados' natural fat content.[11]

LOWERS RISK OF TYPE 2 DIABETES IN WOMEN

In research conducted in Boston and published in 2008 in the *American Journal of Clinical Nutrition*, researchers determined that women who wish to lower their odds of developing type 2 diabetes should couple eating low-carbohydrate foods with foods that contain healthy fats, such as avocados. Women who ate foods such as sugar-sweetened fruit juice, refined sugary cereal, and white bread had a significantly higher risk for type 2 diabetes. Commenting on the research, Thomas Halton, PhD, said that the plant foods with high rates of fat are healthful. But, animal foods with high fats are not. During his research, Dr. Halton and his associates "examined 20 years of dietary survey data from more than 85,000 women."[12]

PROTECTION AGAINST PARKINSON'S DISEASE

A study conducted in the Netherlands and reported in 2005 in *Neurology* reviewed a cohort of 5,289 people aged 55 or older. When the study began, all subjects were free of dementia and Parkinson's disease. During the six years of the study, 51 people were diagnosed with Parkinson's disease. Researchers found that people with higher intakes of unsaturated fats, in food such as avocados, were far less likely to develop Parkinson's disease. In fact, they had more than a 30 percent decrease in risk for this debilitating disease.[13]

Should avocados be included in the diet? Yes, of course. But since they are so high in fats and calories, in general, they should be eaten in moderation.

NOTES

1. Vukovic, Laurel. September 2007. "The Beautiful Side of Avocados: Avocados Look as Good as They Taste and Despite Their High Fat Content Are a Smart Way to Boost Your Health and Beauty." *Better Nutrition* 69(9): 44–45.

2. California Avocado Commission. www.avocado.org.

3. January 10, 2005. "Nutraceuticals Institute at Rutgers University." *The Food Institute Report* 1: 4.

4. Colquhoun, D. M., D. Moores, S. M. Somerset, and J. A. Humphries. 1992. "Comparison of the Effects on Lipoproteins and Apolipoproteins of a Diet High in Monounsaturated Fatty Acids, Enriched with Avocado, and a High-Carbohydrate Diet." *American Journal of Clinical Nutrition* 56: 671–677.

5. Duester, Karen C. April 2001. "Avocado Fruit Is a Rich Source of Beta-Sitosterol." *Journal of the American Dietetic Association* 101(4): 404–405.

6. Ding, Haiming, Young-Woo Chin, Douglas Kinghorn, and Steven M. D'Ambrosio. October 2007. "Chemoprotective Characteristics of Avocado Fruit." *Seminars in Cancer Biology* 17(5): 386–394.

7. September 8, 2007. "Avocados Can Prevent Mouth Cancer." *PTI–The Press Trust of India Ltd.*: NA.

8. Lu, Qing-Yi, James R. Arteaga, Qifeng Zhang, et al. January 2005. "Inhibition of Prostate Cancer Cell Growth by an Avocado Extract: Role of Lipid-Soluble Bioactive Substances." *The Journal of Nutritional Biochemistry* 16(1): 23–30.

9. Naveh, Elinat, Moshe J. Werman, Edmond Sabo, and Ishak Neeman. 2002. "Defatted Avocado Pulp Reduces Body Weight and Total Hepatic Fat but Increases Plasma Cholesterol in Male Rats Fed Diets with Cholesterol." *The Journal of Nutrition* 132: 2015–2018.

10. Schwartz, Gary J., Jin Fu, Giuseppe Astarita, et al. October 8, 2008. "The Lipid Messenger OEA Links Dietary Fat Intake to Satiety." *Cell Metabolism* 8(4): 281–288.

11. Schwartz, Steven J. August 2005. "How Can the Metabolomic Response to Lycopene (Exposures, Durations, Intracellular Concentrations) in Humans Be Adequately Evaluated?" *The Journal of Nutrition* 135: 2040S–2041S.

12. Law, Bridget Murray. July 2008. "Good Fats, Bad Fats, and Diabetes Risk (Type 2)." *Diabetes Forecast* 61(7): 24.

13. de Lau, L. M. L., M. Bornebroek, J. C. M. Witteman, et al. 2005. "Dietary Fatty Acids and the Risk of Parkinson Disease." *Neurology* 64: 2040–2045.

REFERENCES AND RESOURCES
Magazines, Journals, and Newspapers

"Avocados Can Prevent Mouth Cancer." September 8, 2007. *PTI–The Press Trust of India Ltd.*: NA.

Colquhoun, D. M., D. Moores, S. M. Somerset, and J. A. Humphries. 1992. "Comparison of the Effects of Lipoproteins and Apolipoproteins of a Diet High in Mono-unsaturated Fatty Acids, Enriched with Avocado and a High-Carbohydrate Diet." *American Journal of Clinical Nutrition* 56: 671–677.

de Lau, L. M. L., M. Bornebroek, J. C. M. Witteman, et al. 2005. "Dietary Fatty Acids and the Risk of Parkinson Disease." *Neurology* 64: 2040–2045.

Ding, Haiming, Young-Won Chin, Douglas Kinghorn, and Steven M. D'Ambrosio. October 2007. "Chemoprotective Characteristics of Avocado Fruit." *Seminars in Cancer Biology* 17(5): 386–394.

Duester, Karen C. April 2001. "Avocado Fruit Is a Rich Source of Beta-Sitosterol." *Journal of the American Dietetic Association* 101(4): 404–405.

Golub, Catherine. June 2006. "Avocado: A Fruit Unlike Any Other Fruit." *Environmental Nutrition* 29(6): 8.

Halton, Thomas L., Simin Liu, JoAnn Manson, and Frank B. Hu. February 2008. "Low-Carbohydrate-Diet Score and Risk of Type 2 Diabetes in Women." *American Journal of Clinical Nutrition* 87(2): 339–446.

Law, Bridget Murray. July 2008. "Good Fats, Bad Fats, and Diabetes Risk (Type 2)." *Diabetes Forecast* 61(7): 24.

Lu, Qing-Yi, James R. Arteaga, Qifeng Zang, et al. January 2005. "Inhibition of Prostate Cancer Cell Growth by an Avocado Extract: Role of Lipid-Soluble Bioactive Substances." *The Journal of Nutritional Biochemistry* 16(1): 23–30.

Naveh, Einat, Moshe J. Werman, Edmond Sabo, and Ishak Neeman. 2002. "Defatted Avocado Pulp Reduces Body Weight and Total Hepatic Fat but Increases Plasma Cholesterol in Male Rats Fed Diets with Cholesterol." *The Journal of Nutrition* 132: 2015–2018.

"Nutraceuticals Institute at Rutgers University." January 10, 2005. *The Food Institute Report* 1: 4.

Schwartz, Gary J., Jin Fu, Giuseppe Astarita, et al. October 8, 2008. "The Lipid Messenger QEA Links Dietary Fat Intake to Satiety." *Cell Metabolism* 8(4): 281–288.

Schwartz, Steven J. August 2005. "How Can the Metabolic Response to Lycopene (Exposures, Durations, Intracellular Concentrations) in Humans Be Adequately Evaluated?" *The Journal of Nutrition* 135: 2040S–2041S.

Stiefel, Steve. March 2005. "Wholly Guacamole." *Flex* 23(1): 208.

Vukovic, Laurel. September 2007. "The Beautiful Side of Avocados: Avocados Look as Good as They Taste and Despite Their High Fat Content Are a Smart Way to Boost Your Health and Beauty." *Better Nutrition* 69(9): 44–45.

Website

California Avocado Commission. www.avocado.org.

BANANAS

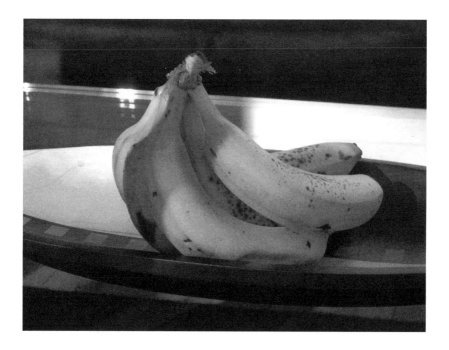

Bananas. It is easy to take them for granted. In the world in which the cost of fruit keeps rising, bananas remain affordable. Originating about 4,000 years ago in Malaysia and today commercially grown in Costa Rica, Mexico, Ecuador, and Brazil, this crescent-shaped fruit, which is most often yellow, also contains fiber, potassium, magnesium, as well as vitamins C and B_6.[1] Over the years, a number of different researchers have found health benefits from bananas.

STROKE

A study published in 2002 in *Neurology* followed 5,600 men and women older than 65 years for four to eight years. During this time, researchers recorded the amount of potassium that the participants consumed, the levels of potassium in their blood, their use of diuretics (medications for high blood pressure, heart failure, and kidney disease), and the number of strokes that the subjects experienced. The researchers found that the risk of stroke was highest among those who had low levels of serum potassium in the blood and low intake of foods, such as bananas, with higher levels of potassium.[2] So, the consumption of bananas may help prevent strokes.

A 2007 issue of *Environmental Nutrition* describes research conducted at the Harvard School of Public Health. Researchers reviewed the diets of more than 43,000 men and found that those with the highest intake of foods high in magnesium and potassium, like bananas, had a reduced risk of stroke. The article noted that, "The Food and Drug Administration now even permits bananas to be marketed with a health claim lauding potassium's link to prevention of high blood pressure and stroke."[3]

Alzheimer's Disease

A study published in 2005 in *Alzheimer's & Dementia: The Journal of the Alzheimer's Association* used data from the Baltimore Longitudinal Study of Aging to review the diets of 579 nondemented people age 60 and over. Over the next several years (the mean follow-up was 9.3 years), 57 people developed Alzheimer's disease. The researchers determined that those who consumed at least the recommended dietary allowance of 400 micrograms of folate, found in bananas, had a 55 percent reduced risk for developing Alzheimer's disease.[4]

In another study published in 2008 in the *Journal of Food Science*, researchers found that when they exposed nerve cells (neurons) to banana, orange, and apple extracts, the antioxidants, or specifically phenolic phytochemicals, in the fruit prevented oxidation. Why is this important? There is a good deal of evidence that brains of people with Alzheimer's are exposed to high levels of oxidative stress. This results in cellular dysfunctions that cause nerve degeneration. Thus, including more foods such as bananas in the diet may protect the brain from the ravages of diseases like Alzheimer's. "These results suggest that fresh apples, bananas, and oranges in our daily diet, along with other fruits may protect neuron cells against oxidative stress-induced neurtoxicity and may play an important role in reducing the risk of neurodegenerative disorders such as Alzheimer's disease."[5]

OSTEOPOROSIS

A University of California, San Francisco, study published in 2002 in *The Journal of Clinical Endocrinology & Metabolism* noted that the consumption of potassium-rich foods, such as bananas, in postmenopausal women helps prevent the loss of calcium from the bones. How does this work? Though salt does not appear to have a similar effect on men or younger women, in postmenopausal women the intake of excess amounts of salt increases the amount of bone minerals excreted in the urine.

In the study, 60 healthy postmenopausal women were placed on a low-salt diet for three weeks. Measurements were taken of their excreted calcium, as well as bone protein and NTx (high levels indicate bone is being broken down or reabsorbed). After three weeks, the subjects were placed on a high salt diet. Half the women were given a potassium supplement; the other half received a placebo. The women remained on the high salt diet for four weeks. The researchers found that the calcium loss in women taking potassium citrate decreased four percent, while it increased 33 percent in those on the placebo. NTx excretion increased 7.5 percent in women on potassium citrate, while it increased 23 percent in women taking the placebo. The researchers note that, "Increased intake of dietary sources of potassium alkaline salts, namely fruit and vegetables, may be beneficial for postmenopausal women at risk for osteoporosis, particularly those consuming a diet generous in sodium chloride."[6]

INSOMNIA

A study conducted in Sydney, Australia, and published in 2007 in *The American Journal of Clinical Nutrition* evaluated how foods that are high on the glycemic index, such as bananas, may assist people dealing with insomnia. Foods like these increase the levels of the amino acid tryptophan in the blood; and, trytophan is well-known to foster drowsiness. People who ate higher glycemic foods about four hours before going to bed required only nine minutes to fall asleep; people who ate lower glycemic foods needed 17.5 minutes to fall asleep. When the high glycemic diet was given one hour before bedtime no such dramatic difference occurred.[7] But, the study only included 12 healthy men between the ages of 18 and 35. And, high glycemic diets may lead to excess weight gain and diabetes. So, they are not a good choice for those who are already overweight or at higher risk for diabetes.

MOOD AND COGNITION

In a Dutch study published in 2002 in *Brain, Behavior, and Immunity*, researchers examined what happens to mood and cognition when the body's levels of tryptophan (which, as previously noted, is found in bananas) are depleted. The subjects consisted of 27 volunteers. Of these, 16 had an immediate relative dealing with major depression. When researchers lowered the level of tryptophan in the bodies of the volunteers, they had problems with memory. In addition, half of the subjects with a family history of depression and nine percent of those without a family history of depression, felt depressed. These findings should be of special interest to those who have a family history of depression and those who have low levels of tryptophan in their bodies, which may be caused by a number of factors such as dieting and undergoing immunotherapy for cancer.[8]

KIDNEY CANCER

In a Swedish study published in 2005 in the *International Journal of Cancer*, researchers obtained dietary information on a group of 61,000 women between the ages of 40 and 76 for 13.4 years. During this time, 122 women developed renal cell carcinoma. The researchers found that certain fruits and vegetables, such as bananas, offered protection against renal cell carcinoma, the most common form of kidney cancer. People who ate bananas four to six times per week had about half the risk of developing this type of cancer as people who did not eat bananas. Some epidemiologists contend that anticancer properties of bananas are a result of their high amounts of potassium.[9]

CHILDHOOD ASTHMA

A study conducted by researchers in London, which was published in 2007 in the *European Respiratory Journal*, investigated whether wheezing was less common in children with higher consumption of fruits such as bananas. Using a questionnaire, the researchers surveyed 2,640 children between the ages of five and ten years. The researchers found that children who ate bananas one or more times per day were less likely to wheeze.[10]

ONE CAVEAT

Bananas, and other foods such as honeydew and zucchini, contain proteins in their pollen that are similar to ragweed pollen. People who react to ragweed pollen may also react to eating these foods, particularly during the ragweed season that begins in August and ends with the first fall frost.

Still, for most people, bananas should be a wonderful, cost-effective part of the diet. And, they should be eaten frequently.

NOTES

1. The George Mateljan Foundation Website. www.whfoods.com.

2. Green, D. M., A. H. Ropper, R. A. Kronmal, et al. 2002. "Serum Potassium Level and Dietary Potassium Intake as Risk Factors for Stroke." *Neurology* 59: 314–320.

3. Hermann, Mindy G. 2007. "Go Bananas! Help Protect Yourself Against High Blood Pressure, Stroke; Boost Immunity." *Environmental Nutrition* 30(2): 8.

4. Corrada, Maria M., Caludia H. Kawas, Judith Hallfrisch, et al. July 2005. "Reduced Risk of Alzheimer's Disease with High Folate Intake: The Baltimore Longitudinal Study of Aging." *Alzheimer's & Dementia: The Journal of the Alzheimer's Association* 1(1): 11–18.

5. Heo, H. J., S. J. Choi, S. G. Choi, et al. 2008. "Effects of Banana, Orange, and Apple on Oxidative Stress-Induced Neurotoxicity in PC12 Cells." *Journal of Food Science* 73(2): H28–H32.

6. Sellmeyer, Deborah E., Monique Schloetter, and Anthony Sebastian. 2002. "Potassium Citrate Prevents Increased Urine Calcium Excretion and Bone Resorption

Induced by a High Sodium Chloride Diet." *The Journal of Clinical Endocrinology & Metabolism* 87(5): 2008–2012.

7. Afaghi, Ahmid, Helen O'Connor, and Chin Moi Chow. February 2007. "High-Glycemic-Index Carbohydrate Meals Shorten Sleep Onset." *The American Journal of Clinical Nutrition* 85(2): 426–430.

8. Riedel, Wim J., Tineke Klaassen, and Jeroen A. J. Schmitt. 2002. "Tryptophan, Mood, and Cognitive Function." *Brain, Behavior, and Immunity* 16(5): 581–589.

9. Rashidkhani, B., P. Lindblad, and A. Wolk. January 20, 2005. "Fruits, Vegetables, and Risk of Renal Cell Carcinoma: A Prospective Study of Swedish Women." *International Journal of Cancer* 113(3): 451–455.

10. Okoko, B. J., P. G. Burney, R. B. Newson, et al. 2007. "Childhood Asthma and Fruit Consumption." *European Respiratory Journal* 29: 1161–1168.

REFERENCES AND RESOURCES
Magazines, Journals, and Newspapers

Afaghi, Ahmed, Helen O'Connor, and Chin Moi Chow. February 2007. "High-Glycemic-Index Carbohydrate Meals Shorten Sleep Onset." *The American Journal of Clinical Nutrition* 85(2): 426–430.

Corrada, Maria M., Claudia H. Kawas, Judith Hallfrisch, et al. July 2005. "Reduced Risk of Alzheimer's Disease with High Folate Intake: The Baltimore Longitudinal Study of Aging." *Alzheimer's & Dementia: The Journal of the Alzheimer's Association* 1(1): 11–18.

Green, D. M., A. H. Ropper, R. A. Kronmal, et al. 2002. "Serum Potassium Level and Dietary Potassium Intake as Risk Factors for Stroke." *Neurology* 59: 314–320.

Heo, H. J., S. J. Choi, S. G. Choi, et al. 2008. "Effects of Banana, Orange, and Apple on Oxidative Stress-Induced Neurotoxicity in PC12 Cells." *Journal of Food Science* 73(2): H28–H32.

Hermann, Mindy G. February 2007. "Go Bananas! Help Protect Yourself Against High Blood Pressure, Stroke; Boost Immunity." *Environmental Nutrition* 30(2): 8.

Okoko, B. J., P. G. Burney, R. B. Newson, et al. 2007. "Childhood Asthma and Fruit Consumption." *European Respiratory Journal* 29: 1161–1168.

Rashidkhani, B., P. Lindblad, and A. Wolk. January 20, 2005. "Fruits, Vegetables, and Risk of Renal Cell Carcinoma: A Prospective Study of Swedish Women." *International Journal of Cancer* 113(3): 451–455.

Riedel, Wim J., Tineke Klaassen, and Jeroen A. J. Schmitt. October 2002. "Tryptophan, Mood, and Cognition." *Brain, Behavior, and Immunity* 16(5): 581–589.

Sellmeyer, Deborah E., Monique Schloetter, and Anthony Sebastian. 2002. "Potassium Citrate Prevents Increased Urine Calcium Excretion and Bone Resorption Induced by a High Sodium Chloride Diet." *The Journal of Clinical Endocrinology & Metabolism* 87(5): 2008–2012.

Website

The George Mateljan Foundation. www.whfoods.com.

BARLEY

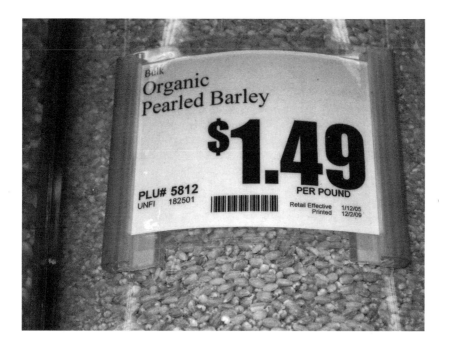

When Americans mention grains, they are usually discussing wheat, oats, rice, or corn. But, of course, there are others. One of these is barley, which is believed to be one of the oldest grains. According to historians, it was used by the ancient Egyptians, and Christopher Columbus brought it to the Americas in 1494.[1]

Today, in the United States, the most common type of barley is pearled. Even though the outer hull and bran have been removed, since barley contains fiber throughout the grain, pearled barley still contains a good deal of soluble and insoluble fiber. In fact, in contrast to a half-cup of cooked brown rice, which contains 1.75 grams of total dietary fiber, a half-cup of cooked barley contains 3 grams of total dietary fiber.[2] But, on the shelves of supermarkets, where it typically sits next to rice and dried peas, it barely has a presence. It may be shocking to hear that most of the barley grown in the United States is used for preparing malt for brewing beer and for animal feed.[3] Should Americans be using more barley? See what the research says.

CARDIOVASCULAR HEALTH

During 2004, researchers at the Diet & Human Performance Laboratory, Beltsville Human Nutrition Research Center, Agricultural Research Service of the U.S. Department of Agriculture, had two important studies published on the lipid-lowering potential of barley. In a study published in the *Journal of the American College of Nutrition*, the researchers attempted to determine if barley, as a source of soluble fiber, would lower the rates of cholesterol in eighteen men between the ages of 28 and 62 who had moderately elevated levels of cholesterol. After five weeks of barley consumption, they found significant improvement in the total and LDL (bad) cholesterol levels. The researchers noted that, "increasing soluble fiber through the consumption of barley in a healthy diet can reduce cardiovascular risk factors."[4]

An article that appeared in *The American Journal of Clinical Nutrition* describes similar research, only this time the researchers studied both men and women with mildly elevated levels of cholesterol. There were nine postmenopausal women, nine premenopausal women, and seven men. Again, after five weeks of barley consumption, the subjects experienced significant reductions in their total and LDL cholesterol. The researchers wrote, "the addition of barley to a healthy diet may be effective in lowering total and LDL cholesterol in both men and women."[5]

In a study published in 2006 in the *Journal of the American Dietetic Association*, the same researchers compared the effects of diets high in predominately insoluble fiber (brown rice and whole wheat) to those with predominately soluble fiber (barley) on the blood pressure readings of men and women with mildly elevated cholesterol levels. Both diets proved to be useful for lowering blood pressure. The researchers noted, "increasing whole-grain foods, whether high in soluble or insoluble fiber, can reduce blood pressure and may help to control weight."[6]

A study published in 2007 in the *British Journal of Nutrition* investigated the effects of the soluble fiber beta-glucan, which is found in abundance in barley, on the cholesterol levels of men and women with higher levels of cholesterol. Researchers found that the inclusion of concentrated barley beta-glucan (BBG) in the diet led to significant reductions in the levels of total and LDL cholesterol. The levels of HDL (good cholesterol) remained unchanged. Commenting on the study, the researchers advised, "food products containing concentrated BBG should be considered an effective option for improving blood lipids."[7]

In a Canadian-based study published in 2006 in *The American Journal of Clinical Nutrition*, researchers attempted to determine if participants in "real world conditions" could effectively lower their levels of elevated cholesterol. The participants were placed on a diet that included a number of cholesterol-lowering foods, such as barley. After twelve months, over 30 percent of the 55 people who completed the study had lowered their cholesterol levels by more than 20 percent. The researchers noted that the results were, "not significantly different from their response to a first-generation statin taken under metabolically controlled conditions."[8]

For the past several years, certain whole-grain barley products have been able to claim that they may be useful in the fight against heart disease. According to the U.S. Food and Drug Administration, soluble fiber foods, such as barley, which contain at least 0.75 gram of soluble fiber per serving, may indicate that, "as part of a diet low in saturated fat and cholesterol, [they] may reduce the risk of heart disease."[9]

BLOOD SUGAR LEVELS

In a study that appeared in 2006 in *Nutrition Research*, twenty men, who were mildly insulin resistant, ate different types of muffins, including muffins that contained varying amounts of soluble-rich barley beta-glucan. The men who ate the muffins with the most barley beta-glucan had the most significant reductions in glucose and insulin responses. The researchers believed that consuming adequate amounts of foods with beta-glucan may help control the rising rates of type 2 diabetes in the United States.[10]

A similar study from Italian researchers was published in 2006 in the *Journal of the American College of Nutrition*. Researchers gave a group of ten healthy volunteers crackers and cookies made from either barley or whole-wheat flour. The barley products contained 3.5 grams of beta-glucan per portion; the dietary fiber in the whole-wheat products was primarily insoluble, and it contained almost no beta-glucan. The researchers found that when compared to the wheat crackers and cookies, the barley products significantly reduced glucose and insulin response.[11]

An intriguing study was published in 2007 in *Diabetes Research and Clinical Practice*. Hoping to understand why imprisonment tended to improve metabolic control in prisoners with type 2 diabetes, researchers conducted a retrospective analysis of the medical charts of 4,385 male prisoners in Fukushima Prison in Japan from 1998 to 2004. In addition to working eight-hour days, five days a week, Japanese prisoners ate diets that were high in dietary fiber that included boiled rice and barley, a food called *mugimeshi*. Because of improvements in their diets and lifestyles, while incarcerated, 5 of 18 prisoners who required insulin and 17 of 34 who were treated with oral hypoglycemic agents were able "to discontinue their treatment and maintain good metabolic control." As a result, the researchers concluded that "a well-regulated lifestyle and long-term intake of high dietary fiber may have beneficial effects on metabolic control in patients with type 2 diabetes."[12]

PREMENOPAUSAL BREAST CANCER

Barley is filled with phytonutrients known as lignans, which are converted in the colon into enterolactone and enterodial, substances with mild estrogen-like properties. In a study published in 2006 in the *European Journal of Cancer Prevention,* German researchers measured the concentrations of enterolactone (and genistein) in plasma samples from 220 premenopausal women and 237 controls. The researchers found that the women with the highest levels of enterolactone had the lowest incidence of premenopausal breast cancer.[13]

ONE CAVEAT

Though barley is a healthy addition to the diet for the vast majority of people, those who are dealing with celiac disease or other forms of gluten intolerance should be very careful to avoid all barley products. Should barley be included in the diet? For most people, it is an excellent addition.

NOTES

1. Bucklan, Erinn. December 2008. "Providing Blood Glucose Stabilization, Cardiovascular Protection, and Cancer Prevention, This Ancient Grain Satisfies More Than Just the Palate." *Life Extension:* NA.

2. USDA National Nutrient Database for Standard Reference Website. http://www.nal.usda.gov/fnic/foodcomp/search/.

3. Schepers, Anastasia. January 2004. "Barley: Ancient Grain, New-Found Nutrition. *Environmental Nutrition* 27(1): 8.

4. Behall, Kay M., Daniel J. Scholfield, and Judith Hallfrisch. 2004. "Lipids Significantly Reduced by Diets Containing Barley in Moderately Hypercholesterolemic Men." *Journal of the American College of Nutrition* 23(1): 55–62.

5. Behall, Kay M., Daniel J. Scholfield, and Judith Hallfrisch. November 2004. "Diets Containing Barley Significantly Reduce Lipids in Mildly Hypercholesterolemic Men and Women." *The American Journal of Clinical Nutrition* 80(5): 1185–1193.

6. Behall, Kay M., Daniel J. Scholfield, and Judith Hallfrisch. September 2006. "Whole-Grain Diets Reduce Blood Pressure in Mildly Hypercholesterolemic Men and Women." *Journal of the American Dietetic Association* 106(9): 1445–1449.

7. Keenan, Joseph M., Melanie Goulson, Tatyana Shamliyan, et al. June 2007. "The Effects of Concentrated Barley Beta-Glucan on Blood Lipids in a Population of Hypercholesterolaemic Men and Women." *British Journal of Nutrition* 97(6): 1162–1168.

8. Jenkins, David J. A., Cyril W. C. Kendall, Dorothea A. Faulkner, et al. March 2006. "Assessment of the Longer-Term Effects of a Dietary Portfolio of Cholesterol-Lowering Foods in Hypercholesterolemia." *The American Journal of Clinical Nutrition* 83(3): 582–591.

9. Worcester, Sharon. July 1, 2006. "Whole Grain Barley Products Can Claim Heart Health Benefits." *Internal Medicine News* 39(13): 39.

10. Behall, Kay M., Daniel J. Scholfield, and Judith G. Hallfrisch. December 2006. "Barley Beta-Glucan Reduces Plasma Glucose and Insulin Responses Compared with Resistant Starch in Men." *Nutrition Research* 26(12): 644–650.

11. Casiraghi, Maria Cristina, Marcella Garsetti, Giulio Testolin, and Furio Brighenti. 2006. "Post-Prandial Responses to Cereal Products Enriched with Barley Beta-Glucan." *Journal of the American College of Nutrition* 25(4): 313–320.

12. Hinata, Masamitsu, Masami Ono, Sanae Midorikawa, and Koji Nakanishi. August 2007. "Metabolic Improvement of Male Prisoners with Type 2 Diabetes in Fukushima Prison, Japan." *Diabetes Research and Clinical Practice* 77(2): 327–332.

13. Piller, Regina, Jenny Chang-Claude, and Jakob Linseisen. June 2006. "Plasma Enterolactone and Genistein and the Risk of Premenopausal Breast Cancer." *European Journal of Cancer Prevention* 15(3): 225–232.

RESOURCES AND REFERENCES
Magazines, Journals, and Newspapers

Behall, Kay M., Daniel J. Scholfield, and Judith Hallfrisch. September 2006. "Whole-Grain Diets Reduce Blood Pressure in Mildly Hypercholesterolemic Men and Women." *Journal of the American Dietetic Association* 106(9): 1445–1449.

Behall, Kay M., Daniel J. Scholfield, and Judith Hallfrisch. December 2006. "Barley Beta-Glucan Reduces Plasma Glucose and Insulin Responses Compared with Resistant Starch in Men." *Nutrition Research* 26(12): 644–650.

Behall, Kay M., Daniel J. Scholfield, and Judith Hallfrisch. November 2004. "Diets Containing Barley Significantly Reduce Lipids in Mildly Hypercholesterolemic Men and Women." *The American Journal of Clinical Nutrition* 80(5): 1185–1193.

Behall, Kay M., Daniel J. Scholfield, and Judith Hallfrisch. 2004. "Lipids Significantly Reduced by Diets Containing Barley in Moderately Hypercholesterolemic Men." *Journal of the American College of Nutrition* 23(1): 55–62.

Bucklan, Erinn. December 2008. "Providing Blood Glucose Stabilization, Cardiovascular Protection, and Cancer Prevention, This Ancient Grain Satisfies More Than Just the Palate." *Life Extension*: NA.

Casiraghi, Maria Christina, Marcella Garsetti, Giulio Testolin, and Furio Brighenti. 2006. "Post-Prandial Responses to Cereal Products Enriched with Barley Beta-Glucan." *Journal of the American College of Nutrition* 25(4): 313–320.

Hinata, Masamitsu, Masami Ono, Sanae Midorikawa, and Koji Nakanishi. August 2007. "Metabolic Improvement of Male Prisoners with Type 2 Diabetes in Fukushima Prison, Japan." *Diabetes Research and Clinical Practice* 77(2): 327–332.

Jenkins, David J. A., Cyril W. C. Kendall, Dorothea A. Faulkner, et al. March 2006. "Assessment of the Longer-Term Effects of a Dietary Portfolio of Cholesterol-Lowering Foods in Hypercholesterolemia." *The American Journal of Clinical Nutrition* 83(3): 582 –591.

Keenan, Joseph M., Melanie Goulson, Tatyana Shamliyan, et al. June 2007. "The Effects of Concentrated Barley Beta-Glucan on Blood Lipids in a Population of Hypercholesterolaemic Men and Women." *British Journal of Nutrition* 97(6): 1162–1168.

Piller, Regina, Jenny Chang-Claude, and Jakob Linseisen. June 2006. "Plasma Enterolactone and Genistein and the Risk of Premenopausal Breast Cancer." *European Journal of Cancer Prevention* 15(3): 225–232.

Schepers, Anastasia. January 2004. "Barley: Ancient Grain, New-Found Nutrition." *Environmental Nutrition* 27(1): 8.

Worcester, Sharon. July 1, 2006. "Whole Grain Barley Products Can Claim Heart Health Benefits." *Internal Medicine News* 39(13): 39.

Website

USDA National Nutrient Database for Standard Reference. http://www.nal.usda.gov/fnic/foodcomp/search/.

BELL PEPPERS

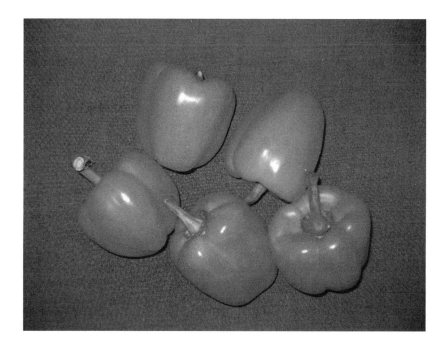

Bell peppers, which are also known as sweet peppers, originated in South America; wild varieties have been dated to 5000 BCE. Thousands of years later, Spanish and Portuguese explorers carried bell peppers to other parts of the world. Today, they are grown in many countries. However, the primary commercial producers are China, Turkey, Spain, Romania, Nigeria, and Mexico.[1]

Bell peppers contain an extraordinary amount of vitamins and nutrients. They have excellent amounts of vitamins A, B_6, and C and very good amounts of dietary fiber, molybdenum, vitamin K, folate, and manganese. Bell peppers have good quantities of potassium, tryptophan, copper, and vitamins B_1 and E. In addition, they contain beta-carotene, a type of carotenoid (highly pigmented fat-soluble compounds naturally present in many foods). Red peppers are particularly nutritious. They have the phytonutrients lycopene, lutein, and zeaxanthin as well as beta-cryptoxanthin, an orange-red carotenoid.[2] But, what have researchers learned?

CANCER
Colorectal Cancer

In a study published in 2007 in *The Journal of Nutrition*, Japanese researchers investigated the association between the intake of folate, vitamins B_6 and B_{12}, and methionine (a sulfur-containing essential amino acid), and the risk of colorectal cancer in a group of middle-aged men and women. The cohort consisted of 81,184 subjects (38,107 men and 43,077 women) who participated in the Japan Public Health Center Prospective Study from 1995–1998. By the end of 2002, there were 526 (335 men, 191 women) diagnosed cases of colorectal cancer. Only vitamin B_6, which is found in abundance in bell peppers, gave a statistically significant benefit to the male subjects. When compared to the men consuming the least amount of vitamin B_6, the men consuming the most vitamin B_6 had a 31 percent reduction in risk for colorectal cancer. The men with higher intakes of alcohol appeared to derive the most benefits. No such results were observed in the women.[3]

The next year, in 2008, *Cancer Epidemiology Biomarkers & Prevention* published a study on the association between intake of dietary and supplemental vitamin B_6 and colorectal cancer. This Scottish study included 2,028 hospital-based people with colorectal cancer and 2,722 population-based controls. The researchers noted, "moderately strong inverse and dose-dependent associations in the whole sample were found between CRC [colorectal cancer] and the intake of dietary and total vitamin B_6." The researchers also conducted a meta-analysis of published studies on the topic. They found that higher intakes of vitamin B_6 reduced the risk of colorectal cancer by 19 percent.[4]

Lung Cancer

In a study published in 2003 in *Cancer Epidemiology Biomarkers & Prevention*, Chinese researchers examined the association between consumption of foods with high amounts of beta-cryptotoxanthin, such as red bell peppers, and lung cancer. Between April 1993 and December 1998, the data were collected from 63,257 men and women between the ages of 45 and 74 who lived in Shanghai, China. During the first eight years of follow-up, medical providers diagnosed 482 cases of lung cancer. The researchers found that when compared to the men and women who ate the least amount of beta-cryptotoxanthin, the men and women who ate the highest amounts had a 27 percent lower risk for developing lung cancer. Even smokers received protection from consumption of foods with beta-cryptotoxanthin. When compared to smokers who ate the least amount of beta-cryptotoxanthin-rich foods, smokers who ate foods with high amounts had a 37 percent lower risk of lung cancer. The researchers wrote that their findings, "lend additional credence to prior experimental and epidemiological data in support of the hypothesis that dietary ß-cryptoxanthin is a chemopreventive agent for lung cancer in humans."[5]

CARDIOVASCULAR HEALTH

In a study published in 2009 in *Circulation*, Boston researchers reviewed the relationship between fasting plasma levels of vitamin B_6 and the rates of heart attacks (myocardial infarctions) in women. The study included 144 women who participated in the ongoing Nurses' Health Study and experienced a heart attack. Each woman was matched to two other Nurses' Health Study women for age, smoking status, and other factors—but without a history of heart attacks. The researchers found a significant association between plasma levels of B_6 and heart attacks. When compared to the women in the lowest quartile of plasma B_6, the women in the highest quartile of B_6 had a 78 percent lower adjusted risk of a heart attack. When the data were analyzed according to age, the women 60 years of age and older who were in the highest quartile of plasma B_6 had a 64 percent lower risk than those in the lowest quartile. The women under 60 who were in the top quartile of plasma B_6 had a 95 percent lower risk of a heart attack.[6]

OSTEOARTHRITIS OF THE KNEE

In a study published in 2007 in *Arthritis Research & Therapy*, Australian researchers examined the association between intake of vitamin C and osteoarthritis of the knee. (As has been noted, bell peppers have excellent amounts of vitamin C.) The researchers selected 293 healthy adults, with a mean age of 59.0 years, who were free of knee pain. Ten years later, the knees of these subjects were examined by magnetic resonance imaging (MRI studies). The researchers found that the subjects who ate high amounts of vitamin C were less likely to have the bone degeneration that leads to knee osteoarthritis. The researchers wrote that, "The present study suggests a beneficial effect of vitamin C intake on the reduction in bone size and the number of bone marrow lesions, both of which are important in the pathogenesis of knee OA [osteoarthritis]." Furthermore, the researchers learned that other antioxidants, including lutein and zeaxanthin, which are found in bell peppers, are protective against the normal age-related wear and tear on the knees.[7]

On the other hand, a study published in 2004 in *Arthritis & Rheumatism* determined that too much vitamin C might exacerbate osteoarthritis of the knee. Researchers from Duke University Medical Center led an investigation into the effects of eight months of treatment with low, medium, and high doses of vitamin C in guinea pigs. (Like humans, guinea pigs are unable to synthesize vitamin C.) The researchers determined that the guinea pigs in the high-dose group suffered the most severe osteoarthritis of the knee and worst cartilage damage.[8]

CATARACTS

In a study published in 2008 in the *Archives of Ophthalmology*, Boston researchers examined the association between intake of the carotenoids lutein and zeaxanthin, found in bell peppers, and the risk of cataracts. The researchers followed 35,551 women for an average of ten years. During that time, there were 2,031 confirmed cases of cataracts. The researchers found that the women with the highest intake of lutein and zeaxanthin (6,716 micrograms per day) had an 18 percent lower risk of developing cataracts than the women with the lowest average intake (1,177 micrograms per day). The researchers commented that their findings showed, "higher dietary intakes of lutein/zeaxzanthin . . . from food and supplements were associated with significantly decreased risk of cataract."[9]

CAVEATS

Roasting bell peppers increases their levels of acidity. That makes them more likely to erode the enamel on teeth. After eating roasted bell peppers, it is best to brush the teeth and/or rinse the mouth with water.

Not all bell peppers have the same antioxidant activity. Red bell peppers have the most. Next are orange bell peppers; followed by yellow. Green peppers are a distant fourth.[10]

Farmers tend to use a good deal of pesticides on conventionally grown bell peppers. It is best to eat peppers that have been grown organically.

Should bell peppers be included in the diet? Certainly. However, as a precaution, people who have diets that are high in vitamin C should eat bell peppers in moderation.

NOTES

1. The George Mateljan Foundation Website. www.whfoods.com.

2. The George Mateljan Foundation Website.

3. Ishihara, Junko, Tetsuya Otani, Manami Inoue, et al. July 2007. "Low Intake of Vitamin B-6 Is Associated with Increased Risk of Colorectal Cancer in Japanese Men." *The Journal of Nutrition* 137: 1808–1814.

4. Theodoratou, Evropi, Susan M. Farrington, Albert Tenesa, et al. 2008. "Dietary Vitamin B_6 Intake and the Risk of Colorectal Cancer." *Cancer Epidemiology Biomarkers & Prevention* 17(1): 171–182.

5. Yuan, Jian-Min, Daniel O. Stram, Kazuko Arakawa, et al. September 2003. "Dietary Cryptoxanthin and Reduced Risk of Lung Cancer: The Singapore Chinese Health Study." *Cancer Epidemiology Biomarkers & Prevention* 12(9): 890–898.

6. Page, John H., Jing Ma, Stephanie E. Chiuve, et al. 2009. "Plasma Vitamin B_6 and Risk of Myocardial Infarction in Women." *Circulation* 120: 649–655.

7. Wang, Yuanyuan, Allison M. Hodge, Anita E. Wluka, et al. 2007. "Effect of Antioxidants on Knee Cartilage and Bone in Healthy, Middle-Aged Subjects: A Cross-Sectional Study." *Arthritis Research & Therapy* 9: R66.

8. Kraus, Virginia B., Janet L. Huebner, Thomas Stabler, et al. 2004. "Ascorbic Acid Increases the Severity of Spontaneous Knee Osteoarthritis in a Guinea Pig Model." *Arthritis & Rheumatism* 50(6): 1822–1831.

9. Christen, William G., Simin Liu, Robert J. Glynn, et al. 2008. "Dietary Carotenoids, Vitamin C and E, and Risk of Cataract in Women: A Prospective Study." *Archives of Ophthalmology* 126(1): 102–109.

10. Sun, T., Z. Xu, C.T. Wu, et al. 2007. "Antioxidant Activities of Different Colored Sweet Bell Peppers (*Capsicum annuum* L.)." *Journal of Food Science* 72(2): S98–S102.

REFERENCES AND RESOURCES
Magazines, Journals, and Newspapers

Christen, William G., Simin Liu, Robert J. Glynn, et al. 2008. "Dietary Carote-noids, Vitamin C and E, and Risk of Cataract in Women: A Prospective Study." *Archives of Ophthalmology* 126(1): 102–109.

Ishihara, Junko, Tetsuya Otani, Manami Inoue, et al. July 2007. "Low Intake of Vita-min B-6 Is Associated with Increased Risk of Colorectal Cancer in Japanese Men." *The Journal of Nutrition* 137: 1808–1814.

Kraus, Virginia B., Janet L. Huebner, Thomas Stabler, et al. June 2004. "Ascorbic Acid Increases the Severity of Spontaneous Knee Osteoarthritis in a Guinea Pig Model." *Arthritis & Rheumatism* 50(6): 1822–1831.

Page, John H., Jing Ma, Stephanie E. Chiuve, et al. 2009. "Plasma Vitamin B_6 and Risk of Myocardial Infarction in Women." *Circulation* 120: 649–655.

Sun, T., Z. Xu, C. T. Wu, et al. 2007. "Antioxidant Activities of Different Colored Sweet Bell Peppers (*Capsicum annuum* L.)." *Journal of Food Science* 72(2): S98–S102.

Theodoratou, Evropi, Susan M. Farrington, Albert Tenesa, et al. 2008. "Dietary Vitamin B_6 Intake and Risk of Colorectal Cancer." *Cancer Epidemiology Bio-markers & Prevention* 17(1): 171–182.

Wang, Yuanyuan, Allison M. Hodge, Anita E. Wluka, et al. 2007 "Effect of Antiox-idants on Knee Cartilage and Bone in Healthy, Middle-Aged Subjects: A Cross-Sectional Study." *Arthritis Research & Therapy* 9: R66.

Yuan, Jian-Min, Daniel O. Stram, Kazuko Arakawa, et al. September 2003. "Dietary Cryptoxanthin and Reduced Risk of Lung Cancer: The Singapore Chinese Health Study." *Cancer Epidemiology Biomarkers & Prevention* 12(9): 890–898.

Website

The George Mateljan Foundation. www.whfoods.com.

BLACK BEANS

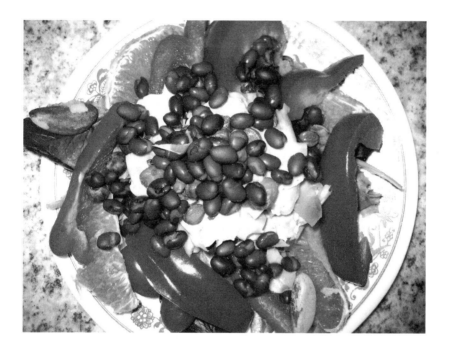

One of the reasons people sometimes give for their failure to eat a healthful diet is the expense. These people maintain that eating better is just too costly, especially during difficult economic times. But that is not necessarily true. For example, black beans are often cited as a wonderful example of an inexpensive, nutritious food.

Black beans are believed to be helpful in lowering cholesterol levels, and their high amount of fiber prevents sugar from rising rapidly after a meal. That makes them desirable for people with diabetes. Black beans are considered an excellent source of the trace mineral molybdenum, which is used to detoxify sulfites. They are thought to be a good source of dietary fiber, folate, trypto-phan, manganese, protein, magnesium, vitamin B_1, phosphorus, and iron.[1]

Black beans, which are also known as *Phaselus vulgaris*, are popular in a number of different countries including Brazil, Mexico, Cuba, Guatemala, and the Dominican Republic. They are widely eaten in many other countries, including the United States.[2] But what does the research say?

OVERALL HEALTH

In a study published in 2003 in the *Journal of Agricultural and Food Chemistry*, Michigan State University researchers tested the antioxidant activity of 12 types of dry beans. Antioxidants destroy free radicals, which have been linked to illnesses associated with aging, such as heart disease and cancer. Black beans were found to have the highest amounts of antioxidants. They were followed by red, brown, yellow, and white beans—in that order. Darker-colored beans tended to have more antioxidants than the lighter varieties.

One group of antioxidants, known as anthocyanins, was the most active antioxidant in the black beans. In fact, in a startling finding, researchers determined that the amount of anthocyanins per 100-gram (g) serving of black beans was about ten times the amount of overall antioxidants in an equivalent amount of oranges and about the same amount found in an equivalent serving of cranberries, grapes, and apples. The researchers studied dry beans; when cooked, beans lose some of these anthocyanins. Still, the researchers thought that the cooked beans probably retained a considerable amount of anthocyanins.[3]

The results of a similar study, conducted at North Dakota State University, were published in 2007 in the *Journal of Food Science*. Black beans, as well as lentils, black soybeans, red kidney beans, and pinto beans, were found to have more antioxidants than yellow and green peas, chickpeas, and yellow soybeans. In addition, the extracts of black beans (and lentils, black soybeans, and red kidney beans) helped slow the amount of time it took to make LDL (or "bad") cholesterol. In so doing, black beans have the potential to prevent the development of atherosclerosis.[4]

CANCER PREVENTION

In a Brazilian study published in 2003 in *Food and Chemical Toxicology*, researchers attempted to evaluate the protective effect that cooked and dehydrated black beans may have on the bone marrow and peripheral blood cells of exposed mice. When the researchers fed the mice a 20 percent black bean diet, they found that the mice experienced a reduction in precancerous cells. This was seen even in those mice that were given an agent to promote the growth of cancer cells. Hoping to identify the component of the beans that impart this protection, the researchers tested anthocyanin. However, when administered at the highest dosage (50 milligrams per kilogram of body weight), the anthocyanin caused DNA damage. The researchers concluded that the interactions of the combination of elements that go into creating black beans are better than any of the beans' individual components.[5]

In a study published in July 2006 in *The Journal of Nutrition*, researchers lead by Dr. Elaine Lanza, head of the Colon Cancer Prevention Group at the National Cancer Institute, investigated more than 2,000 men and women over the age of 35 who were diagnosed with precancerous polyps during the six months before the study began. Over the four years of the study, the subjects were asked questions about their diets. Many tried dietary changes to prevent the growth of more polyps. Those who added the most beans to their diets, including black beans, had a significantly reduced risk of recurrence of advanced polyps.[6]

CARDIOVASCULAR HEALTH

A study published in 2006 in the *Archives of Internal Medicine* examined the association of intake of protein and blood pressure readings. Included in the study were 4,680 people, aged 40 to 59 years, from China, Japan, the United Kingdom, and the United States. No significant relationships were found between animal protein intake and blood pressure or between total protein intake and blood pressure. However, researchers found a significant inverse relationship between the consumption of vegetable protein, such as black beans, and blood pressure. For every 2.8 percent increase in vegetable protein intake—about $3/4$ cup of black beans for someone on a 2,000-calorie diet—there was an average drop of 2.14 millimeters (mm) in systolic pressure and 1.35 mm in diastolic pressure.[7]

WEIGHT CONTROL

In a study published in 2009 in *The Journal of Nutrition*, researchers at the Brigham Young University College of Health and Human Performance in Provo, Utah, examined how the intake of fiber, such as that found in black beans, could influence the control of weight gain in women. The cohort of 252 women completed baseline and follow-up assessments 20 months apart. The researchers found that, "increasing dietary fiber significantly reduces the risk of gaining weight and fat in women, independent of several potential confounders, including physical activity, dietary fat intake, and others." Why does fiber have such a strong influence? "Fiber's influence seems to occur primarily through reducing energy intake over time."[8]

DIABETES PREVENTION

In a study published in 2009 in the *Archives of Pediatrics & Adolescent Medicine*, researchers at the Keck School of Medicine at the University of Southern California in Los Angeles attempted to determine if reducing the amount of dietary sugar and increasing the amount of dietary fiber, such as that found in black beans, could help prevent the development of type 2 diabetes in Latino adolescents, who are often overweight and at increased risk for diabetes.

The researchers divided 54 overweight teens (average age 15.5) into three groups. One group had one nutrition class per week; a second group had one nutrition class per week and two sessions of strength training per week; a third group served as the control.

At the end of the 16-week study, researchers observed that 55 percent of the adolescents had decreased their sugar intake by an average of 47 g per day, the amount of sugar contained in a can of soda. Fifty-nine percent of the adolescents had increased their fiber intake by an average of five g per day, an amount equal to one-half cup of beans. The adolescents who decreased their intake of sugar averaged a 33 percent decrease in insulin secretion; those who increased their fiber intake had a 10 percent reduction in visceral adipose tissue volume. Both of these factors decrease the risk of type 2 diabetes. The researchers noted that the adolescents who made these relatively modest changes in their diets "showed improvements in key risk factors for type 2 diabetes, specifically in insulin secretion and visceral fat."[9]

CAVEATS

Dry and canned black beans are equally nutritious. Yet, in some instances, canned black beans may contain higher amounts of salt. Whenever possible, those beans should be avoided. To further reduce the salt in canned beans, they should be rinsed with tap water.

Should black beans be included in the diet? Of course. However, they should be added gradually. Eating too many black beans too quickly may result in gastrointestinal upset.

NOTES

1. The George Mateljan Foundation Website. www.whfoods.com.

2. The George Mateljan Foundation Website.

3. Beninger, Clifford W. and George L. Hosfield. 2003. "Antioxidant Activity of Extracts, Condensed Tannin Fractions, and Pure Flavonoids from *Phaseolus vulgaris* L. Seed Coat Color. *Journal of Agricultural and Food Chemistry* 51(27): 7879–7883.

4. Xu, B. J., S. H. Yuan, and S. K. Chang. September 2007. "Comparative Studies on the Antioxidant Activities of Nine Common Food Legumes Against Copper-Induced Human Low-Density Lipoprotein Oxidation in Vitro." *Journal of Food Science* 72(7): S522-S527.

5. Azevedo, L., J. C. Gomes, P. C. Stringheta et al. 2003. "Black Bean (*Phaseolus vulgaris* L.) as a Protective Agent Against DNA Damage in Mice." *Food and Chemical Toxicology* 41(12): 1671–1676.

6. Lanza, Elaine, Terryl J. Hartman, Paul S. Albert et al. July 2006. "High Dry Bean Intake and Reduced Risk of Advanced Colorectal Adenoma Recurrence Among Participants in the Polyp Prevention Trial." *The Journal of Nutrition* 136: 1896–1903.

7. Elliott, Paul, Jeremiah Stamler, Alan R. Dyer et al. January 9, 2006. "Association Between Protein Intake and Blood Pressure." *Archives of Internal Medicine* 166(1): 79–87.

8. Tucker, Larry A. and Kathryn S. Thomas. March 2009. "Increasing Total Fiber Intake Reduces Risk of Weight and Fat Gains in Women." *The Journal of Nutrition* 139(3): 576–581.

9. Ventura, Emily, Jaimie Davis, Courtney Byrd-Williams et al. April 2009. "Reduction in Risk Factors for Type 2 Diabetes Mellitus in Response to a Low-Sugar, High-Fiber Dietary Intervention in Overweight Latino Adolescents." *Archives of Pediatrics & Adolescent Medicine* 163(4): 320–327.

REFERENCES AND RESOURCES
Magazines, Journals, and Newspapers

Azevedo, L., J. C. Gomes, P. C. Stringheta et al. 2003. "Black Bean (*Phaselus vulgaris* L.) as a Protective Agent Against DNA Damage in Mice." *Food and Chemical Toxicology* 41(12): 1671–1676.

Beninger, Clifford W. and George L. Hosfield. 2003. "Antioxidant Activity of Extracts, Condensed Tannin Fractions, and Pure Flavonoids from *Phaselous vulgaris* L. Seed Coat Color Genotypes." *Journal of Agricultural and Food Chemistry* 51(27): 7879–7883.

Elliott, Paul, Jeremiah Stamler, Alan R. Dyer et al. January 9, 2006. "Association Between Protein Intake and Blood Pressure." *Archives of Internal Medicine* 166(1): 79–87.

Lanza, Elaine, Terryl J. Hartman, Paul S. Albert et al. July 2006. "High Dry Bean Intake and Reduced Risk of Advanced Colorectal Adenoma Recurrence Among Participants in the Polyp Prevention Trial." *American Society for Nutrition* 136: 1896–1903.

Tucker, Larry A. and Kathryn S. Thomas. March 2009. "Increasing Total Fiber Reduces Risk of Weight and Fat Gains in Women." *The Journal of Nutrition* 139(3): 576–581.

Ventura, Emily, Jaimie Davis, Courtney Byrd-Williams et al. April 2009. "Reduction in Risk Factors for Type 2 Diabetes Mellitus in Response to a Low-Sugar, High-Fiber Dietary Intervention in Overweight Latino Adolescents." *Archives of Pediatrics & Adolescent Medicine* 163(4): 320–327.

Winham, Donna, Densie Webb, and Amy Barr. September–October 2008. "Beans and Good Health." *Nutrition Today* 43(5): 201–209.

Xu, B. J., S. H. Yuan, and S. K. Chang. September 2007. "Comparative Studies on the Antioxidant Activities of Nine Common Food Legumes Against Copper-Induced Human Low-Density Lipoprotein Oxidation in Vitro." *Journal of Food Science* 72(7): S522–S527.

Website

The George Mateljan Foundation. www.whfoods.com.

BLUEBERRIES

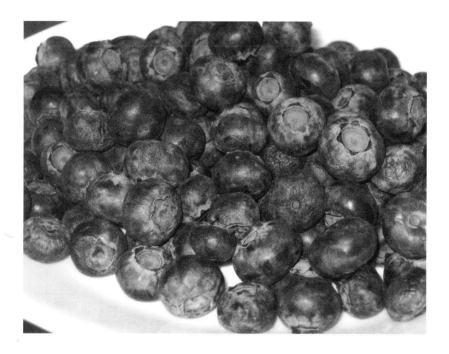

James Joseph, PhD, a nutrition researcher at the Human Nutrition Research Center on Aging at Tufts University, begins his days by drinking a glass of pomegranate juice and eating a cup of wild blueberries. According to a 2008 article in *Psychology Today*, after studying blueberries, otherwise known as vaccinium, for years, Dr. Joseph is convinced that they help the brain and the body fight the seemingly endless number of problems associated with aging. While blueberries contain traditional nutrients, such as carbohydrates, fiber, vitamins C and E, and manganese, they also have anthocyanidins (dark flavonoid phytochemicals), which fight oxidative stress and inflammation. "Cumulatively, the berries produce antioxidant effects, neutralizing cellular damage created by free radicals of oxygen and blocking pathways by which oxidative stress damages cells. Perhaps more important, they function as anti-inflammatory agents to preserve cardiovascular as well as brain integrity."[1]

In a 2004 interview with the *Seattle Post-Intelligencer*, Dr. Joseph said that the old neurons in the brain are like couples who have been married a long time—they no longer communicate. Blueberries change that dynamic. They enable neurons to once again converse. "Blueberries have compounds that boost neuron signals and help turn back on systems in the brain that can lead to using other proteins to help with memory or other cognitive skills."[2]

In his research on rats and mice, Dr. Joseph has found that rats that eat blueberries have fewer cases of Alzheimer's disease and lower instances of arthritis-related inflammation. He and his colleagues have also determined that blueberries may be useful for those undergoing radiation therapy. They reduce the effects on cognitive and motor skills and may "even eliminate radiation-induced nausea."[3] Rats that were fed a diet containing two percent blueberry extracts before undergoing radiation did far better than those rats who received no blueberries before their radiation treatments. "Irradiation causes deficits in behavior and signaling in rats which were ameliorated by an antioxidant diet." Possibly, "the polyphenols in these fruits might be acting in different brain regions."[4]

Dr. Joseph has even observed that blueberries tend to work best when eaten with certain high-fat foods such as walnuts, which contain polyphenols and omega-3 fatty acids. Working together, the blueberries and walnuts make nerve cell membranes more responsive. As a result, "the efficacy of all transactions" is improved. In addition, the combination of blueberries and walnuts "may help block inflammation at the cellular level, a process now implicated in cardiovascular disease, Alzheimer's disease, and other degenerative processes of aging."[5]

CARDIOVASCULAR HEALTH

A Canadian study lead by Wilhelmina Kalt, PhD, a researcher with Agriculture and Agri-Food Canada, published in 2008 in the *British Journal of Nutrition*, reported that pigs who were fed a 2-percent blueberry diet experienced reductions of total, LDL, and HDL cholesterol. The two-percent blueberry diet is equivalent to two cups of blueberries in the human diet. Why is this significant? Pigs and humans have similar levels of LDL. They are also prone to diet-related vascular disease and atherosclerotic plaques in the carotid artery and aorta. Furthermore, their heart rate and blood pressure resemble human heart rate and blood pressure.[6] A 2008 article in *Grocer* states that as a result of her research, Dr. Kalt advises people to eat at least four ounces of blueberries every day.[7]

CANCER

In a 2006 study published in the *Journal of Agricultural and Food Chemistry*, Navindra Seeram, PhD, assistant director of the UCLA Center for Human Nutrition and assistant professor at the David Geffen School of Medicine at UCLA, reported that the extracts of common berries, such as blueberries, which are filled with antioxidants, inhibit the growth of in vitro mouth, prostate, breast, and colon cancer cells. Dr. Seeram and his colleagues also determined that higher amounts of berries inhibit larger numbers of cancer cells. "With increasing concentration of berry extract, increasing inhibition of cell proliferation in all of the cell lines were observed, with different degrees of potency between cell lines."[8]

Another study, published in 2007 in *Clinical Cancer Research*, describes research conducted by scientists at Rutgers University and the U.S. Department of Agriculture (USDA) on the relationship between pterostilbene, a naturally occurring antioxidant in blueberries, and colon cancer. During the study, rats were given a compound to induce colon cancer. Half of the rats were then placed on a balanced diet; the other half were given the same diet, but it was supplemented with pterostilbene. At the end of eight weeks, when compared to the control group, the rats that had consumed supplemental pterostilbene had 57 percent fewer pre-cancerous colonic lesions. Researchers concluded that the "study suggests that pterostilbene, a compound present in blueberries, is of great interest for the prevention of colon cancer."[9]

Agnes Rimando, PhD, a researcher with Natural Products Utilization Research in Mississippi, a division of the USDA Agriculture Research Service, has found similar results. In her studies, Dr. Rimando has noted that pterostilbene may well impair the ability of enzymes to activate chemical carcinogens. So cells that might otherwise turn cancerous do not.[10]

ANTI-AGING AND GENERAL WELL-BEING

It has been well established that there is a strong relationship between oxidative stress and chronic illness and aging. Moreover, the antioxidants in blueberries are known to fight that oxidative stress. A research study published in 2007 in the *Journal of the American College of Nutrition* found that it is not only important for people to eat blueberries and other antioxidant foods. It is also significant *when* they eat them. To reduce oxidative stress throughout the day, the researchers recommend eating blueberries or other antioxidant foods with each meal.[11]

A 2006 study published in *Neurobiology of Aging* addressed the fact that as people age, the heat shock proteins in the brain, which, like antioxidants, support healthy brain functions, decline. Could eating blueberries reverse this decline? For ten weeks, researchers fed a blueberry-enhanced diet to young and old rats and compared them to a control group of old rats, who were fed a diet without blueberries.

As expected, after ten weeks the brains of the young rats were found to contain large amounts of heat shock proteins, and the brains of the old rats who did not eat blueberries had low amounts of heat shock proteins. However, the heat shock proteins of the old rats who ate blueberries were completely restored. Researchers concluded that blueberries may well play a serious role in protecting against the neurodegenerative processes that often are associated with aging.[12]

A 2005 article in *Nutrition Today* summarizes the many reasons for including blueberries in the diet. "The blueberry is becoming more widely recognized for its flavor, nutrition, and health benefits. Both production and consumption in the United States have more than doubled in the last 20 years. Not only are blueberries ranked among the highest in antioxidant activity when compared to other fruits and vegetables, they are also one of the richest sources of anthocyanins."[13] And, there is very strong evidence that the consumption of anthocyanins reduces the risk the heart disease, cancer, and other problems associated with aging.

NOTES

1. Marano, Daniel A. May–June 2008. "The Smartest Food: Phytochemical-Rich Berries Can Multiply Their Own Brain-Saving Effects When Eaten with Certain Fat-Rich Foods." *Psychology Today* 41(3): 59–60.

2. Condor, Bob. September 6, 2004. "Living Well: Blueberries Trigger Neurons That Keep the Brain Sharp." *Seattle Post-Intelligencer*, available at http://seattle pinwsource.com/health.

3. "Eating Blueberries to Battle Alzheimer's: 'Getting the Blues' May Also Help Lower Cholesterol and Reduce the Side Effects of Radiation Treatment." December 2004. *Tufts University Health & Nutrition Letter* 22(10): 3.

4. Shukitt-Hale, Barbara, Amanda N. Carey, Daniel Jenkins, et al. August 2007. "Beneficial Effects of Fruit Extracts on Neuronal Function and Behavior in a Rodent Model of Accelerated Aging." *Neurobiology of Aging* 28(8): 1187–1194.

5. Marano, Daniel A.

6. "Research: Diets with Blueberries Show Promise in Lowering Cholesterol." June 26, 2008. *Food & Beverage Close-Up*: NA.

7. "Blueberries Reduce Cholesterol in Pigs." August 23, 2008. *Grocer* 231(7869): 54s.

8. Seeram, N. P., L. S. Adams, Y. Zhang, et al. December 13, 2006. "Blackberry, Black Raspberry, Blueberry, Cranberry, Red Raspberry, and Strawberry Extracts Inhibit Growth and Stimulate Apoptosis of Human Cancer." *Journal of Agricultural and Food Chemistry* 54(25): 9329–9239.

9. Suh, Nanjoo, Shiby Paul, Xiangpei Hao, et al. January 1, 2007. "Pterostilbene, An Active Constituent of Blueberries, Suppresses Aberrant Crypt Foci Formation in the Azoxymethane-Induced Colon Carcinogenesis Model in Rats." *Clinical Cancer Research* 13: 350–355.

10. Pons, Luis. November–December 2006. "Pterostilbene's Healthy Potential: Berry Compound May Inhibit Breast Cancer and Heart Disease." *Agricultural Research* 54(11–12): 6–7.

11. Prior, Ronald L., Liwei Gu, Xianli Wu, et al. April 2007. "Plasma Antioxidant Capacity Changes Following a Meal as a Measure of the Ability of a Food to Alter In Vivo Antioxidant Status." *Journal of the American College of Nutrition* 26(2): 170–181.

12. Galli, Rachel L., Donna F. Bielinski, Aleksandra Szprengiel, et al. February 2006. "Blueberry Supplemented Diet Reverses Age-Related Decline in Hippocampal HSP70 Neuroprotection." *Neurobiology of Aging* 27(2): 344–350.

13. Lewis, Nancy and Jaime Ruud. March/April 2005. "Blueberries in the American Diet." *Nutrition Today* 40(2): 92–96.

REFERENCES AND RESOURCES
Magazines, Journals, and Newspapers

"Blueberries Reduce Cholesterol in Pigs." August 23, 2008. *Grocer* 231(7869): 54.

Bone, Kerry. February 12, 2008. "Blue is the Healthy Color: The Health Benefits of Anthocyanins." *Dynamic Chiropractic* 26(4): S25–S26.

Condor, Bob. September 6, 2004. "Living Well: Blueberries Trigger Neurons That Keep the Brain Sharp." *Seattle Post-Intelligencer*, available at http://seattlepinwsource.com/health.

"Eating Blueberries to Battle Alzheimer's: 'Getting the Blues' May Also Help Lower Cholesterol and Reduce the Side Effects of Radiation Treatment." December 2004. *Tufts University Health & Nutrition Letter* 22(11): 3.

Galli, Rachel L., Donna F. Bielinski, Aleksandra Szprengiel, et al. February 2006. "Blueberry Supplemented Diet Reverses Age-Related Decline in Hippocampal HSP70 Neuroprotection." *Neurobiology of Aging* 27(2): 344–350.

Kalt, W., Kim Foote, and S. A. E. Fillmore. July 2008. "Effect of Blueberry Feeding on Plasma Lipids in Pigs." *British Journal of Nutrition* 100 (1): 70–78.

Lewis, Nancy and Jaime Ruud. March/April 2005. "Blueberries in the American Diet." *Nutrition Today* 40(2): 92–96.

Marano, Daniel A. May–June 2008. "The Smartest Food: Phytochemical-Rich Berries Can Multiply Their Own Brain-Saving Effects When Eaten with Certain Fat-Rich Foods." *Psychology Today* 41(3): 59–60.

Pons, Luis. November–December 2006. "Pterostilbene's Healthy Potential: Berry Compound May Inhibit Breast Cancer and Heart Disease." *Agricultural Research* 54(11-12): 6–7.

Prior, Ronald L., Liwei Gu, Xianli Wu, et al. April 2007. "Plasma Antioxidant Capacity Changes Following a Meal as a Measure of the Ability of a Food to Alter In Vivo Antioxidant Status." *Journal of the American College of Nutrition* 26(2): 170–181.

"Research: Diets with Blueberries Show Promise in Lowering Cholesterol." June 26, 2008. *Food & Beverage Close-Up*: NA.

Seeram, N. P., L. S. Adams, Y. Zhang, et al. December 13, 2006. "Blackberry, Black Raspberry, Blueberry, Cranberry, Red Raspberry, and Strawberry Extracts Inhibit Growth and Stimulate Apoptosis of Human Cancer Cells in Vitro." *Journal of Agricultural and Food Chemistry* 54(25): 9329–9339.

Shukitt-Hale, Barbara, Amanda N. Carey, Daniel Jenkins, et al. August 2007. "Beneficial Effects of Fruit Extracts on Neuronal Function and Behavior in a Rodent Model of Accelerated Aging." *Neurobiology of Aging* 28(8): 1187–1194.

Shukitt-Hale, Barbara, Rachel L. Galli, Vanessa Meterko, et al. March 2005. "Dietary Supplementation with Fruit Polyphenolics Ameliorates Age-Related Deficits in Behavior and Neuronal Markers of Inflammation and Oxidative Stress." *AGE* 27(1): 49–57.

Suh, Naajoo, Shiby Paul, Xingpei Hao, et al. January 1, 2007. "Pterostilbene, An Active Constituent of Blueberries, Suppresses Aberrant Crypt Foci Formation in the Azoxymethane-Induced Colon Carcinogenesis Model in Rats." *Clinical Cancer Research* 13: 350–355.

Websites

U.S. Highbush Blueberry Council. www.blueberry.org.
Wild Blueberries. www.wildblueberries.com.

BRAZIL NUTS

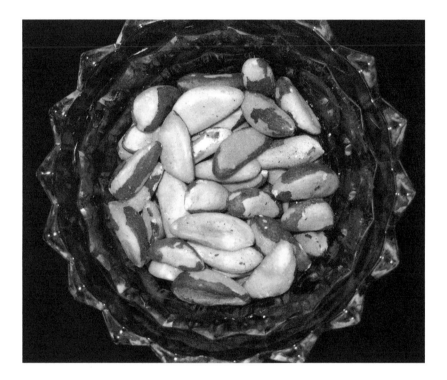

Selenium is an essential trace element that is found in a number of different foods. But, of all the foods that contain selenium, Brazil nuts pack the most punch. Thus, while one medium whole egg has 14 micrograms of selenium and one ounce of cheddar cheese has four micrograms of selenium, one ounce of dried Brazil nuts contains 544 micrograms of selenium.[1]

Throughout the world, other than Brazil nuts, plant foods are considered the primary dietary source for selenium. However, the amount of selenium in a specific food is very much a function of the amount of selenium in the soil. In the United States, the soils in the Dakotas and in the high plains of northern Nebraska contain high levels of selenium. People who live in those regions tend to have higher intakes of this element. On the other hand, the soils in sections of China and Russia have essentially no selenium.[2]

The research on Brazil nuts and selenium is not always consistent. Nevertheless, it is still interesting to review.

PROSTATE CANCER

A study published in 2001 in *The Journal of Urology* reviewed the relationship between the amount of selenium in the blood and the risk for developing prostate cancer. The research was completed using men listed on the Baltimore Longitudinal Study of Aging. These included "52 with known prostate cancer and 96 age matched controls with no detectable prostatic disease." The researchers found that low rates of selenium in the blood are "associated with a 4 to 5-fold increased risk of prostate cancer."[3]

A few years later, in 2004, another study on the relationship between levels of blood selenium and prostate cancer was published in *JNCI: Journal of the National Cancer Institute*. These researchers, who used data from men enrolled in the Physician's Health Study, found "that higher levels of selenium may slow prostate cancer tumor progression."[4]

However, a 2009 article in *JAMA, The Journal of the American Medical Association* noted dramatically different results from studies involving 35,533 generally healthy men from 427 sites in the United States, Canada, and Puerto Rico. The men were randomly assigned to one of four groups: selenium (200 micrograms per day), vitamin E (400 IU/day), selenium and vitamin E, and placebos. Although follow-up was originally planned for seven to twelve years, after 5.46 years, the researchers found no statistically significant differences between the four groups. The researchers concluded that selenium (and vitamin E) "did not prevent prostate cancer in this population of relatively healthy men."[5]

COGNITIVE FUNCTION

A study published in 2007 in the *American Journal of Epidemiology* describes a cross-sectional survey of 2,000 people, aged 65 years and older, who live in two different provinces in rural China. More than 70 percent of the people surveyed had lived in the same villages since birth. To determine selenium levels, nail samples were collected. (Nails are used because they grow slowly and steadily and give a sense of the amount of selenium over a period of time.) The subjects were given a battery of tests including the Community Screening Instrument for Dementia (CSID), the Indiana University Token Test, and the Consortium to Establish a Registry for Alzheimer's Disease (CERAD). The researchers found that people with lower levels of selenium had lower rates of cognitive function. In fact, their rates tended to be comparable to those of people ten years older. The researchers said that, "results in this geographically stable cohort support the hypothesis that a lifelong low selenium level is associated with lower cognitive function."[6]

BLADDER CANCER

A study published in 2009 in *Cancer Prevention Research*, a journal of the American Association for Cancer Research, said that, in some instances, selenium may play a role in preventing bladder cancer. Researchers analyzed data from 857 cases of bladder cancer and 1,191 general population controls. While they found no relationship between levels of selenium in toenails and bladder cancer, the researchers observed that there is the possibility that in certain molecular phenotypes of tumors and certain subgroups of the population (such as women and moderate smokers), selenium may play some form of preventive role.[7]

OSTEOARTHRITIS (OA)

At the 2005 American College of Rheumatology Annual Scientific Meeting, Joanne Jordan, MD, a rheumatologist at the University of North Carolina at Chapel Hill, presented a study she completed on the incidence of osteoarthritis (OA) and the level of selenium in toenail chippings. Dr. Jordan and her colleagues measured the amount of selenium in the toenails of 940 people. They found that the people with the lowest levels of selenium were more likely to develop osteoarthritis. Moreover, "the lower the selenium level, the more severe the OA."[8]

BARRETT'S ESOPHAGUS

In a study conducted at the Fred Hutchinson Cancer Research Center and the University of Washington and published in 2003 in *JNCI Journal of the National Cancer Institute*, researchers attempted to determine if higher levels of selenium may inhibit the progression of the precancerous condition known as Barrett's esophagus into esophageal cancer. Although only five to ten percent of people with Barrett's esophagus actually develop esophageal cancer, those who do have a grim prognosis. More than 90 percent die within five years.

During the study, medical histories, blood tests, and esophageal tissue were taken from 399 Barrett's esophagus patients. The researchers found that people with the lowest levels of selenium in the blood had the highest risk of developing esophageal cancer. In fact, they had a two- to three-fold increased risk of developing changes leading to esophageal cancer compared to those with selenium levels in the middle or high range.[9]

PREECLAMPSIA

In a study that was published in 2003 in the *American Journal of Obstetrics and Gynecology*, researchers at the University of Surrey in the United Kingdom attempted to determine if there was an association between low levels of selenium and preeclampsia, a serious condition that may occur during pregnancy. (Preeclampsia is characterized by high blood pressure and protein in the urine.

Other symptoms include swelling, sudden weight gain, vision changes, and headaches.)

The researchers obtained toenail clippings from 53 preeclmaptic patients and 53 matched pregnant controls. After they were analyzed, researchers found the "median toenail selenium concentrations in the preeclamptic subjects were significantly lower than in their matched controls." In addition, "within the preeclamptic group, lower selenium status was significantly associated . . . with more severe expression of disease, as measured by delivery before 32 weeks."[10]

MUSCLE STRENGTH

In a study published in 2007 in the *American Journal of Clinical Nutrition*, researchers investigated the association between low plasma selenium and muscle strength in 891 men and women 65 years of age or older. They found that the seniors with the lowest levels of blood selenium were about 95 percent more likely to have poor knee and grip strength than those with the highest levels.[11]

Should Brazil nuts be included in the diet? For the vast majority of people who are not allergic to Brazil nuts, of course. However, higher intakes may cause selenium toxicity, with symptoms such as nausea, vomiting, hair loss, skin lesions, and abnormalities of the fingernails. Men and women 19 years and older should consume no more than 400 micrograms per day. Since the average Brazil nut contains between 70 and 90 micrograms of selenium, most people should eat a maximum of four Brazil nuts per day.[12]

NOTES

1. Fahey, Jed, Marianna Fordyce-Baum, Orville Levander, et al. December 2007. *Dietary Supplement Fact Sheet: Selenium.* National Institutes of Health, Office of Dietary Supplements: NA.

2. Fahey, Jed, Marianna Fordyce-Baum, Orville Levander, et al.: NA.

3. Brooks, James D., E. Jeffrey Metter, Daniel W. Chan, et al. December 2001. "Plasma Selenium Level Before Diagnosis and the Risk of Prostate Cancer Development." *The Journal of Urology* 166(6): 2034–2038.

4. Li, Haojie, Meir J. Stampfer, Edward L. Giovannucci, et al. 2004. "A Prospective Study of Plasma Selenium Levels and Prostate Cancer Risk." *JNCI: Journal of the National Cancer Institute* 96(9): 696–703.

5. Lippman, Scott M., Eric A. Klein, Phyllis J. Goodman, et al. January 7, 2009. "Effect of Selenium and Vitamin E on Risk of Prostate Cancer and Other Cancers." *JAMA, The Journal of the American Medical Association* 301(1): 39–51.

6. Gao, Sujuan, Yinlong Jin, Kathleen S. Hall, et al. 2007. "Selenium Level and Cognitive Function in Rural Elderly Chinese." *American Journal of Epidemiology* 165(8): 955–965.

7. Wallace, Kristin, Karl T. Kelsey, Alan Schned, et al. January 1, 2009. "Selenium and Risk of Bladder Cancer: A Population-Based Case-Control Study." *Cancer Prevention Research* 2: 70–73.

8. Kreimer, Susan and Mary Anne Dunkin. February 1, 2008. "Can Your Nails Help Diagnose Arthritis or Osteoporosis?" Website of Arthritis Foundation. www.arthritis.org.

9. Rudolph, Rebecca E., Thomas L. Vaughan, Alan R. Kristal, et al. May 21, 2003. "Serum Selenium Levels in Relation to Markers of Neoplastic Progression Among Persons with Barrett's Esophagus." *JNCI: Journal of the National Cancer Institute* 95(10): 750–757.

10. Rayman, Margaret P., Peter Bode, and Christopher W. G. Redman. November 2003. "Low Selenium Status Is Associated with the Occurrence of the Pregnancy Disease Preeclampsia in Women from the United Kingdom." *American Journal of Obstetrics and Gynecology* 189(5): 1343–1349.

11. Lauretani, Fulvio, Richard D. Semba, Stefania Bandinelli, et al. August 2007. "Association of Low Plasma Selenium Concentrations with Poor Muscle Strength in Older Community-Dwelling Adults: The InCHIANTI Study." *The American Journal of Clinical Nutrition* 86(2): 347–352.

12. The George Mateljan Foundation Website. www.whfoods.com.

RESOURCES AND REFERENCES
Magazines, Journals, and Newspapers

Brooks, James D., E. Jeffrey Metter, Daniel W. Chan, et al. December 2001. "Plasma Selenium Level Before Diagnosis and the Risk of Prostate Cancer." *The Journal of Urology* 166(6): 2034–2038.

Fahey, Jed, Marianna Fordyce-Baum, Orville Levander, et al. December 2007. *Dietary Supplement Fact Sheet: Selenium.* National Institutes of Health, Office of Dietary Supplements: NA.

Gao, Sujuan, Yinlong Jin, Kathleen S. Hall, et al. 2007. "Selenium Level and Cognitive Function in Rural Elderly Chinese." *American Journal of Epidemiology* 165(8): 955– 965.

Lauretani, Fulvio, Richard D. Semba, Stefania Bandinelli, et al. August 2007. "Association of Low Plasma Selenium Concentrations with Poor Muscle Strength in Older Community-Dwelling Adults: The InCHIANTI Study." *The American Journal of Clinical Nutrition* 86(2): 347–352.

Li, Haojie, Meir J. Stampfer, Edward L. Giovannucci, et al. 2004. "A Prospective Study of Plasma Selenium Levels and Prostate Cancer Risk." *JNCI: Journal of the National Cancer Institute* 96(9): 696–703.

Lippman, Scott M., Eric A. Klein, Phyllis J. Goodman, et al. January 7, 2009. "Effect of Selenium and Vitamin E on Risk of Prostate Cancer and Other Cancers." *JAMA, The Journal of the American Medical Association* 301(1): 39–51.

Rayman, Margaret P., Peter Bode, and Christopher W. G. Redman. November 2003. "Low Selenium Status Is Associated with the Occurrence of the Pregnancy Disease Preeclampsia in Women from the United Kingdom." *American Journal of Obstetrics and Gynecology* 189(5): 1343–1349.

Rudolph, Rebecca E., Thomas L. Vaughan, Alan R. Kristal, et al. May 21, 2003. "Serum Selenium Levels in Relation to Markers of Neoplastic Progression Among Persons with Barrett's Esophagus." *JNCI: Journal of the National Cancer Institute* 95(10): 750–757.

Wallace, Kristin, Karl T. Kelsey, Alan Schned, et al. January 1, 2009. "Selenium and Risk of Bladder Cancer: A Population-Based Case-Control Study." *Cancer Prevention Research* 2: 70–73.

Websites

Arthritis Foundation. www.arthritis.org.
The George Mateljan Foundation. www.whfoods.com.

BROCCOLI

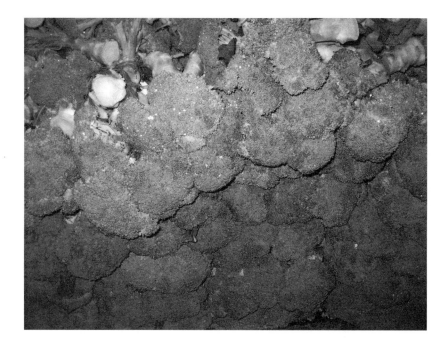

While broccoli has long been considered an extremely healthful food, life has not always been easy for this cruciferous vegetable. Two decades ago, it became particularly difficult early in the presidency of George H. W. Bush. For it was then that President Bush declared that although he has always hated broccoli, when he was a child, his mother made him eat it. Now that he was the leader of the free world, he would no longer eat any broccoli. In fact, he would not allow it to be served in the White House.[1]

Though he was quite adamant, perhaps the former president should have reconsidered what he was saying. Broccoli is believed to be an excellent source of vitamins C, K, and A; folate; and dietary fiber. It is a very good source of manganese, tryptophan, potassium, vitamins B_6 and B_2, phosphorus, magnesium, protein, and omega-3 fatty acids. In addition, broccoli is a good source of vitamins B_1, B_3, and B_5, iron, calcium, zinc, and vitamin E.[2] But, it is necessary to investigate the research.

CANCER
Bladder Cancer

In a Texas study published in 2007 in the *International Journal of Cancer*, researchers compared the diets of 697 newly diagnosed bladder cancer patients to 708 healthy controls matched by age, gender, and ethnicity. It soon became apparent that the patients with bladder cancer ate far fewer cruciferous vegetables, such as broccoli, than the healthy subjects. In fact, when compared to the subjects who ate the least amount of cruciferous vegetables, the subjects who ate the most cruciferous vegetables had a 29 percent reduced risk of developing bladder cancer. Interestingly, broccoli and other cruciferous vegetables provided the most protection to those at the highest risk—men, smokers, and older people. The researchers noted that like other cruciferous vegetables, broccoli contains isothiocyanates (ITCs), nonnutrient compounds that fight cancer.[3]

In a 2008 study published in *Cancer Epidemiology Biomarkers & Prevention*, researchers at the Roswell Park Cancer Institute in Buffalo, New York, conducted a case-control study of 275 patients with bladder cancer and 825 cancer-free controls. They found "a strong and statistically significant inverse association between bladder cancer risk and raw cruciferous vegetable intake." The inverse relationship was also significant among smokers. However, no such association was found with cooked cruciferous vegetables. The researchers noted that these inconsistent findings may be because cooking may "substantially reduce or destroy isothiocyanates."[4]

Commenting on these results in a 2008 article in *Oncology News International*, Li Tang, MD, PhD, noted, "Raw cruciferous vegetables such as broccoli, cabbage, and cauliflower are better than their cooked counterparts in terms of bladder cancer prevention. Intake of three or more helpings of such vegetables per month may reduce the risk of bladder cancer by 37 percent. Smokers, even heavy smokers, may benefit from the intake of raw cruciferous vegetables. Risk reduction for smokers was 40 percent to 54 percent."[5]

In a New Zealand study that was published in 2008 in *Cancer Research*, researchers induced bladder cancer in rats. Then, they had the rats eat freeze-dried aqueous extract of broccoli sprouts. The researchers found that, "the incidence, multiplicity, size, and progression of bladder cancer were all inhibited by the extract, while the extract itself caused no histologic chances in the bladder."[6]

Prostate Cancer

In a study published in 2007 in *JNCI: Journal of the National Cancer Institute*, researchers used the Prostate, Lung, Colorectal, and Ovarian Cancer Screening Trial data to evaluate the association between prostate cancer risk and intake of fruits and vegetables. Of the 29,361 men in the cohort, 1,338 were found to have prostate cancer during the 4.2 years follow-up. Though the researchers did not find an association between vegetable and fruit consumption and overall risk of prostate cancer, they did observe a relationship between higher intakes of vegetables, especially broccoli and cauliflower, and reduced risk of extraprostatic prostate cancer or prostate cancer that has spread outside the prostate.[7]

CARDIOVASCULAR HEALTH

In a study published in 2008 in the *Journal of Agricultural and Food Chemistry*, researchers fed one group of six rats broccoli; another group of six rats was the control. At the end of 30 days, the researchers gave the rats experimental heart attacks. When compared to the control rats, after the heart attacks, the rats that had been fed broccoli had lower amounts of dead heart muscle and heart muscle cells. They also experienced positive changes to proteins and chemicals that protect the heart.[8]

SKIN HEALTH

In a study published in 2007 in the *Proceedings of the National Academy of Sciences of the United States*, researchers described applying broccoli sprout extract to the skin of hairless mice and later to the skin of six human volunteers. In the mouse study, after application of the extract, the mice were exposed to ultraviolet radiation. Other mice served as controls. The researchers found that the mice that were treated with the extract developed significantly fewer skin cancer tumors than the controls. And, the tumors that the treated mice did develop were smaller than those on the control mice.

In the human studies, the researchers selected two locations on the backs of each of the volunteers, who ranged in age from 28 to 53 years. One to three days before exposing the backs to ultraviolet radiation, broccoli sprout extract was applied topically to one of the locations. The researchers found that the areas treated with broccoli sprout extract had an average of 37.7 percent less redness and inflammation than the areas that had not been treated. Still, the reaction to the extract varied widely from person to person.[9]

ANTI-AGING

In a study published in 2008 in *The Journal of Allergy and Clinical Immunology*, UCLA researchers found that when sulforaphane, a chemical found in broccoli, was directly administered to old mice, the mice's decline in cellular immune function was reversed. Similar results were obtained when they gathered individual immune cells from old mice, treated them, and then returned the treated cells to the recipient animals. Additionally, the researchers learned that when dendritic cells, which introduce foreign substances and infectious agents to the immune system, were exposed to sulforaphane, they enhanced the immune function of the aged mice.[10]

Thus, it is possible that sulforaphane has the potential to reinvigorate the immune system of older people so that they may better prevent the illnesses associated with aging. According to Andre E. Nel, one of the researchers, "This is a radical new way of thinking about how to increase the immune function of elderly people to possibly protect against viral infections and cancer."[11]

ONE CAVEAT

In a study published in 2008 in the *Journal of Agricultural and Food Chemistry*, Dutch researchers recruited eight men to consume 200 grams of crushed raw or cooked broccoli with a warm meal. After the meal, blood and urine samples were taken every hour. The men who ate the raw broccoli were found to have significantly higher amounts of sulforaphane in their blood and urine. The researchers noted that, "the consumption of raw broccoli results in faster absorption, higher bioavailability, and higher peak plasma amounts of sulforaphane, compared to cooked broccoli."[12] So, raw broccoli is a better choice than cooked broccoli. But, when raw broccoli is not available, cooked broccoli is still an excellent food.

Should broccoli be a regular part of the diet? Definitely.

NOTES

1. Stone, Jett. July–August 2008. "Broccoli Rave: Forget Face-Lifts and Fake Knees. Scientist Have Seen the Fountain of Youth—and It's Broccoli." *Psychology Today* 41(4):61.

2. The George Mateljan Foundation Website. www.whfoods.com.

3. Zhoa, Hua, Jie Lin, H. Barton Grossman, et al. May 15, 2007. "Dietary Isothiocyanates, GSTM1, GSTT1, NAT2 Polymorphisms and Bladder Cancer Risk." *International Journal of Cancer* 120(10): 2208–2213.

4. Tang, L., G. R. Zirpoli, K. Guru, et al. April 2008. "Consumption of Raw Cruciferous Vegetables Is Inversely Associated with Bladder Cancer Risk." *Cancer Epidemiology Biomarkers & Prevention* 17(4): 938–944.

5. Kelly, Janis. January 2008. "Broccoli Sprout Extract Might Lower Bladder Cancer Risk." *Oncology News International* 17(1): 18.

6. Munday, Rex, Paulette Mhawech-Fauceglia, Christine M. Munday, et al. March 1, 2008. "Inhibition of Urinary Bladder Carcinogenesis by Broccoli Sprouts." *Cancer Research* 68(5): 1593–1600.

7. Kirsh, Victoria A., Ulrike Peters, Susan T. Mayne et al. 2007. "Prospective Study of Fruit and Vegetable Intake and Risk of Prostate Cancer." *JNCI: Journal of the National Cancer Institute* 99(15): 1200–1209.

8. Mukherjee, Subhendu, Hiranmoy Gangopadhyay, and Dipak K. Das. 2008. "Broccoli: A Unique Vegetable That Protects Mammalian Hearts Through the Redox Cycling of the Thioredoxin Superfamily." *Journal of Agricultural and Food Chemistry* 56(2): 609–617.

9. Talalay, Paul, Jed W. Fahey, Zachary R. Healy, et al. October 30, 2007. "Sulforaphane Mobilizes Cellular Defenses That Protect Skin Against Damage by UV Radiation." *Proceedings of the National Academy of Sciences of the United States* 104(44): 17500–17505.

10. Kim, Hyon-Jeen, Berenice Barajas, Meiying Wang, and Andre E. Nel. May 2008. "Nrf2 Activation by Sulforaphane Restores the Age-Related Decrease of T_H1 Immunity: Role of Dendritic Cells." *The Journal of Allergy and Clinical Immunology* 121(5): 1255–1261.e7.

11. Stone, Jett. July–August 2008: 61.

12. Vermeulen, Martijn, Ineke W. A. A. Klöpping-Ketelaars, Robin van den Berg, and Wouter H. J. Vaes. 2008. "Bioavailability and Kinetics of Sulforaphane in Humans After Consumption of Cooked Verses Raw Broccoli." *Journal of Agricultural and Food Chemistry* 56(22): 10505–10509.

REFERENCES AND RESOURCES
Magazines, Journals, and Newspapers

Kelly, Janis. January 2008. "Broccoli Sprout Extract Might Lower Bladder Cancer Risk." *Oncology News International* 17(1): 18.

Kim, Hyon-Jeen, Berenice Barajas, Meiying Wang, and Andre E. Nel. May 2008. "Nrf2 Activation by Sulforaphane Restores the Age-Related Decrease of T_H1 Immunity: Role of Dendritic Cells." *The Journal of Allergy and Clinical Immunology* 121(5): 1255–1261.e7.

Kirsh, Victoria A., Ulrike Peters, Susan T. Mayne, et al. 2007. "Prospective Study of Fruit and Vegetable Intake and Risk of Prostate Cancer." *JNCI: Journal of the National Cancer Institute* 99(15): 1200–1209.

Mukherjee, Subhendu, Hiranmoy Gangopadhyay, and Dipak K. Das. 2008. "Broccoli: A Unique Vegetable That Protects Mammlian Hearts Through the Redox Cycling of the Thioredoxin Superfamily." *Journal of Agricultural and Food Chemistry* 56(2): 609–617.

Munday, Rex, Paulette Mhawech-Fauceglia, Christine M. Munday, et al. March 1, 2008. "Inhibition of Urinary Bladder Carcinogenesis by Broccoli Sprouts." *Cancer Research* 68(5): 1593–1600.

Stone, Jett. July–August 2008. "Broccoli Rave: Forget Face-Lifts and Fake Knees. Scientists Have Seen the Fountain of Youth—and It's Broccoli." *Psychology Today* 41(4): 61.

Talalay, Paul, Jed W. Fahey, Zachary R. Healy, et al. October 30, 2007. "Sulforaphane Mobilizes Cellular Defenses That Protect Skin Against Damage by UV Radiation." *Proceedings of the National Academy of Sciences* 104(44): 17500–17505.

Tang, L., G. R. Zirpoli, K. Guru, et al. April 2008. "Consumption of Raw Cruciferous Vegetables Is Inversely Associated with Bladder Cancer Risk." *Cancer Epidemiology Biomarkers & Prevention* 17(4): 938–944.

Vermeulen, Martijn, Ineke W. A. A. Klöpping-Ketelaars, Robin van den Berg, and Wouter H. J. Vaes. 2008. "Bioavailability and Kinetics of Sulforaphane in Humans After Consumption of Cooked Verses Raw Broccoli." *Journal of Agricultural and Food Chemistry* 56(22): 10505–10509.

Zhao, Hua, Jie Lin, H. Barton Grossman, et al. May 15, 2007. "Dietary Isothiocyanates, GSTM1, GSTT1, NAT2 Polymorphisms and Bladder Cancer Risk." *International Journal of Cancer* 120(10): 2208–2213.

Website

The George Mateljan Foundation. www.whfoods.com.

BUCKWHEAT

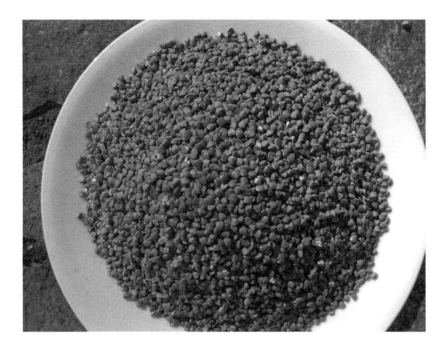

A native of Asia and northern Europe, buckwheat was widely cultivated in China from the 10th until the 13th century. During the 14th and 15th centuries, it was also grown in Europe and Russia. The Dutch brought buckwheat to the United States in the 17th century.

Buckwheat is considered a very good source of manganese and a good source of magnesium and dietary fiber. Though most of the fiber is insoluble, which supports the gastrointestinal tract, buckwheat also contains soluble fiber, which lowers cholesterol levels and slows digestion, making one feel fuller for longer periods of time. Additionally, buckwheat has amino acids, protein, copper, selenium, zinc, as well as the flavonols rutin and quercetin.[1]

It is interesting to note that buckwheat is not a wheat or cereal grain. Though it looks like and is prepared as a grain, buckwheat is the fruit of a broadleaved plant, which is related to rhubarb.[2]

By itself, buckwheat has no gluten. So, it is a good choice for people who have a gluten sensitivity or celiac disease. However, buckwheat is frequently used in breads, pasta, and pancakes. And, depending upon the other ingredients, it may or may not be gluten-free. For example, buckwheat may be combined with wheat flour to make soba noodles, which are not gluten-free.

Buckwheat does not appear to be a favored grain for many Americans. That might change as more people hear what some of the researchers have learned.

CARDIOVASCULAR HEALTH

Wisconsin researchers knew that dietary protein, such as soy protein, is able to lower cholesterol levels. They were also aware that animal studies had determined that buckwheat protein raises the amount of cholesterol contained in fecal excretion and lowers the amount of serum cholesterol in rodents. So, they decided to use a human intestinal cell model to understand how buckwheat protein alters the absorption of cholesterol.

In an in vitro study published in 2007 in the *Journal of Agricultural and Food Chemistry*, the researchers found that buckwheat protein had a strong ability to bind with cholesterol. In so doing, it significantly reduced the absorption of cholesterol by up to 47 percent. Intestinal cholesterol that is not absorbed is secreted out of the body, thus reducing the amount of circulating cholesterol in the blood. As a result, the regular consumption of buckwheat helps to remove more cholesterol from the blood and lowers levels of serum cholesterol.[3] In a study published in 2007 in the *Journal of Food Science*, Japanese researchers investigated the effects of giving rats fed a cholesterol-enriched diet either common buckwheat protein or tartary buckwheat protein. The researchers found that the common buckwheat protein product and tartary buckwheat protein product reduced cholesterol levels by 32 and 25 percent, respectively. The researchers concluded that if buckwheat is proven to be similarly effective in humans, it may well be useful to the millions of people dealing with elevated levels of cholesterol.[4]

In a South Korean study published in 2008 in the *Annals of Nutrition and Metabolism*, researchers fed 40 male rats an obesogenic diet (a diet that fosters obesity) for four weeks. Then, the rats were divided into four groups. For the next four weeks, each group was fed a diet containing one of the following foods: white rice, adlay, buckwheat, or waxy barley. The researchers found that the rats eating the adlay-buckwheat- and waxy-barley-enhanced diets had greater improvement in the levels of triglycerides than the rats eating the white rice-enhanced diet. The rats eating the buckwheat- and waxy barley-supplemented diets had lower levels of total cholesterol and LDL (or bad) cholesterol and higher levels of HDL (good) cholesterol than the rats on the white rice-added diet. The rats fed buckwheat and waxy barley had a larger aortic lumen (opening) than those on adlay and white rice. The researchers noted that the "consumption of BW [buckwheat]- and WB [waxy barley]-containing diets significantly improved several cardiovascular risk factors induced by obesity in experimental rats."[5]

MANAGEMENT OF DIABETES

In a study published in 2003 in the *Journal of Agricultural and Food Chemistry*, Canadian researchers found evidence that buckwheat may be useful for people dealing with diabetes. The researchers began with about 40 rats with chemically induced type 1 diabetes. The rats were given either a single dose of buckwheat extract or a placebo. After 90 minutes and 120 minutes, the rats' glucose levels were measured. While there was no glucose reduction in the rats that were given the placebo, the rats that had buckwheat seed extract experienced lowered blood glucose levels by 12 to 19 percent.

According to the researchers, buckwheat is able to lower glucose levels because it contains high amounts of a compound known as chiroinositol, which makes cells more sensitive to insulin.[6]

CANCER

A National Cancer Institute study published in 2008 in *Lung Cancer* noted that in rural Xuanwei County, China, there is a high incidence of lung cancer. This is thought to be a direct result of the burning of smoky coal indoors to cook and heat the poorly ventilated homes. "Thus, residents could be exposed to carcinogenic coal emissions not only via inhalation but also via ingestion of these foodstuffs."

Researchers conducted a population-based case-control study of these groups that included 498 people with lung cancer and 498 controls. They found that intake of rice, green vegetables, mushrooms, and fresh meat was associated with an increased risk for lung cancer. Conversely, the consumption of buckwheat, corn, radishes, peppers, melons, pickled vegetables, and salt-preserved meat was related to a reduced risk for lung cancer. So, at least in this study, buckwheat is among several foods that are believed to decrease the risk for lung cancer.[7]

In a study published in 2007 in the *International Journal of Epidemiology*, researchers used the data from the UK Women's Cohort Study to review the association between dietary fiber, such as the fiber in buckwheat, and the incidence of breast cancer. The cohort included 35,972 pre-menopausal and post-menopausal women. In pre-menopausal women, a statistically significant relationship was found between total fiber intake and risk of breast cancer. In fact, pre-menopausal women who ate more than 30 grams of fiber per day halved their risk of developing breast cancer. When compared to pre-menopausal women who eat less than 20 grams of fiber per day, they had a 52 percent lower risk of breast cancer. Fiber from whole grains, like buckwheat, offers the most protection. The pre-menopausal women who ate at least 13 grams per day of whole-grain fiber had a 41 percent lower risk of breast cancer than the pre-menopausal women who ate less than 4 grams per day. No such statistically significant associations were seen in post-menopausal women.

OVERALL HEALTH

In a 2007 cross-sectional study in *Clinical and Experimental Pharmacology and Physiology*, researchers from Shanghai, China, sampled a total of 3,542 people from two adjacent counties of Inner Mongolia, China. One group consumed buckwheat seed as a staple food; the other group consumed corn. The researchers hoped to find an association between rates of hypertension (high blood pressure), abnormal concentrations of blood lipids, and hyperglycemia (high levels of blood sugars) and the consumption of these staple foods. The researchers found statistically significant differences between the two groups. The group who ate buckwheat seed had better blood pressure, lipid, and sugar levels than the corn-consuming group. The researchers suggested that buckwheat might help prevent these medical problems.[8]

Should buckwheat be included in the diet? Unless someone has a buckwheat intolerance or allergy, which is believed to be relatively uncommon in the United States, buckwheat should be part of the diet.

NOTES

1. The George Mateljan Foundation Website. www.whfoods.com.

2. Schepers, Anastasia. October 2004. "Beyond Pancakes: Buckwheat Boasts Nutrient Arsenal." *Environmental Nutrition* 27(10): 8.

3. Metzger, Brandon T., David M. Barnes, and Jess D. Reed. 2007. "Insoluble Fraction of Buckwheat (*Fogopyrum esculentum Moench*) Protein Possessing Cholesterol-Binding Properties That Reduce Micelle Cholesterol Solubility and Uptake by Caco-2 Cells." *Journal of Agricultural and Food Chemistry* 55(15): 6032–6038.

4. Tomotake, H., N. Yamamoto, H. Kitabayashi, et al. 2007. "Preparation of Tartary Buckwheat Protein and Its Improving Effect on Cholesterol Metabolism in Rats and Mice Fed Cholesterol-Enriched Diet." *Journal of Food Science* 72(7): S528–S533.

5. Son, B. K., J. Y. Kim, and S. S. Lee. 2008. "Effect of Adlay, Buckwheat, and Barley on Lipid Metabolism and Aorta Histopathology in Rats Fed an Obesogenic Diet." *Annals of Nutrition and Metabolism* 52(3): 181–187.

6. Kawa, Julianne M., Carla G. Taylor, and Roman Przybylski. 2003. "Buckwheat Concentrate Reduces Serum Glucose in Streptozotocin-Diabetic Rats." *Journal of Agricultural and Food Chemistry* 51(25): 7287–7291.

7. Shen, M., R. S. Chapman, X. He, et al. September 2008. "Dietary Factors, Food Contamination and Lung Cancer Risk in Xuanwei, China." *Lung Cancer* 61(3): 275–282.

8. Zhang, H. W., Y. H. Zhang, M. J. Lu, et al. September 2007. "Comparison of Hypertension, Dyslipidaemia and Hyperglycaemia Between Buckwheat Seed-Consuming and Non-Consuming Mongolian-Chinese Population in Inner Mongolia, China." *Clinical and Experimental Pharmacology and Physiology* 34(9): 838–844.

REFERENCES AND RESOURCES
Magazines, Journals, and Newspapers

Cade, Janet Elizabeth, Victoria Jane Burley, and Darren Charles Greenwood. April 2007. "Dietary Fibre and Risk of Breast Cancer in the UK Women's Cohort Study." *International Journal of Epidemiology* 36: 431–438.

Kawa, Julianne M., Carla G. Taylor, and Roman Przybylski. 2003. "Buckwheat Concentrate Reduces Serum Glucose in Streptozotocin-Diabetic Rats." *Journal of Agricultural and Food Chemistry* 51(25): 7287–7291.

Metzger, Brandon T., David M. Barnes, and Jess D. Reed. 2007. "Insoluble Fraction of Buckwheat (*Fagopyrum esculentum Moench*) Protein Possessing Cholesterol-Binding Properties That Reduce Micelle Cholesterol Solubility and Uptake by Caco-2 Cells." *Journal of Agricultural and Food Chemistry* 55(15): 6032–6038.

Schepers, Anastasia. October 2004. "Beyond Pancakes: Buckwheat Boasts Nutrient Arsenal." *Environmental Nutrition* 27(10): 8.

Shen, M., R. S. Chapman, X. He, et al. September 2008. "Dietary Factors, Food Contamination and Lung Cancer Risk in Xuanwei, China." *Lung Cancer* 61(3): 275–282.

Son, B. K., J. Y. Kim, and S. S. Lee. 2008. "Effect of Adlay, Buckwheat and Barley on Lipid Metabolism and Aorta Histopathology in Rats Fed an Obesogenic Diet." *Annals of Nutrition and Metabolism* 52(3): 181–187.

Tomotake, H., N. Yamamoto, H. Kitabayashi, et al. 2007. "Preparation of Tartary Buckwheat Protein Product and Its Improving Effect on Cholesterol Metabolism in Rats and Mice Fed Cholesterol-Enriched Diet." *Journal of Food Science* 72(7): S528–S533.

Zhang, H. W., Y. H. Zhang, M. J. Lu, et al. September 2007. "Comparison of Hypertension, Dyslipidaemia and Hyperglycaemia Between Buckwheat Seed-Consuming and Non-Consuming Mongolian-Chinese Populations in Inner Mongolia, China." *Clinical and Experimental Pharmacology and Physiology* 34(9): 838–844.

Website

The George Mateljan Foundation. www.whfoods.com.

CABBAGE

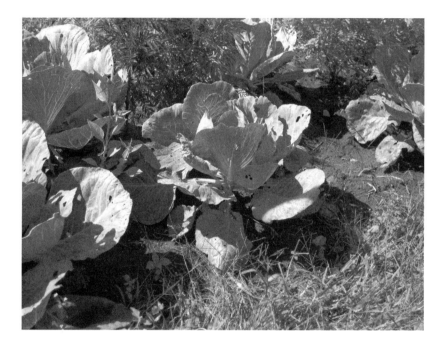

Historically, cabbage has been considered both a food and a medicine. In its early years, it grew in the wild and looked more like kale leaves with no head.

It is believed that cabbage was brought to Europe around 600 BCE by Celtic nomads. Later, cabbage was much revered by the ancient Greeks and Romans. In time, cabbage spread across Europe and became particularly popular in Germany, Poland, and Russia. Today, cabbage is primarily grown in Russia, Poland, China, and Japan.[1] There are three main types—green, red, and Savoy. (Savoy has a milder and more delicate flavor than green and red cabbage.)

Cabbage is an incredibly nutritious food. It is an excellent source of vitamins K and C and a very good source of dietary fiber, manganese, vitamin

B_6, folate, and omega-3 fatty acids. Cabbage is considered a good source of vitamins A, B_1, and B_2, calcium; potassium; and protein. In addition, cabbage contains phytochemicals such as glucosinolates, isothiocyanates, and indole-3-carbinol, which are thought to have anti-cancer properties.[2] But, it is important to review the research, the vast majority of which centers on these anti-cancer properties.

CANCER
Breast Cancer

A 2006 article in *JNCI: Journal of the National Cancer Institute* describes research conducted by Dorothy Rybaczyk Pathak, PhD, on the Polish immigrant communities around Chicago and Detroit. The research has included hundreds of Polish-American women and women who were born in Poland and immigrated to the United States. According to Dr. Pathak, within one generation, the rates of breast cancer among the women tripled. What appears to be the culprit? Dr. Pathak thinks it is closely associated with the consumption of cabbage.

Dr. Pathak and her fellow researchers divided their subjects into one of three cabbage consuming categories: low consumers (1.5 servings or less per week), moderate consumers (1.5 to 3 servings per week), and high consumers (more than three servings per week). Because it is believed that heating reduces the bioavailability of the glucosinolates in cabbage, only servings of raw and briefly cooked cabbage were considered in the calculation.

In a truly striking finding, when compared to the adolescents and women who ate 1.5 or fewer servings of raw or short-cooked cabbage or sauerkraut (chopped or shredded cabbage fermented in its own juice) per week, the women who ate more than three servings of these foods had a 72 percent reduced risk of breast cancer. Interestingly, the inverse relationship was strongest when high amounts of cabbage were eaten during adolescence, even when lower amounts were consumed in adulthood. However, high consumption of cabbage in adulthood was also associated with a lower risk for breast cancer. In the article, Dr. Pathak is quoted, "This is a unique population. Poles consume cabbage in many forms, and a lot of it—three times more than Americans. Working with the migrant population allowed us to study the effect of a wide range of exposures to cabbage that can't be found in the U.S. population."[3]

In a study published in 2008 in *Carcinogenesis*, researchers from Santa Barbara, California, and Urbana, Illinois, noted that cabbage and other cruciferous vegetables contain a type of isothiocyanate known as sulforaphane or SFN. They found that sulforaphane inhibits the growth of cancer cells, much like the anticancer drugs taxol and vincristine, and results in cell death. But, sulforaphane is weaker than those anticancer drugs and less toxic. The researchers noted that, "it is important to determine whether SFN might facilitate or interfere with conventional chemotherapy." Why? "If it does not interfere, an attractive possibility is that SFN may be useful not only for prevention of cancer but also for treatment of cancer along with the commonly used conventional drugs."[4]

In a 2008 study published in the *Proceedings of the National Academy of Sciences*, University of California, Berkeley, researchers reported that the compound indole-3-carbinol found in cabbage fights breast cancer cells. During their investigation, the researchers learned that indole-3-carbinol lowers the level of activity of the enzyme elastase, which has been associated with rapidly advancing breast cancer. When elastase is present in higher amounts, patients are more likely to have less of a response to chemotherapy and endocrine therapy and are less likely to survive. The researchers theorize that indole-3-carbinol or related compounds may become "targeted therapies of human breast cancers where high elastase levels are correlated with poor prognosis."[5] Thus, some form of indole-3-carbinol or a related phytochemical may someday be included in the treatment for breast cancer, especially when there are high levels of elastase.

Bladder Cancer

In a study published in 2007 in the *International Journal of Cancer*, researchers from the University of Texas M. D. Anderson Cancer Center in Houston analyzed the diets of 697 patients with newly diagnosed bladder cancer and 708 healthy people, matched by age, gender, and ethnicity. The researchers found that the average consumption of cruciferous vegetables, such as cabbage, was significantly lower in the people with bladder cancer than those who were healthy. In fact, when compared to the people who ate the least amount of cruciferous vegetables, the people who ate the most had a 29 percent lower risk for the disease. The protective elements of these vegetables were also evident in those who are at greatest risk for bladder cancer: men, smokers, and people who are at least 64 years old.[6]

Pancreatic Cancer

In a study published in 2009 in the *JNCI: Journal of the National Cancer Institute*, researchers from Texas Tech University Health Sciences Center in Amarillo investigated the effects of one type of isothiocyanate, known as benzyl isothiocyanate, on cultures of pancreatic cancer cells and on a mouse model of pancreatic cancer. The researchers found that when pancreatic cancer cells were exposed to benzyl isothiocyanate, there were high amounts of cell death (apoptosis). Moreover, the healthy pancreatic cells were unaffected by the treatments.[7]

Polyps

In a study published in 2006 in *Carcinogenesis*, researchers in New Jersey and South Korea examined the use of sulforaphane on mice that are bred to develop intestinal polyps, the precursor to colorectal cancer. The researchers found that when these mice were fed sulforaphane, their tumors were smaller and grew at a slower rate. When the mice did develop polyps, many of the polyps self-destructed. And, the mice that were fed higher doses of sulforaphane had a lower risk of ever developing polyps than those on the lower dose. The researcher concluded that sulforaphane has a chemoprotective activity.[8]

CARDIOVASCULAR HEALTH

In a study published in 2007 in *The Journal of Nutrition*, Hawaiian researchers determined that a very small amount of indole-3-carbinol is able to reduce the liver's secretion of apolipoprotein B-100 (apoB), the primary transporter of LDL (bad) cholesterol to tissues. Since LDL has been associated with plaque formation in the blood vessels, lowering the amount of LDL is a clear cardiovascular benefit.[9]

In another study published in 2008 in *Diabetes*, researchers from England's University of Warwick determined that sulforaphane triggered the production of a protein known as nrf2 that supports blood vessel health. When sulforaphane was present, the activation of nrf2 doubled. This support takes place even in blood vessels that have been damaged, a case more likely in people with diabetes. Furthermore, blood vessel damage is a significant cause of morbidity and mortality in people with diabetes.[10]

ONE CAVEAT

Members of the cabbage family contain goitrogens, naturally occurring substances that some contend may interfere with the proper functioning of the thyroid gland. Since cooking probably helps to inactivate the goitrogens, people with known thyroid disease, such as hypothyroidism, may wish to avoid eating raw cabbage. People should discuss this issue with healthcare providers.

Should cabbage be included in the diet? In most instances, absolutely.

NOTES

1. The George Mateljan Foundation Website. www.whfoods.com.

2. The George Mateljan Foundation Website.

3. Nelson, Nancy J. 2006. "Migrant Studies Aid the Search for Factors Linked to Breast Cancer Risk." *JNCI: Journal of the National Cancer Institute* 98(7): 436–438.

4. Azarenko, Olga, Tatiana Okouneva, Keith W. Singletary, et al. 2008. "Suppression of Microtubule Dynamic Instability and Turnover in MCF7 Breast Cancer Cells by Sulforaphane." *Carcinogenesis* 29(12): 2360–2368.

5. Nguyen, Hanh H., Ida Aronchik, Gloria A. Brar, et al. December 16, 2008. "The Dietary Phytochemical Indole-3-Carbinol Is a Natural Elastase Enzymatic Inhibitor That Disrupts Cyclin E Protein Processing." *Proceedings of the National Academy of Sciences* 105(50): 19750–19755.

6. Zhao, Hua, Jie Lin, H. Barton Grossman, et al. 2007. "Dietary Isothiocyanates, GSTM1, GSTT1, NAT2 Polymorphisms and Bladder Cancer Risk." *International Journal of Cancer* 120(10): 2208–2213.

7. Sahu, Ravi P. and Sanjay K. Srivastava. 2009. "The Role of STAT-3 in the Induction of Apoptosis in Pancreatic Cancer Cells by Benzyl Isothiocyanate." *JNCI: Journal of the National Cancer Institute* 101(3): 176–193.

8. Hu, Rong, Tin Oo Khor, Guoxiang Shen, et al. 2006. "Cancer Chemoprevention of Intestinal Polyposis in ApcMin/+ Mice by Sulforaphane, a Natural Product Derived from Cruciferous Vegetable." *Carcinogenesis* 27(10): 2038–2046.

9. Maiyoh, Geoffrey K., Joan E. Kuh, Adele Casaschi, and Andre G. Theriault. October 2007. "Cruciferous Indole-3-Carbinol Inhibits Apolipoprotein B Secretion in HepG2 Cells." *The Journal of Nutrition* 137: 2185–2189.

10. Xue, Mingzhan, Qingwen Qian, Antonysunil Adaikalakoteswari, et al. October 2008. "Activation of NF-E2-Related Factor-2 Reverses Biochemical Dysfunction of Endothelial Cells Induced by Hyperglycemia Linked to Vascular Disease." *Diabetes* 57(10): 2809–2817.

REFERENCES AND RESOURCES
Magazines, Journals, and Newspapers

Azarenko, Olga, Tatiana Okouneva, Keith W. Singletary, et al. 2008. "Suppression of Microtubule Dynamic Instability and Turnover in MCF7 Breast Cancer Cells by Sulforaphane." *Carcinogenesis* 29(12): 2360–2368.

Hu, Rong, Tin Oo Khor, Guoxiang Shen, et al. 2006. "Cancer Chemoprevention of Intestinal Polyposis in ApcMin/+ Mice by Sulforaphane, a Natural Product Derived from Cruciferous Vegetable." *Carcinogenesis* 27(10): 2038–2046.

Maiyoh, Geoffrey K., Joan E. Kuh, Adele Casaschi, and Andre G. Theriault. October 2007. "Cruciferous Indole-3-Carbinol Inhibits Apolipoprotein B Secretion in HepG2 Cells." *The Journal of Nutrition* 137: 2185–2189.

Nelson, Nancy J. 2006. "Migrant Studies Aid the Search for Factors Linked to Breast Cancer Risk." *JNCI: Journal of the National Cancer Institute* 98(7): 436–438.

Nguyen, Hanh H., Ida Aronchik, Gloria A. Brar, et al. December 16, 2008. "The Dietary Phytochemical Indole-3-Carbinol is a Natural Elastase Enzymatic Inhibitor That Disrupts Cyclin E Protein Processing." *Proceedings of the National Academy of Sciences* 105(50): 19750–19755.

Sahu, Ravi P. and Sanjay K. Srivastava. 2009. "The Role of STAT-3 in the Induction of Apoptosis in Pancreatic Cancer Cells by Benzyl Isothiocyanate." *JNCI: Journal of the National Cancer Institute* 101(3): 176–193.

Xue, Mingzhan, Qingwen Qian, Antonysunil Adaikalakoteswari, et al. October 2008. "Activation of NF-E2-Related Factor-2 Reverses Biochemical Dysfunction of Endothelial Cells Induced by Hyperglycemia Linked to Vascular Disease." *Diabetes* 57(10): 2809–2817.

Zhao, Hua, Jie Lin, H. Barton Grossman, et al. 2007. "Dietary Isothiocyanates, GSTM1, GSTT1, NAT2 Polymorphisms and Bladder Cancer Risk." *International Journal of Cancer* 120(10): 2208–2213.

Website

The George Mateljan Foundation. www.whfoods.com.

CAPERS

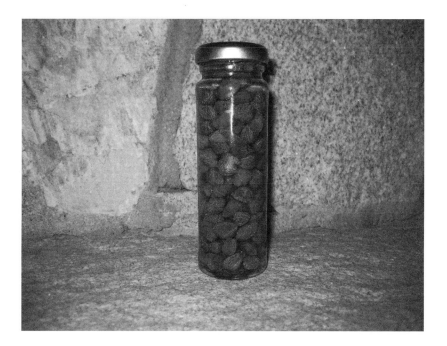

Since they are so tiny and used more often as a garnish and/or seasoning, it may be challenging for some to think about the healthfulness of capers. But, they are an integral part of the much discussed Mediterranean diet, and there is some compelling research on these pickled flower buds of a perennial spiny bush known as *Capparis spinosa*.

Moreover, while capers have no fat, they do contain protein, vitamins A and E, niacin, calcium, and manganese. They are also a very good source of dietary fiber, vitamins C and K, riboflavin, folate, iron, magnesium, and copper.[1] Above all, they have large amounts of quercetin, a powerful anti-oxidant flavonoid.

On the negative side, the capers that are commercially available tend to contain large amounts of sodium. Still, a good deal of this may be rinsed off in a colander before the capers are consumed. Though the research on capers is somewhat limited, it is important to review.

CANCER PREVENTION
Prostate Cancer

In a laboratory study published in 2001 in *Carcinogenesis*, Mayo Clinic researchers in Rochester, Minnesota, determined that quercetin was able to block the androgen (hormone) activity in androgen-responsive human prostate cell lines. By blocking this activity, the growth of prostate cancer cells may be prevented or stopped. The researchers suggest that quercetin has the potential "to become a chemopreventive and/or chemotherapeutic agent for prostate cancer."[2]

Colon Cancer

In a laboratory study published in 2005 in *Nutrition Journal*, researchers from the University of Georgia treated human colon adenocarcinoma cells with quercetin. Following treatment, the researchers found a "decreased expression of three proteins and the increased expression of one protein." According to the researchers, "such changes in the levels of these particular proteins could underlie the chemoprotective action of quercetin toward colon cancer."[3]

In a study published in *The Journal of Nutrition*, researchers from Texas A & M University investigated how laboratory rats with or without the early stages of colon cancer responded to diets supplemented with quercetin. The researchers found that the rats fed the quercetin had a better ability to maintain an equilibrium between the growth of healthy new cells and the death of cells that have completed their work. Those rats had lower rates of new cancer cells and higher rates of cells undergoing cell death, a process known as apoptosis. Thus, the rats that took supplemental quercetin had better colon health.

These same researchers also examined Cox-1 and Cox-2, two enzymes that are present in colon cancer. They found that the rats that consumed quercetin had lower levels of these enzymes in their bodies. Though more research is clearly needed, the researchers speculated that quercetin may suppress tumor development.[4]

CARDIOVASCULAR HEALTH

In a study published in 2007 in *The Journal of Nutrition*, Utah researchers attempted to determine if the intake of quercetin supplementation over a 28-day period could lower blood pressure in people with elevated levels, a condition known as hypertension. The randomized, double-blind, placebo-controlled, crossover study included 19 men and women with prehypertension and 22 men and women with stage 1 hypertension. Quercetin supplementation did not alter the blood pressure levels of the subjects with prehypertension. However, following treatment, the subjects with stage 1 hypertension had reduced levels of systolic, diastolic, and mean arterial pressures. The researchers noted that, "these data are the first to our knowledge to show that quercetin supplementation reduces blood pressure in hypertensive subjects."[5]

In a study published online in 2009 in the British Journal of Nutrition, researchers investigated the effects of quercetin supplementation on cardiovascular health factors such as blood pressure, lipid metabolism, markers of oxidative stress, inflammation, and body composition in 93 overweight or obese subjects between the ages of 25 and 65. All of the subjects exhibited traits of metabolic syndrome, which placed them at added risk for cardiovascular disease. During two six-week study periods, which were separated by a five-week washout period, subjects received either a daily 150-mg quercetin supplement or a placebo. The researchers determined that the subjects who took quercetin had a lowering of their levels of systolic blood pressure as well as a reduction in plasma oxidized LDL concentrations. They concluded that "quercetin may provide protection against CVD [cardiovascular disease]."[6]

Several years earlier, in a study that appeared in 2005 in the Journal of Ethnopharmacology, Moroccan researchers investigated the effect of oral doses of caper extracts on the lipid metabolism of normal and diabetic rats. Levels of plasma triglyceride were measured after one week and then again after two weeks. In both instances, the normal and diabetic rats had a significant decrease in plasma triglyceride concentrations. Meanwhile, levels of plasma cholesterol were measured in the normal rats after four days and again after a week. In both cases, the normal rats had lowered cholesterol levels. The levels of cholesterol of the diabetic rats were measured after four days and again after two weeks. Again, there were significant reductions. After four days of the caper extract, the diabetic rats also had a significant decrease in body weight. The researchers noted that it appeared that the extract of capers "exhibits a potent lipid lowering activity in both normal and severe hyperglycemic rats after repeated oral administration of CS [Capparis spinosa L. or capers] aqueous extract."[7]

OVERALL HEALTH

In an Italian study published in 2007 in the Journal of Agricultural and Food Chemistry, researchers added caper extracts to grilled turkey red muscle meat. Then, after simulating digestion, they analyzed the byproducts. The researchers learned that the capers, even when used in only small amounts, helped prevent pro-oxidants, molecules that attack healthy cells and have been associated with an increased risk of cardiovascular disease and cancer. The researchers noted that capers may well be beneficial for health, especially for those people who eat foods that are higher in fat and red meat.[8]

REDUCED RISK FOR INFLUENZA

In a study published in 2008 in the *American Journal of Physiology—Regulatory, Integrative and Comparative Physiology*, South Carolina researchers randomly assigned mice to one of four treatment groups: exercise-placebo, exercise-quercetin, control-placebo, or control-quercetin. The mice that exercised ran to fatigue on a treadmill for three consecutive days. Researchers determined that the mice that exercised were at increased risk for the flu. Yet, the mice that exercised and took quercetin had about the same rate of illness as those who did not exercise. The severity of illness among the mice that did not exercise was about the same as the mice that did exercise but took quercetin. The researchers noted that the short-term use of quercetin may "lessen the impact of stressful exercise on susceptibility to respiratory infection."[9]

INCREASED ENDURANCE

In another study from South Carolina, which was published in 2009 in the *American Journal of Physiology*, researchers determined that mice who received seven days of quercetin supplementation had more mitochondria in their muscle and brain cells. That gave the mice more energy and enabled them to run significantly longer before exhaustion than the mice fed placebos. The researchers commented that the "benefits of quercetin on fitness without exercise training may have important implications for enhancement of athletic and military performance and may also extend to prevention and/or treatment of chronic diseases."[10]

Are capers a healthy addition to the diet? From the previously noted studies, they certainly appear to be.

NOTES

1. Nutrition Data Website. www.nutritiondata.com.

2. Xing, Nianzeng, Yi Chen, Susan H. Mitchell, and Charles Y. F. Young. March 2001. "Quercetin Inhabits the Expression and Function of the Androgen Receptor in LNCaP Prostate Cancer Cells." *Carcinogenesis* 22(3): 409–414.

3. Mouat, Michael F., Kumar Kolli, Ronald Orlando, et al. 2005. "The Effects of Quercetin on SW480 Human Colon Carcinoma Cells: A Proteomic Study." *Nutrition Journal* 4: 11.

4. Warren, Cynthia A., Kimberly J. Paulhill, Laurie A. Davidson, et al. January 2009. "Quercetin May Suppress Rat Aberrant Crypt Foci Formation by Suppressing Inflammatory Mediators That Influence Proliferation and Apoptosis." *The Journal of Nutrition* 139(1): 101–105.

5. Edwards, Randi L., Tiffany Lyon, Sheldon E. Lewis, et al. November 2007. "Quercetin Reduces Blood Pressure in Hypertensive Subjects." *The Journal of Nutrition* 137: 2405–2411.

6. Egert, Sarah, Anja Bosy-Westphal, Jasmin Seiberl, et al. October 2009. "Quercetin Reduces Systolic Blood Pressure and Plasma Oxidised Low-Density Lipoprotein Concentrations in Overweight Subjects with a High-Cardiovascular

Disease Risk Phenotype: A Double-Blinded, Placebo-Controlled Cross-Over Study."
British Journal of Nutrition 102: 1065–1074.
    7. Eddouks, M., A. Lemhadri, and J. B. Michel. April 26, 2005. "Hypolipi-
demic Activity of Aqueous Extract of *Capparis spinosa* L. in Normal and Diabetic
Rats." *Journal of Ethnopharmacology* 98(3): 345–350.
    8. Tesoriere, L., D. Butera, C. Gentile, and M. A. Livrea. 2007. "Bioactive
Components of Caper (*Capparis spinosa* L.) from Sicily and Antioxidants Effects in
a Red Meat Simulated Gastric Digestion." *Journal of Agricultural and Food Chemistry*
55(21): 8465–8471.
    9. Davis, J. M., E. A. Murphy, J. L. McClellan, et al. August 2008. "Quercetin
Reduces Susceptibility to Influenza Infection Following Stressful Exercise." *American
Journal of Physiology—Regulatory, Integrative and Comparative Physiology* 295;
R505–R509.
    10. Davis, J. Mark, E. Angela Murphy, Martin D. Carmichael, and Ben Davis.
April 2009. "Quercetin Increases Brain and Muscle Mitochondrial Biogenesis and
Exercise Tolerance." *The American Journal of Physiology* 296(4): R1071–R1077.

REFERENCES AND RESOURCES
Magazines, Journals, and Newspapers

Davis, J. M., E. A. Murphy, J. L. McClellan, et al. August 2008. "Quercetin Reduces
    Susceptibility to Influenza Infection Following Stressful Exercise." *American Journal
    of Physiology—Regulatory, Integrative, and Comparative Physiology* 295: R505–R509.
Davis, J. Mark, E. Angela Murphy, Martin D. Carmichael, and Ben Davis. April
    2009. "Quercetin Increases Brain and Muscle Mitochondrial Biogenesis and
    Exercise Tolerance." *The American Journal of Physiology* 296(4): R1071–R1077.
Eddouks, M., A. Lemhadri, and J. B. Michel. April 26, 2005. "Hypolipidemic Activ-
    ity of Aqueous Extract of *Capparis spinosa* L. in Normal and Diabetic Rats."
    Journal of Ethnopharmacology 98(3): 345–350.
Edwards, Randi L., Tiffany Lyon, Sheldon E. Litwin, et al. November 2007.
    "Quercetin Reduces Blood Pressure in Hypertensive Subjects." *The Journal of
    Nutrition* 137: 2405–2411.
Egert, Sarah, Anja Bosy-Westphal, Jasmin Seiberl, et al. October 2009. "Quercetin
    Reduces Systolic Blood Pressure and Plasma Oxidised Low-Density Lipoprotein
    Concentrations in Overweight Subjects with a High Cardiovascular Disease
    Risk Phenotype: A Double-Blinded, Placebo-Controlled Cross-Over Study."
    British Journal of Nutrition 102: 1065–1074.
Mouat, Michael F., Kumar Kolli, Ronald Orlando, et al. 2005. "The Effects of
    Quercetin on SW480 Human Colon Carcinoma Cells: A Proteomic Study."
    Nutrition Journal 4: 11.
Tesoriere, L., D. Butera, C. Gentile, and M. A. Livrea. 2007. "Bioactive Compo-
    nents of Caper (Capparis spinosa L.) from Sicily and Antioxidant Effects in a
    Red Meat Simulated Gastric Digestion." *The Journal of Agricultural and Food
    Chemistry* 55(21): 8465–8471.
Warren, Cynthia A., Kimberly J. Paulhill, Laurie A. Davidson, et al. January 2009.
    "Quercetin May Suppress Rat Aberrant Crypt Foci Formation by Suppressing
    Inflammatory Mediators That Influence Proliferation and Apoptosis." *The
    Journal of Nutrition* 139(1): 101–105.

Xing, Nianzeng, Yi Chen, Susan H. Mitchell, and Charles Y. F. Young. March 2001. "Quercetin Inhibits the Expression and Function of the Androgen Receptor in LNCaP Prostate Cancer Cells." *Carcinogenesis* 22(3): 409–414.

Website

Nutrition Data. www.nutritiondata.com.

CARROTS

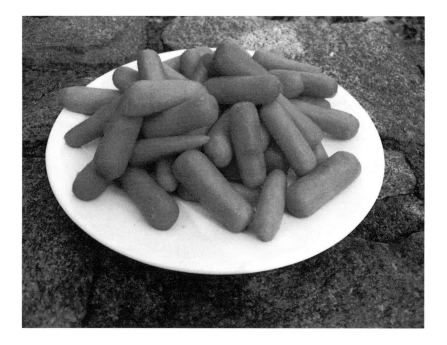

They are ubiquitous. Just about every market has at least some variety of carrots. There are big carrots and little tiny baby ones—and every size in-between.

Carrots are traditionally known for fostering eye health, and research is now showing that they may well be useful for preventing and treating other medical concerns. So what does the research report?

CARDIOVASCULAR HEALTH

In a study published in 2006 in *The Journal of Nutrition*, researchers divided a group of mice, which were bred to develop atherosclerosis, into two groups. Half were fed a vegetable-free diet; the others were fed a diet including vegetables, such as carrots and peas. At the end of 16 weeks, the researchers measured the cholesterol in the blood vessels. They found that the mice that were fed the vegetable-enriched diet had plaques that were 38 percent smaller. There was also a 37 percent reduction in serum amyloid, which means there was a reduction in inflammation. "The results indicate that a diet rich in green and yellow vegetables inhibits the development of atherosclerosis and may therefore lead to a reduction in the risk of coronary heart disease."[1]

A study of 3,061 Japanese men and women between the ages of 39 and 80 was published in 2006 in the *Journal of Epidemiology*. During the almost 12-year follow-up period, there were a total of 80 deaths from cardiovascular disease. Researchers found that high levels of alpha- and beta-carotene (contained in carrots) in the body were related to a reduced risk for cardiovascular disease mortality.[2]

In a study published in 2008 in *The Journal of Nutrition*, researchers followed 559 men, with an average age of 72, for 15 years. Over the course of that time, 197 of the men died from cardiovascular disease. The men with higher intakes of alpha- and beta-carotenes (from carrots) had significantly lower rates of death from cardiovascular disease. The researchers concluded that the dietary intake of carrots was inversely associated with mortality from cardiovascular disease in elderly men.[3]

CANCER PREVENTIVE

A study published in 2005 in the *Journal of Agricultural and Food Chemistry* examined the association between colorectal cancer in rats and the consumption of raw carrots or falcarinol, a natural fungal disease pesticide found in carrots. (In the human diet, the only source of falcarinol is carrots.)

Researchers divided 24 rats with precancerous colorectal tumors into three groups. The first group was fed regular rat food plus ten percent freeze-dried carrots; the second group was fed rat food plus falcarinol (the amount equal to the freeze-dried carrots); and the third group was fed only standard rat food. After 18 weeks, the researchers found that the rats that were fed carrots or falcarinol were one-third less likely to develop colorectal cancer tumors than those fed the standard rat food. The researchers concluded that, "The present study provides a new perspective on the known epidemiological associations between high intake of carrots and reduced incidence of cancers."[4]

Researchers at the Anderson Cancer Center at the University of Texas, Houston studied the association between the consumption of foods containing phytoestrogens, such as carrots, and lung cancer. In a 2005 article in JAMA, *The Journal of the American Medical Association*, the researchers compared the dietary histories of 1,674 people with lung cancer to 1,735 healthy people. The results were dramatic. After controlling for smoking status and other known risk factors, the incidence of lung cancer in people with the highest levels of phytoestrogen consumption was 46 percent lower that the people with the lowest levels of phytoestrogen consumption. While acknowledging that, "there are limitations and concerns regarding case-control studies of diet and cancer," the researchers note that, "these data provide further support for the limited but growing epidemiologic evidence that phytoestrogens are associated with a decrease in risk of lung cancer."[5]

PREVENTION OF DIABETES

A study published in 2006 in the *Journal of Epidemiology* found that the antioxidant pigments in carotenoids found in foods like carrots (and tomatoes and dark leafy greens) may help prevent people from developing diabetes. Researcher analyzed data from 4,493 subjects, between the ages of 18 and 30, who participated in the Coronary Artery Risk Development Young Adults Study. During the 16 years that the group was followed, 148 people developed diabetes. Nonsmokers who had diets high in carotenoids were found to be far less likely to develop diabetes. In fact, they had about half the risk. People who smoked appeared to derive no such benefit.[6]

LOWERS RISK FOR BENIGN PROSTATIC HYPERPLASIA (ENLARGED PROSTATE)

A study published in 2007 in *The American Journal of Clinical Nutrition* examined the role that fruits and vegetables, such as carrots and cantaloupes, may play in helping men prevent the often uncomfortable condition known as benign prostatic hyperplasia (BPH). Researchers compared about 6,000 men between the ages of 46 and 81 who had surgery for or symptoms of benign prostatic hyperplasia to more than 18,000 men who had not experienced prostate problems. The study participants who ate an average of at least one-and-a-half daily servings of beta-carotene foods, such as carrots and cantaloupes, had a 13 percent lower risk of an enlarged prostate than those who ate only about one serving per week. The researchers noted that their "findings are consistent with the hypothesis that a diet rich in vegetables may reduce the occurrence of BPH."[7]

LOWERS RISK FOR AGE-RELATED MACULAR DEGENERATION (ARMD OR AMD)

A Dutch study published in 2005 in *JAMA, The Journal of the American Medical Association* included more than 4,000 people aged 55 years or older. (AMD, a disorder in which there is a loss of central vision, is the leading cause of blindness in this age group.) During the eight years of the study, researchers compared changes in eye health of the participants with their intake of nutrients including foods with beta-carotene, such as carrots. Researchers found that the participants who consumed an above-median intake of foods that contain beta-carotene, as well as vitamins C, E, and zinc, had a 35 percent lower risk of AMD.[8]

In another study, of women in Iowa, Wisconsin, and Oregon, which was published in 2006 in the *Archives of Ophthalmology*, researchers examined the association between the intake of lutein and zeaxanthin, two carotenoids, and the incidence of age-related macular degeneration. They found that in healthy women younger than 75 years, diets rich in these two carotenoids may have some protective value.[9]

Another study, published in 2007 in the *Archives of Ophthalmology*, found similar results. The study, which included 4,519 people between the ages of 60 and 80, observed an inverse relationship intake between the consumption of dietary carotenoids, such as carrots, vitamin A, alpha-tocopherol, and vitamin C with AMD. Those with the highest consumption of these nutrients were least likely to develop AMD.[10]

Obviously, carrots are an excellent addition to the diet. But, people should not go overboard. When eaten in excess, carrots may cause hypercarotenemia, a condition in which sections of skin and the whites of the eye turn orange and yellow. The cure is very easy—eat fewer carrots.

NOTES

1. Adams, Michael R., Deborah L. Golden, Haiying Chen, et al. July 2006. "A Diet Rich in Green and Yellow Vegetables Inhibits Atherosclerosis in Mice." *The Journal of Nutrition* 136: 1886–1889.

2. Ito, Yoshinori, Mio Kurata, Koji Suzuki, et al. 2006. "Cardiovascular Disease Mortality and Serum Carotenoid Levels: A Japanese Population-Based Follow-Up Study." *Journal of Epidemiology* 16(4): 154–160.

3. Buijsse, Brian, Edith J. M. Feskens, Lemogang Kwape, et al. February 2008. "Both Alpha- and Beta-Carotene, but Not Tocopherols and Vitamin C, Are Inversely Related to 15-Year Cardiovascular Mortality in Dutch Elderly Men." *The Journal of Nutrition* 138: 344–350.

4. Kobk-Larsen, Morten, Lars P. Christensen, Werner Vach, et al. 2005. "Inhibitory Effects of Feeding with Carrots of (−)-Falcarinol on Development of Azoxymethane-Induced Preneoplastic Lesions in the Rat Colon." *Journal of Agricultural and Food Chemistry* 53(5): 1823–1827.

5. Schabath, Matthew B., Ladia M. Hernandez, Xifeng Wu, et al. September 28, 2005. "Dietary Phytoestrogens and Lung Cancer Risk." *JAMA, The Journal of the American Medical Association* 294(12): 1493–1504.

6. Hozawa, Atsushi, David R. Jacobs, Michael W. Steffes, et al. May 2006. "Associations of Serum Carotenoid Concentrations with the Development of Diabetes and with Insulin Concentration: Interaction with Smoking. The Coronary Artery Risk Development in Young Adults (CARDIA) Study." *American Journal of Epidemiology* 163(10): 929–937.

7. Rohrmann, Sabine, Edward Giovannucci, Walter C. Willett, and Elizabeth Platz. February 2007. "Fruit and Vegetable Consumption, Intake of Micronutrients, and Benign Prostatic Hyperplasia in U.S. Men." *The American Journal of Clinical Nutrition* 85(2): 523–529.

8. van Leeuwen, Redmer, Sharmila Boekhoorn, Johannes R. Vingerling, et al. December 28, 2005. "Dietary Intake of Antioxidants and Risk of Age-Related Macular Degeneration." *JAMA, The Journal of the American Medical Association* 294(24): 3101–3107.

9. Moeller, Suzen M., Niyati Parekh, Lesley Tinker, et al. "Associations Between Intermediate Age-Related Macular Degeneration and Lutein and Zeaxanthin in the

Carotenoids in Age-Related Eye Disease Study (CAREDS)." *Archives of Ophthalmology* 124(8): 1151–1162.

    10. SanGiovanni, John Paul, Emily Y. Chew, Traci E. Clemons, et al. September 2007. "The Relationship of Dietary Carotenoid and Vitamin A, E, and C Intake with Age-Related Macular Degeneration in a Case-Control Study." *Archives of Ophthalmology* 125(9): 1225–1232.

REFERENCES AND RESOURCES
Magazine, Journals, and Newspapers

Adams, Michael R., Deborah L. Golden, Haiying Chen, et al. July 2006. "A Diet Rich in Green and Yellow Vegetables Inhibits Atherosclerosis in Mice." *The Journal of Nutrition* 136: 1886–1889.

Buijsse, Brian, Edith J. M. Feskens, Lemogang Kwape, et al. February 2008. "Both Alpha- and Beta-Carotene, but Not Tocopherols and Vitamin C, Are Inversely Related to 15-Year Cardiovascular Mortality in Dutch Elderly Men." *The Journal of Nutrition* 138: 344–350.

Hozawa, Atsushi, David R. Jacobs, Jr., Michael W. Steffes, et al. May 2006. "Associations of Serum Carotenoid Concentrations with the Development of Diabetes and with Insulin Concentration: Interaction with Smoking. The Coronary Artery Risk Development in Young Adults (CARDIA) Study." *American Journal of Epidemiology* 163(10): 929–937.

Ito, Yoshinori, Mio Kurata, Koji Suzuki, et al. 2006. "Cardiovascular Disease Mortality and Serum Cholesterol Levels: A Japanese Population-Based Follow-Up Study." *Journal of Epidemiology* 16(4): 154–160.

Kobk-Larsen, Morten, Lars P. Christensen, Werner Vach, et al. 2005. "Inhibitory Effects of Feeding with Carrots or (−)-Falcarinol on Development of Azoxymethane-Induced Preneoplastic Lesions in the Rat Colon." *Journal of Agriculture and Food Chemistry* 53(5): 1823–1827.

Moeller, Suzen M., Niyati Parekh, Lesley Tinker, et al. August 2006. "Associations Between Intermediate Age-Related Macular Degeneration and Lutein and Zeaxanthin in the Carotenoids in Age-Related Eye Disease Study (CAREDS)." *Archives of Ophthalmology* 124(8): 1151–1162.

Rohrmann, Sabine, Edward Giovannucci, Walter C. Willett, and Elizabeth A. Platz. February 2007. "Fruit and Vegetable Consumption, Intake of Micronutrients, and Benign Prostatic Hyperplasia in U.S. Men." *The American Journal of Clinical Nutrition* 85(2): 523–529.

SanGiovanni, John Paul, Emily Y. Chew, Traci E. Clemons, et al. September 2007. "The Relationship of Dietary Carotenoid and Vitamin A, E, and C Intake with Age-Related Macular Degeneration in a Case-Control Study." *Archives of Ophthalmology* 125(9): 1225–1232.

Schabath, Matthew B., Ladia M. Hernandez, Xifeng Wu, et al. September 28, 2005. "Dietary Phytoestrogens and Lung Cancer Risk." *JAMA, The Journal of the American Medical Association* 294(12): 1493–1504.

an Leeuwen, Redmer, Sharmila Boekhoorn, Johannes R. Vingerling, et al. December 28, 2005. "Dietary Intake of Antioxidants and Risk of Age-Related Macular Degeneration." *JAMA, The Journal of the American Medical Association* 294(24): 3101–3107.

Website

The George Mateljan Foundation. www.whfoods.com.

CELERY

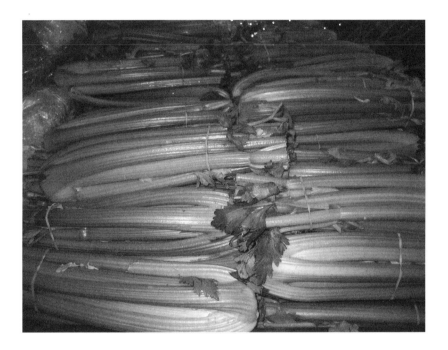

Initially available only in the wild, celery is thought to have originated in the Mediterranean regions of northern Africa and southern Europe. But, it is also believed to be native to areas extending east to the Himalayas.

At first, celery was considered a medicine. These medicinal properties are noted in the *Odyssey*, which was written by the Greek poet Homer in the 9th century BCE. In ancient Greece, celery leaves were fashioned into laurels and adorned on athletes, and in ancient Rome, celery was used as a seasoning.

By the Middle Ages, celery had become a food that was cooked. It was not until the 18th century that it was consumed as a raw vegetable in Europe. In the 19th century, celery finally made its way to the United States.[1]

Celery contains excellent amounts of vitamins K and C. It has very good amounts of potassium, folate, dietary fiber, molybdenum, manganese, and vitamin B_6. In addition, celery has good amounts of calcium, vitamins A, B_1, and B_2, magnesium, tryptophan, phosphorus, and iron.[2] But, what have the researchers learned?

CANCER

In a study published in 2008 in the *Proceedings of the National Academy of Sciences*, two University of California, Riverside, researchers found that the ingestion of apigenin, a class of flavonoid, a phytonutrient (plant compound) with high antioxidant activity that is found in celery, improves the response of cancer cells to chemotherapy. How is this accomplished? The researchers determined that apigenin activates a tumor suppressor known as p53 and transports it into the nucleus of the cancer cell. There it stops cell growth and causes cell death. The researchers noted that, "apigenin specifically restores p53 nuclear localization and this provides a molecular basis of using apigenin for targeting cancers caused by abnormal cytoplasm localization of wild-type p53."[3]

Ovarian Cancer

In a population-based study that was published in 2009 in the *International Journal of Cancer*, Harvard researchers reviewed the association between intake of apigenin and incidence of ovarian cancer. The cohort consisted of 1,141 women with ovarian cancer and 1,183 matched controls. The average age of the participants was 51.

When compared to the women with the lowest intake of apigenin, the women with the highest intake had a "borderline significant decrease" in risk of ovarian cancer. Interestingly, the researchers found that no such benefit was obtained from consuming four other flavonoids—myricetin, kaempferol, quercetin, and luteolin. Moreover, they found no association "between total flavonoid intake and ovarian cancer risk."[4]

Prostate Cancer

In a study published in 2005 in *The FASEB Journal*, researchers from Case Western Reserve University in Cleveland, Ohio, fed mice doses of 20 and 50 micrograms (mcg) of apigenin daily for a total of eight weeks. After the first two weeks of supplementation, they implanted prostate tumors in the mice. In a second protocol, the tumors were implanted two weeks before the supplementation was started. The researchers found that in both versions of the study, the apigenin slowed the growth of prostate tumor cells. Furthermore, the apigenin did not appear to have any adverse side effects. The researchers noted that their findings "present the possibility that apigenin . . . may be useful in the prevention or treatment of prostate cancer."[5]

Added Anti-Cancer Benefit

In an in vitro study published in 2004 in *Carcinogenesis,* researchers found that when apigenin was consumed with foods containing sulforaphane, a chemical found in all brassica vegetables such as broccoli, it offers far greater protection against cancer cells. Though both apigenin and sulforaphane act in different ways, they have a "synergistic effect."[6]

ASTHMA

In a study published in 2006 in the *Journal of Agricultural and Food Chemistry,* Japanese researchers supplemented the diets of mice with apigenin for two weeks and measured the levels of immune and inflammatory markers. When compared to a control group of mice, the researchers found that the apigenin suppressed the levels of immunoglobulin E (IgE) by 50 percent. IgE is associated with the expression of asthma and other allergies; higher levels of IgE increase the risk of asthma and allergies. The researchers noted that their results suggest that "a diet containing apigenin can reduce serum IgE."[7]

PREVENTING BONE LOSS AND SUPPORTING WEIGHT LOSS

In a study published in 2008 in *Life Sciences,* South Korean researchers attempted to determine if apigenin protects bones in estrogen-deficient rats from which the ovaries had been removed. The researchers used three-month-old Sprague-Dawley rats that were either sham-operated (a placebo surgical procedure) or ovariectomized and fed a diet that fosters bone loss for seven weeks. Then, for 15 weeks, the rats were fed 10 mg/kg apigenin three times per week. The researchers found that the apigenin increased mineral content and density of the bones and had a positive effect on bone turnover. In addition, apigenin decreased body weight and dietary consumption. They concluded that the "data suggest that apigenin should be considered for use in the treatment of osteoporosis."[8]

CARDIOVASCULAR HEALTH

In a study published in 2007 in the *Proceedings of the National Academy of Sciences,* researchers examined the cardiovascular effects of the consumption of nitrite, which is found in celery, on mice. While a control group of mice ate a standard diet, for seven days researchers added 50 mg/L nitrite to the drinking water of another group of mice. All of the mice then had simulated heart attacks, followed by 24 hours of reperfusion (the restoration of blood flow to an organ or tissue—in this case the heart). As might be anticipated, the hearts of the mice on nitrite supplementation had higher levels of nitrite. Of more significance is the fact that when compared to the control mice, the hearts of the mice on nitrite had a 48 percent reduction in heart muscle damage. The mice on a high-nitrite diet were also more likely to survive a heart attack. Their survival rate was 77 percent; the mice on a nitrite-deficient diet survived only 58 percent of the time. When the researchers conducted a similar trial with nitrate, the nitrate supplemented mice had higher amounts of nitrate in their heart muscle and less heart muscle damage, though the reduction in damage was less than was obtained from nitrite. The researchers concluded that, "nitrite and nitrate may serve as essential nutrients for optimal cardiovascular health and may provide a treatment modality for cardiovascular health."[9]

PROTECTION AGAINST INFLAMMATORY BRAIN DISEASES

In two studies—an in vitro study and a second study on mice—published together in 2008 in the *Proceedings of the National Academy of Sciences*, researchers from the University of Illinois at Urbana-Champaign examined the association between consumption of luteolin, a flavonoid found in high concentrations in celery (and green pepper) and brain inflammation. The researchers treated microglia brain cells with different concentrations of luteolin. They then exposed the cells to a substance that caused inflammation. When compared to untreated cells, luteolin inhibited inflammation by as much as 90 percent. In the in vivo trial on mice, the researchers gave the mice different concentrations of luteolin. After 21 days, they were injected with the same inflammation triggering substance. Luteolin was found to decrease the levels of inflammation. In fact, the mice that were given the highest concentrations of luteolin had the most protection in the hippocampus, the area of the brain concerned with memory and learning. Thus, the researchers speculated that luteolin may be useful in the prevention of brain diseases such as Alzheimer's and dementia.[10]

Should celery be included in the diet? Certainly. And, it is a good idea to consume it with at least one brassica vegetable.

NOTES

1. The George Mateljan Foundation Website. www.whfoods.com.

2. The George Mateljan Foundation Website.

3. Cai, Xin and Xuan Liu. November 4, 2008. "Inhibition of Thr-55 Phosphorylation Restores p53 Nuclear Localization and Sensitizes Cancer Cells to DNA Damage." *Proceedings of the National Academy of Sciences* 105: 16958–16963.

4. Gates, Margaret A., Allison F. Vitonis, Shelley S. Tworoger, et al. April 2009. "Flavonoid Intake and Ovarian Cancer Risk in a Population-Based Case-Control Study." *International Journal of Cancer* 124(8): 1918–1925.

5. Shukla, Sanjeev, Anil Mishra, Pingfu Fu, et al. December 2005. "Up-Regulation of Insulin-Like Growth Factor Binding Protein-3 by Apigenin Leads to Growth Inhibition and Apoptosis of 22Rv1 Xenograft in Athymic Nude Mice." *The FASEB Journal* 19(14): 2042–2044.

6. Švehlíková, Vanda, Shuran Wang, Jana Jakubíková, et al. September 2004. "Interactions Between Sulforaphane and Apigenin in the Induction of UGT1A1 and GSTA1 in Caco-2 Cells." *Carcinogenesis* 25(9): 1629–1637.

7. Yano, Satomi, Daisuke Umeda, Norihide Maeda, et al. 2006. "Dietary Apigenin Suppresses IgE and Inflammatory Cytokines Production in C57BL/6N Mice." *Journal of Agricultural and Food Chemistry* 54(14): 5203–5207.

8. Park, J. A., S. K. Ha, T. H. Kang, et al. June 20, 2008. "Protective Effect of Apigenin on Ovariectomy-Induced Bone Loss in Rats." *Life Sciences* 82(25–26): 1217–1223.

9. Bryan, Nathan S., John W. Calvert, John W. Elrod, et al. November 27, 2007. "Dietary Nitrite Supplementation Protects Against Myocardial Ischemia-Reperfusion Injury." *Proceedings of the National Academy of Sciences* 104: 19144–19149.

10. Jang, Saebyeol, Keith W. Kelley, and Rodney W. Johnson. 2008. "Luteolin Reduces IL-6 Production in Microglia by Inhibiting JNK Phosphorylation and Activation of AP-1." *Proceedings of the National Academy of Sciences* 105: 7534–7539.

REFERENCES AND RESOURCES
Magazines, Journals, and Newspapers

Bryan, Nathan S., John W. Calvert, John W. Elrod, et al. November 27, 2007. "Dietary Nitrite Supplementation Protects Against Myocardial Ischemia-Reperfusion Injury." *Proceedings of the National Academy of Sciences* 104: 19144–19149.

Cai, Xin and Xuan Liu. November 4, 2008. "Inhibition of Thr-55 Phosphorylation Restores p53 Nuclear Localization and Sensitizes Cancer Cells to DNA Damage." *Proceedings of the National Academy of Sciences* 105: 16958–16963.

Gates, Margaret A., Allison F. Vitonis, Shelley S. Tworoger, et al. April 2009. "Flavonoid Intake and Ovarian Cancer Risk in a Population-Based Case-Control Study." *International Journal of Cancer* 124(8): 1918–1925.

Jang, Saebyeol, Keith W. Kelley, and Rodney W. Johnson. 2008. "Luteolin Reduces IL-6 Production in Microglia by Inhibiting JNK Phosphorylation and Activation of AP-1." *Proceedings of the National Academy of Sciences* 105: 7534–7539.

Park, J. A., S. K. Ha, T. H. Kang, et al. June 20, 2008. "Protective Effect of Apigenin on Ovariectomy-Induced Bone Loss in Rats." *Life Sciences* 82(25-26): 1217–1223.

Shukla, Sanjeev, Anil Mishra, Pingfu Fu, et al. December 2005. "Up-Regulation of Insulin-Like Growth Factor Binding Protein-3 by Apigenin Leads to Growth Inhibition and Apoptosis of 22Rv1 Xenograft in Athymic Nude Mice." *The FASEB Journal* 19(14): 2042–2044.

Švehlíková, Vanda, Shuran Wang, Jana Jakubíková, et al. September 2004. "Interactions Between Sulforaphane and Apigenin in the Induction of UGT1A1 and GSTA1 in CaCo-2 Cells." *Carcinogenesis* 25(9): 1629–1637.

Yano, Satomi, Daisuke Umeda, Norihide Maeda, et al. 2006. "Dietary Apigenin Suppresses IgE and Inflammatory Cytokines Production in C57BL/6N Mice." *Journal of Agricultural and Food Chemistry* 54(14): 5203–5207.

Website

The George Mateljan Foundation. www.whfoods.com.

CHERRIES

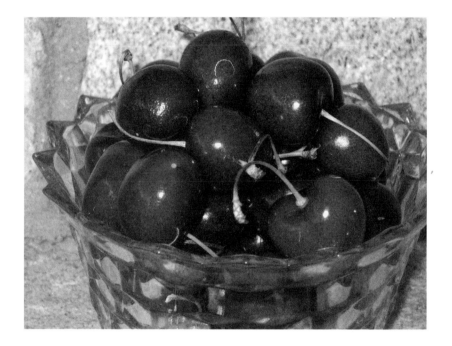

From the time little children learn their very first history lessons about the founding of the United States, they hear about cherries. Wasn't George Washington known for cutting down his father's cherry tree? The story is told so often because this young child, who grew up to become the first president of the United States, did not attempt to shy away from the truth. He told his father exactly what he had done.

While the story of George Washington and the cherry tree may or may not be true, today cherries are also believed to be an extraordinarily healthful fruit. Some think that they should be considered a type of "superfood." They have been said to be useful for inflammation, pain, cancer prevention, and sleep regulation; they also may have anti-aging properties. But, does the research support these claims?

REDUCTION IN INFLAMMATION AND PAIN

In a study conducted at Johns Hopkins Hospital in Baltimore and published in 2004 in *Behavioural Brain Research*, researchers tested the use of anthocyanins (antioxidant flavonoids) extracted from tart cherries on inflammation-induced pain in rats. They also examined how the effects of anthocyanins compared to benefits obtained from using the non-steroidal anti-inflammatory drug indomethacin and how the consumption of anthocyanins affected motor coordination. The researchers found that the highest dose of anthocyanins (400 mg/kg) obtained results comparable to indomethacin (5 mg/kg). And, even at the highest dose, anthocyanins did not alter motor coordination. The researchers concluded that, "tart cherry anthocyanins may have a beneficial role in the treatment of inflammatory pain."[1]

Meanwhile, researchers at the University of Vermont found an association between the consumption of tart cherry juice blend and the prevention of muscle damage. In a study published in 2006 in the *British Journal of Sports Medicine*, fourteen male college students drank twelve ounces of a cherry juice blend or a placebo twice daily for eight consecutive days. In order to create muscle damage, on the fourth day, the students completed two sets of twenty negative-rep bicep curls. Both before the workout and four days after the workout, researchers measured arm strength and muscle pain. When the study was repeated two weeks later, the subjects who first drank the juice drank the placebo and those who drank the placebo drank the juice. The exercises were repeated on the opposite arm. The researchers found that, "strength loss and pain were significantly less in the cherry juice trial verses placebo. . . . Strength loss average over the four days after eccentric exercise [exercise in which the contracting muscle is forcibly lengthened] was 22 percent with the placebo but only four percent with the cherry juice."[2]

A study published in 2003 in *The Journal of Nutrition* reviewed the association between consumption of Bing sweet cherries and the amount of uric acid (urate) in the blood. (Higher levels of uric acid in the blood are directly correlated with gout.) After an overnight fast, ten healthy women between the ages of 22 and 40 years consumed two servings of Bing sweet cherries (280 g). Blood and urine samples were taken before eating the cherries and at 1.5 hours, 3 hours, and 5 hours after eating the cherries. Three hours after eating the cherries there were significant decreases in uric acid levels. Though not significant, there were also decreases in levels of inflammation.[3]

CANCER

In a Michigan State University study published in 2003 in *Cancer Letters*, researchers fed a diet containing tart cherries, anthocyanins, or cyanidin (a breakdown product of anthocyanins) to mice that were predisposed to have a high risk for colon cancer. A second group of similar mice served as the control group. The researchers found that the mice that consumed tart cherries, anthocyanins (which is found in tart cherries), or cyanidin developed fewer and smaller colon cancers. "These results suggest that tart cherry anthocyanins and cyanidin may reduce the risk of colon cancer."[4]

A Swedish study, published in 2004 in the *Journal of Agricultural and Food Chemistry*, investigated the effects of ten different extracts of fruits and berries, including cherries, on breast and colon cancer cells. The extracts were found to decrease the proliferation of both types of cancer cells, "and the effect was concentration dependent."[5]

CARDIOVASCULAR HEALTH, METABOLIC SYNDROME, AND TYPE 2 DIABETES

During the 2007 Experimental Biology Annual Meeting, researchers from the University of Michigan Cardiovascular Center and the University of Michigan Cardioprotection Research Laboratory noted that the intake of cherries may reduce the risk of cardiovascular disease, metabolic syndrome, and type 2 diabetes. In the research, one group of rats was fed a diet that consisted of one percent whole tart cherry powder; another group of rats was fed a diet that was ten percent whole tart cherry powder. A control group of rats was fed a diet without cherry powder, but with the same amount of carbohydrates and calories. After 90 days, the rats fed cherry powder had lower levels of total cholesterol, triglycerides, insulin, and fasting glucose levels. "All of these measures are factors that are linked to metabolic syndrome." According to the lead researcher of the study, Steven F. Bolling, MD, a cardiac surgeon, "Metabolic syndrome is a cluster of traits that can greatly increase your risk of heart disease, stroke and type 2 diabetes . . . Lifestyle changes have been shown to lower the odds of developing metabolic syndrome, and there is tremendous interest in studying the impact of particular foods that are rich in antioxidants, such as cherries."[6]

SLEEP REGULATION AND ANTI-AGING

Researchers are learning more about how the body benefits from an increased intake of melatonin, a powerful antioxidant that is made in the body's pineal gland. Though the body naturally produces melatonin, it may not produce all that it requires. Furthermore, as the body ages, it produces less. Melatonin is known to play an integral role in helping to regulate biorhythm and sleep patterns. Tart cherries are one of the very few known food sources of melatonin. And, melatonin researchers, such as Russel J. Reiter, PhD, from the University of Texas Health and Science Center, believe that tart cherries may be useful for those with sleep problems and those dealing with jet lag. In fact, Dr. Reiter advises plane travelers to eat dried cherries one hour before going to sleep. "After arrival, consume cherries one hour before desired sleep each night for at least three consecutive evenings."[7]

In a study that was published in 2007 in *Basic & Clinical Pharmacology & Toxicology*, Dr. Reiter and other researchers investigated what would happen if they administered melatonin for seven days to a diurnal animal (one that is active during the day and sleeps at night). They selected ringdoves, pigeons with whitish patches on each side of the neck and wings edged with white. The researchers studied both young ringdoves, between the ages of two and three years, and old ringdoves, between the ages of ten and twelve years. Three different melatonin doses were used: 0.25, 2.5, and 5 mg/kg body weight. "The results showed that the administration of whichever melatonin dose decreased both diurnal and nocturnal old ringdove activity, the reduction being larger at night. The young animals also reduced their nocturnal activity with all three melatonin concentrations, whereas their diurnal activity only decreased with the 2.5- and 5-mg/kg body weight treatments." The researchers concluded that, "treatment with melatonin may be appropriate to improve nocturnal rest, and beneficial as a therapy for sleep disorders."[8]

And, a study on mice published in 2007 in *Free Radical Research*, which included Dr. Reiter and his Texas colleagues and researchers at the University of Granada in Spain, determined that melatonin helps to neutralize the oxidation and inflammation associated with aging. The researchers even recommended that around age 30 or 40, people begin a daily consumption of melatonin.[9]

Should cherries be part of the diet? Absolutely.

NOTES

1. Tall, J. M., N. P. Seeram, C. Zhao, et al. August 12, 2004. "Tart Cherry Anthocyanins Suppress Inflammation-Induced Pain Behavior in Rat." *Behavioural Brain Research* 153(1): 181–188.

2. Connolly, D. A. J., M. P. McHugh, and O. I. Padilla-Zakour. June 2006. "Efficacy of a Tart Cherry Juice Blend in Preventing the Symptoms of Muscle Damage." *British Journal of Sports Medicine* 40: 679–683.

3. Jacob, Robert A., Giovanna M. Spinozzi, Vicky A. Simon, et al. June 2003. "Consumption of Cherries Lowers Plasma Urate in Healthy Women." *The Journal of Nutrition* 133: 1826–1829.

4. Kang, S. Y., N. P. Seeram, M. G. Nair, and L. D. Bourquin. May 8, 2003. "Tart Cherry Anthocyanins Inhibit Tumor Development in Apc(Min) Mice and Reduce Proliferation of Human Colon Cells." *Cancer Letters* 194(1): 13–19.

5. Olsson, Marie E., Karl-Erik Gustavsson, Staffan Andersson, et al. 2004. "Inhibition of Cancer Cell Proliferation In Vitro by Fruit and Berry Extracts and Correlations with Antioxidant Levels." *Journal of Agricultural and Food Chemistry* 52(24): 7264–7271.

6. Medical News Today. www.medicalnewstoday.com/articles/69375.php.

7. Cherry Marketing Institute. www.choosecherries.com/health/sleep.aspx.

8. Paredes, Sergio D., Ma Pilar Terron, Vicente Valero, et al. April 2007. "Orally Administered Melatonin Improves Nocturnal Rest in Young and Old Ringdoves (*Streptopelia risoria*)." *Basic & Clinical Pharmacology & Toxicology* 100(4): 258–268.

9. Rodriguez, Maria I., Miguel Carretero, Germaine Escames, et al. January 2007. "Chronic Melatonin Treatment Prevents Age-Dependent Cardiac Mitochondrial Dysfunction in Senescence-Accelerated Mice." *Free Radical Research* 41(1): 15–24.

RESOURCES AND REFERENCES
Magazines, Journals, and Newspapers

Connolly, D. A. J., M. P. McHugh, and O. I. Padilla-Zakour. June 2006. "Efficacy of a Tart Cherry Juice Blend in Preventing the Symptoms of Muscle Damage." *British Journal of Sports Medicine* 40: 679–683.

Jacob, Robert A., Giovanna M. Spinozzi, Vicky A. Simon, et al. June 2003. "Consumption of Cherries Lowers Plasma Urate in Healthy Women." *The Journal of Nutrition* 133: 1826–1829.

Kang, S. Y., N. P. Seeram, M. G. Nair, and L. D. Bourquin. May 8, 2003. "Tart Cherry Anthocyanins Inhibit Tumor Development in Apc(Min) Mice and Reduce Proliferation of Human Colon Cells." *Cancer Letters* 194(1): 13–19.

Olsson, Marie E., Karl-Erik Gustavsson, Staffan Andersson, et al. 2004. "Inhibition of Cancer Cell Proliferation In Vitro by Fruit and Berry Extracts and Correlations with Antioxidant Levels." *Journal of Agricultural and Food Chemistry* 52(24): 7264–7271.

Paredes, Sergio D., Ma Pilar Terron, Vincente Valero, et al. April 2007. "Orally Administered Melatonin Improves Nocturnal Rest in Young and Old Ringdoves (*Streptopelia risoria*)." *Basic & Clinical Pharmacology & Toxicology* 100(4): 258–268.

Rodriguez, Maria I., Miguel Carretero, Germaine Escames, et al. January 2007. "Chronic Melatonin Treatment Prevents Age-Dependent Cardiac Mitochondrial Dysfunction in Senescence-Accelerated Mice." *Free Radical Research* 41(1): 15–24.

Tall, J. M., N. P. Seeram, C. Zhao, et al. August 12, 2004. "Tart Cherry Anthocyanins Suppress Inflammation-Induced Pain Behavior in Rat." *Behavioural Brain Research* 153(1): 181–188.

Websites

Cherry Marketing Institute. http://choosecherries.com.
Medical News Today. www.medicalnewstoday.com.

CHICKPEAS

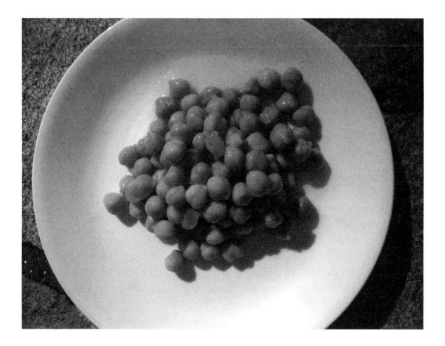

Though chickpeas, which are also known as garbanzo beans, originated in the Middle East about 7,000 years ago, they were not actually cultivated in the Mediterranean basin until around 3000 BCE. From the Mediterranean basin, their cultivation spread to India and Ethiopia.

Chickpeas were popular during the ancient Egyptian, Greek, and Roman civilizations. During the 16th century, Spanish and Portuguese explorers introduced them to the subtropics, and people from India brought them along when they moved to other countries. Today, the major commercial producers of chickpeas are India, Pakistan, Turkey, Ethiopia, and Mexico.[1]

Chickpeas have excellent amounts of molybdenum and manganese. They have very good amounts of folate and good amounts of dietary fiber, tryptophan, protein, copper, phosphorus, and iron.[2] But, what have the researchers learned?

CARDIOVASCULAR HEALTH

In a randomized crossover study published in 2006 in the *Annals of Nutrition & Metabolism*, Australian researchers supplemented the diets of 47 men and women with either chickpeas or wheat. After a period of at least five weeks, the subjects were placed on the alternate supplementation. The dietary plan that included chickpeas had a little less protein and fat and more carbohydrates than the plan that included wheat. When compared to the subjects on the wheat supplementation, the subjects on chickpea supplementation experienced significant reductions in cholesterol levels—a 3.9 percent drop in total cholesterol and a 4.6 percent drop in LDL ("bad") cholesterol. The researchers noted that, "inclusion of chickpeas in an intervention diet results in lower serum total and low-density lipoprotein cholesterol levels as compared with a wheat-supplemented diet."[3]

A study published in 2003 in the *Archives of Internal Medicine* followed close to 10,000 subjects for an average of 19 years. When the study began, none of the subjects had evidence of cardiovascular disease. During the years of the study, there were 1,843 cases of incident coronary heart disease and 3,762 cases of incident cardiovascular disease. Compared to the subjects who ate the least amount of fiber, the subjects who ate the most fiber, such as the soluble and insoluble fiber in chickpeas, had 12 percent less coronary heart disease and 11 percent less cardiovascular disease. The subjects who ate the most water-soluble fiber had a 15-percent reduction in the risk for coronary heart disease and a 10-percent reduction in the risk for cardiovascular disease.[4]

In order to determine the association between the intake of folate and the risk for hypertension (high blood pressure), a study published in 2005 in *JAMA, The Journal of the American Medical Association*, examined the findings of two prospective cohort studies. (As has been noted, chickpeas have very good amounts of folate.) The two cohorts included 156,063 women between the ages of 27 and 70. One cohort—known as the "younger women"—included women between the ages of 27 and 44; the other cohort—known as the "older women"—included women between the ages of 43 and 70. At baseline, no one had a history of hypertension. During the eight years of follow-up, there were 7,373 cases of hypertension among the younger women and 12,347 cases of hypertension among the older women. The researchers found that, "higher total folate intake was associated with a decreased risk of incident hypertension, particularly in younger women."[5]

Another study on the association between intake of folate and reductions in blood pressure was conducted by Italian researchers and published in 2009 in the *European Journal of Clinical Nutrition*. In this trial, 15 postmenopausal women received daily doses of 15 milligrams of 5-methyltetrahydrofolate (5-MTHF), the predominant naturally circulating form of folate. A second group of 15 postmenopausal women served as the placebo group; they received no 5-MTHF. At the end of three weeks, the researchers observed that the women who took the folate had average reductions of 4.5 millimeters of mercury (mmHg) in systolic blood pressure and 5.3 mmHg in diastolic blood pressure. The blood pressure readings of the women in the placebo group remained the same. The women in the folate group also had reductions in levels of homocysteine of 11.8 micromoles per liter; this is in contrast to the women in the placebo group who had reductions of 8.7 micromoles per liter. Studies have shown an association between increased levels of the amino acid homocysteine and increased risk for cardiovascular disease. The researchers concluded that higher amounts of folate may be useful for maintaining the cardiovascular health of postmenopausal women.[6]

A 2009 article in *Chemistry and Industry* reported on research conducted on chickpeas, beans, peas, and lentils at the University of Manitoba in Canada. The cohort consisted of 25 subjects who had peripheral artery disease, the build-up of fatty tissues in the arteries of the legs. After including one-half cup of chickpeas, beans, peas, and lentils in their daily diets for eight weeks the subjects had "tremendous" improvement in the blood flow of the legs. Additionally, the researchers observed a 10 percent increase in flexibility of blood vessels and a 5 percent reduction in the levels of LDL cholesterol.[7]

In a double-blind, placebo-controlled study published in 2008 in *European Heart Journal,* Hong Kong researchers attempted to determine if isoflavone, a chemical found in chickpeas, could improve arterial functioning in people who have suffered an ischemic stroke, a stroke caused by a blood clots or other types of obstruction. Fifty patients took isoflavone supplement; fifty-two took placebos. At the end of 12 weeks, compared to the people taking placebos, the subjects on isoflavone supplementation had improvements in arterial function. The researchers noted that, "these findings may have important implication for the use of isoflavone for secondary prevention in patients with cardiovascular disease, on top of conventional interventions."[8]

COLORECTAL CANCER

In a study published in 2009 in the *European Journal of Clinical Nutrition,* Korean researchers compared data from 596 men and women with colorectal cancer to data from 509 people who did not have this disease. The researchers found that the subjects who had the highest intake of folate had 53, 58, and 52 percent reduced risks of colorectal cancer, colon cancer, and rectal cancer, respectively. When the researchers focused on the gender of the participants, they found that it was actually only the women who benefited from the high intake of folate. The researchers noted that, "a statistically significant relationship between higher dietary folate intake and reduced risk of CRC [colorectal cancer], colon cancer and rectal cancer in women. A significant association is indicated between higher total folate intake and reduced risk of rectal cancer in women."[9]

ASTHMA

In a study published in 2009 in *The Journal of Allergy and Clinical Immunology*, researchers from Baltimore, Maryland, investigated the relationship between levels of serum folate and the prevalence of allergy and asthma symptoms. After reviewing the medical records of more than 8,000 people between the ages of 2 and 85, the researchers found that subjects with high amounts of folate in their blood had fewer allergies, less wheezing, and lower rates of asthma. Additionally, the people with higher rates of folate had lower levels of immunoglobulin E (IgE), the primary antibody associated with allergic responses. Moreover, when compared to the people with the highest rates of folate, the people with the lowest folate levels had a 40 percent higher risk for wheezing and a 30 percent higher risk for elevated levels of IgE. Those with the lowest levels also had a 31 percent higher risk of allergic symptoms and a 16 percent higher risk of having asthma.[10]

Are chickpeas a valuable addition to the diet? They certainly appear to be.

NOTES

1. The George Mateljan Foundation Website. www.whfoods.com.

2. The George Mateljan Foundation Website.

3. Pittaway, J. K., K. D. K. Ahuja, M. Cehun, et al. 2006. "Dietary Supplementation with Chickpeas for at Least 5 Weeks Results in Small but Significant Reductions in Serum Total and Low-Density Lipoprotein Cholesterols in Adult Women and Men." *Annals of Nutrition & Metabolism* 50(6): 512–518.

4. Bazzano, Lydia A., Jiang He, Lorraine G. Ogden, et al. September 8, 2003. "Dietary Fiber Intake and Reduced Risk of Coronary Heart Disease in U.S. Men and Women." *Archives of Internal Medicine* 163(16): 1897–1904.

5. Forman, John P., Eric B. Rimm, Meir J. Stampfer, et al. January 19, 2005. "Folate Intake and the Risk of Incident Hypertension Among U.S. Women." *JAMA, The Journal of the American Medical Association* 293(3): 320–329.

6. Cagnacci, A., M. Cannoletta, and A. Volpe. 2009. "High-Dose Short-Term Folate Administration Modifies Ambulatory Blood Pressure in Postmenopausal Women. A Placebo-Controlled Study." *European Journal of Clinical Nutrition* 63: 1266–1268.

7. "Beans, Beans Good for Your Heart." May 25, 2009. *Chemistry and Industry* 10: 8.

8. Chan, Yap-Hang, Kui-Kai Lau, Kai-Hang Yiu, et al. 2008. "Reduction of C-Reactive Protein with Isoflavone Supplement Reverses Endothelial Dysfunction in Patients with Ischaemic Stroke." *European Heart Journal* 29(22): 2800–2807.

9. Kim, J., D. H. Kim, B. H. Lee, et al. 2009. "Folate Intake and the Risk of Colorectal Cancer in a Korean Population." *European Journal of Clinical Nutrition* 63: 1057–1064.

10. Matsui, Elizabeth and William Matsui. 2009. "Higher Serum Folate Levels Are Associated with a Lower Risk of Atopy and Wheeze." *The Journal of Allergy and Clinical Immunology* 123(6): 1253–1259.

REFERENCES AND RESOURCES
Magazines, Journals, and Newspapers

Bazzano, Lydia A., Jiang He, Lorraine G. Ogden, et al. September 8, 2003. "Dietary Fiber Intake and Reduced Risk of Coronary Heart Disease in U.S. Men and Women." *Archives of Internal Medicine* 163(16): 1897–1904.

"Beans, Beans Good for Your Heart." May 25, 2009. *Chemistry and Industry* 10: 8.

Cagnacci, A., M. Cannoletta, and A. Volpe. 2009. "High-Dose Short-Term Folate Administration Modifies Ambulatory Blood Pressure in Postmenopausal Women: A Placebo-Controlled Study." *European Journal of Clinical Nutrition* 63: 1266–1268.

Chan, Yap-Hang, Kui-Kai Lau, Kai-Hang Yiu, et al. 2008. "Reduction of C-Reactive Protein with Isoflavone Supplement Reverses Endothelial Dysfunction in Patients with Ischaemic Stroke." *European Heart Journal* 29(22): 2800–2807.

Forman, John P., Eric B. Rimm, Meir J. Stampfer, et al. January 19, 2005. "Folate Intake and the Risk of Incident Hypertension Among U.S. Women." *JAMA, The Journal of the American Medical Association* 293(3): 320–329.

Kim, J., D. H. Kim, B. H. Lee, et al. 2009. "Folate Intake and the Risk of Colorectal Cancer in a Korean Population." *European Journal of Clinical Nutrition* 63: 1057–1064.

Matsui, Elizabeth C. and William Matsui. June 2009. "Higher Serum Folate Levels Are Associated with a Lower Risk of Atopy and Wheeze." *The Journal of Allergy and Clinical Immunology* 123(6): 1253–1259.

Pittaway, J. K., K. D. K. Ahuja, M. Cehun, et al. 2006. "Dietary Supplementation with Chickpeas for at Least 5 Weeks Results in Small but Significant Reductions in Serum Total and Low-Density Lipoprotein Cholesterols in Adult Women and Men." *Annals of Nutrition & Metabolism* 50(6): 512–518.

Website

The George Mateljan Foundation. www.whfoods.com.

CHOCOLATE

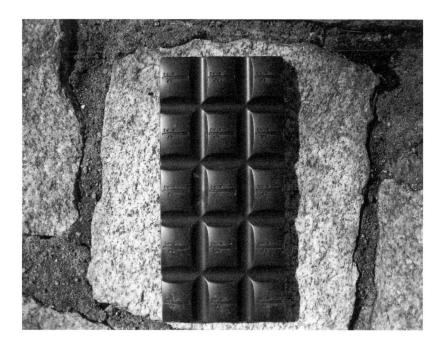

Until recent years, a discussion of healthier foods would not include chocolate. In fact, chocolate was generally viewed as a food that should be eaten rarely, especially among those who were attempting to maintain a healthier lifestyle.

Then, in August 2003, JAMA, *The Journal of the American Medical Association*, reported the results of research at the Medical College of the University of Cologne in Germany. Researchers studied 13 people, six men and seven women, between the ages of 55 and 64, who had recently been diagnosed with mild cases of high blood pressure. For two weeks, half the subjects ate a daily 100-gram dark chocolate bar and the other half ate a 100-gram white chocolate bar. People who ate the dark chocolate bar experienced a drop in blood pressure—an average of five points for systolic (top number) and two points for diastolic (bottom number). Those who ate the white chocolate had no change in blood pressure.[1]

The same month, *Nature* reported the findings of researchers at Italy's National Institute for Food and Nutrition. The researchers felt that the antioxidants in chocolate may well support cardiovascular health. However, when chocolate is consumed with milk, the milk interferes with the absorption of the antioxidants, thereby negating any potential benefits.[2] The researchers concluded that people should consume dark chocolate that has no milk.

Not surprisingly, these two studies, both in prestigious publications, received a good deal of attention. What more could a chocolate lover want? There was now some evidence that eating chocolate, or at least dark chocolate, was healthful. A 2008 article in *Choice*, which is published by the largest consumer organization in Australia, notes that "it's extraordinary that chocolate could even be considered a remotely healthy food. Even dark chocolate, which is considered healthier than milk chocolate, has on average more than 40 percent fat, including about 26 percent saturated fat, and almost 30 percent sugar."[3]

So how can chocolate be healthful? The *Choice* article states that chocolate contains about 5 to 8 percent protein and minerals such as iron, copper, magnesium, and zinc. "But its main saving grace is that it contains high levels of flavonoids—chemicals that help to protect plants from disease and insects. Gram for gram, cocoa contains higher levels of flavonoids than other . . . sources such as red wine, tea, apples, and berries."[4]

CARDIOVASCULAR BENEFITS

Over the years, the supposed healthfulness of chocolate has been studied extensively. One interesting report appeared in 2005 in *The American Journal of Clinical Nutrition*. Italian researchers randomly divided 15 healthy young adults into two groups. For 15 days, each group ate either daily 100-gram dark chocolate bars that contained about 500 mg of polyphenols or daily 90-gram white chocolate bars. Then, for seven days, none of the subjects ate any chocolate. After that, each group ate the other type of chocolate for an additional 15 days. The findings were significant. The researchers noted that, "Dark, but not white, chocolate decreases blood pressure and improves insulin sensitivity in healthly persons."[5] (Insulin sensitivity is the body's ability to use glucose, a type of sugar.)

In a 2007 article in *The Practitioner*, cardiologist Peter Savill described ten randomized controlled trials. Five attempted to determine the association between cocoa and blood pressure, and five tried to find a relationship between tea and blood pressure. Generally, the participants in the cocoa trials ate 100 grams of flavanol-rich chocolate per day for at least two weeks. People in the tea trials drank four to six cups of tea per day for a median duration of four weeks. Dr. Savill commented that, "the magnitude of blood pressure reduction in the cocoa group is impressive and comparable with that seen in trials of antihypertensive drug monotherapy." At the same time, people who participated in the tea trials saw "no significant effect on blood pressure."[6]

A study published in *The Journal of Nutrition* in 2008 evaluated the association between consumption of dark chocolate and serum C-reactive protein (a measure of inflammation—higher amounts may be seen in individuals at higher risk for cardiovascular disease). Researchers found that people who ate moderate amounts of dark chocolate had lower levels of C-reactive protein in their blood. The average reduction was 17 percent. "Our findings suggest that regular consumption of small doses of dark chocolate may reduce inflammation."[7]

In a 2008 study of 45 overweight adults with a mean age of 53 that appeared in *The American Journal of Clinical Nutrition,* researchers randomly assigned the subjects to consume either a solid dark chocolate bar containing 22 grams of cocoa powder or a cocoa-free placebo bar. In a second phase of the study, subjects were randomly assigned to consume either sugar-free cocoa containing 22 grams of cocoa powder, sugar cocoa containing 22 grams of cocoa powder, or a placebo. When compared to the placebo, both the solid dark chocolate and the liquid cocoa improved endothelial (lining of blood vessels) function and lowered blood pressure. "Endothelial function improved significantly more with sugar-free than regular cocoa."[8]

POTENTIAL ANTI-CANCER BENEFITS

A research study published in 2008 in *Cell Cycle* indicates that chocolate may be a tool against cancer cells. Researchers at Georgetown University School of Medicine found that a synthetic cocoa derivative (GECGC) actually slowed the rate of growth and increased the rate of destruction of in vitro human cancer cells. Moreover, it accomplished this without having an effect on normal cells. The researchers concluded that "synthesized GECGC has a selective anti-proliferative effect on human cancer cells and warrants further evaluation as a preventive and chemotherapeutic reagent to human malignancies."[9]

SOME HAVE THEIR DOUBTS

Not everyone believes that chocolate is a healthful food. First, it is important to realize that processing changes the natural flavanol antioxidants found in cocoa. A 2008 report published in the *Journal of Agricultural and Food Chemistry* contends that when cocoa is processed with alkali, a common practice known as Dutch processing or Dutching, "the flavanols are substantially reduced." Still, the cocoa does preserve some flavanol antioxidants.[10]

There is also the problem of the high calorie ingredients in chocolate bars. The United States is already dealing with record levels of overweight and obese adults and children. A 2007 editorial in *Critical Care Nurse* notes that, "Although some of the proposed benefits of chocolate consumption (eg, lowering blood pressure) are positive and linear, neither is limitless because processed cocoa products such as candy bars, cookies, and cakes are typically laden with substantial calorie load, which can readily offset their antioxidant benefits."[11]

The previously noted 2008 article in *Choice* raises more concerns. The favorable results of the studies may have been "overemphasized," and what is statistically significant does not, necessarily, have clinical importance. Additionally, "much of the research is conducted or sponsored by the chocolate or cocoa industry, which leaves it open to potential bias."[12]

Two additional studies have found potential problems for regular consumers of chocolate. A study published in 2008 in the *American Journal of Clinical Nutrition* examined the association of chocolate consumption and bone density in women between the ages of 70 and 85. Researchers found that the more chocolate the women ate, the lower their bone density. Researchers hypothesized that the oxalate (naturally occurring organic acids found in humans, plants, and animals) contained in the chocolate prevents the absorption of calcium and the high sugar fosters the excretion of calcium.[13]

In another study, also published in 2008 in the *American Journal of Clinical Nutrition*, researchers attempted to determine a relationship between the short-term consumption of chocolate and cocoa and neuropsychological functioning and cardiovascular health. While no association was found between chocolate and cocoa and neuropsychological or cardiovascular variables, during the midpoint and end of the study, the people who consumed the chocolate and cocoa were found to have significantly higher pulse rates.[14] Clearly, that is a negative finding.

In all probability, the chocolate studies will continue. Wouldn't it be nice if researchers could find definitive proof that many illnesses could be prevented or cured by simply eating dark chocolate? Until that day, chocolate should comprise only a tiny fraction of the diet. And, when it is time for a small piece, stick to dark chocolate.

Or, as a 2008 article in *Nutrition Bulletin* states, "Overall, chocolate should still remain as a treat, rather than a health food."[15]

NOTES

1. Taubert, Dirk, Reinhard Berkels, Renate Roesen, et al. August 27, 2003. "Chocolate and Blood Pressure in Elderly Individuals with Isolated Systolic Hypertension." *JAMA, The Journal of the American Medical Association* 290(8): 1029–1030.

2. Serafini, Mauro, Rossana Bugianesi, Giuseppe Maiani, et al. August 28, 2003. "Plasma Antioxidants from Chocolate." *Nature* 424(6952): 1013.

3. "Food of the Gods Enriches Us All: Research Shows That a Little Chocolate Is Good for Your Heart Health, While Fair Trade and Organic Chocolate Is Good for Your Heart Strings as Well as Your Taste Buds, According to Our Expert and Lay Tasters." November 2008. *Choice*: 12–16.

4. "Food of the Gods Enriches Us All." November 2008. *Choice*: 12–16.

5. Grassi, Davide, Cristina Lippi, Stefano Necozione, et al. March 2005. "Short-Term Administration of Dark Chocolate Is Followed by a Significant Increase in Insulin Sensitivity and a Decrease in Blood Pressure in Healthy Persons." *The American Journal of Clinical Nutrition* 81(3): 611–614.

6. Savill, Peter. June 29, 2007. "Cardiovascular Disease: Chocolate Shown to Reduce Pressure." *The Practitioner*: 11

7. di Giuseppe, Romina, Augusto Di Castelnuovo, Floriana Centritto, et al. October 2008. "Regular Consumption of Dark Chocolate Is Associated with Low Serum Concentrations of C-Reactive Protein in a Healthy Italian Population." *The Journal of Nutrition* 138(10): 1939–1945.

8. Faridi, Zubaida, Valentine Yanchou Njike, Suparna Dutta, et al. July 2008. "Acute Dark Chocolate and Cocoa Ingestion and Endothelial Function: A Randomized Controlled Crossover Trial." *The American Journal of Clinical Nutrition* 88(1): 58–63.

9. Kim, Min, Xiaofang Wu, Insun Song, et al. June 1, 2008. "Selective Cytotoxicity of Synthesized Procyanidin 3-o-Galloylepicatechin-4b,8-3-o-Galloylcatechin to Human Cancer Cells." *Cell Cycle* 7(11): 1648–1657.

10. Miller, Kenneth B., William Jeffrey Hurst, Mark J. Payne, et al. September 24, 2008. "Impact of Alkalization on the Antioxidant and Flavanol Content of Commercial Cocoa Powders." *Journal of Agricultural and Food Chemistry* 56(18): 8527–8533.

11. Alspach, Grif. February 2007. "The Truth Is Often Bittersweet . . .: Chocolate Does a Heart Good." *Critical Care Nurse* 27(1): 11–15.

12. "Food of the Gods Enriches Us. . . .": 12–16.

13. Hodgson, Jonathan M., Amada Devine, Valerie Burke, et al. January 2008. "Chocolate Consumption and Bone Density in Older Women." *American Journal of Clinical Nutrition* 87(1): 175–180.

14. Crews Jr., W. David, David W. Harrison, and James W. Wright. April 2008. "A Double-Blind, Placebo-Controlled, Randomized Trial of the Effects of Dark Chocolate and Cocoa on Variables Associated with Neuropsychological Functioning and Cardiovascular Health: Clinical Findings from a Sample of Healthy, Cognitively Intact Older Adults." *American Journal of Clinical Nutrition* 87(4): 872–880.

15. Aisbitt, Bridget. June 2008. "Chocolate: The Dark Side?" *Nutrition Bulletin* 33(2): 114–116.

REFERENCES AND RESOURCES
Magazines, Journals, and Newspapers

Aisbitt, Bridget. June 2008. "Chocolate: The Dark Side?" *Nutrition Bulletin* 33(2): 114–116.

Alspach, Grif. February 2007. "The Truth Is Often Bittersweet . . .: Chocolate Does a Heart Good." *Critical Care Nurse* 27(1): 11–15.

Bland, Philip. December 17, 2007. "Mental Health: Chocolate May Alleviate Depression." *The Practitioner*: 15.

Crews Jr., W. David, David W. Harrison, and James W. Wright. April 2008. "A Double-Blind, Placebo-Controlled, Randomized Trial of the Effects of Dark Chocolate and Cocoa on Variables Associated with Neuropsychological

Functioning and Cardiovascular Health: Clinical Findings from a Sample of Healthy, Cognitively Intact Older Adults." *American Journal of Clinical Nutrition* 87(4): 872–880.

di Giuseppe, Romina, Augusto Di Castelnuovo, Floriana Centritto, et al. October 2008. "Regular Consumption of Dark Chocolate is Associated with Low Serum Concentrations of C-Reactive Protein in a Healthy Italian Population." *The Journal of Nutrition* 138(10): 1939 –1945.

Faridi, Zubaida, Valentine Yanchou Njike, Suparna Dutta, et al. July 2008. "Acute Dark Chocolate and Cocoa Ingestion and Endothelial Function: A Randomized Controlled Crossover Trial." *The American Journal of Clinical Nutrition* 88(1): 58–63.

"Food of the Gods Enriches Us All: Research Shows That a Little Chocolate Is Good for Your Heart Health, While Fair Trade and Organic Chocolate Is Good for your Heart Strings as Well as Your Taste Buds, According to Our Expert and Lay Tasters." November 2008. *Choice*: 12–16.

Fraga, Cesar G. March 2005. "Chocolate, Diabetes, and Hypertension." *The American Journal of Clinical Nutrition* 81(3): 541–542.

Grassi, Davide, Cristina Lippi, Stefano Necozione, et al. March 2005. "Short-Term Administration of Dark Chocolate is Followed by a Significant Increase in Insulin Sensitivity and a Decrease in Blood Pressure in Health Persons." *The American Journal of Clinical Nutrition* 81(3): 611–614.

Hodgson, Jonathan M., Amanda Devine, Valerie Burke, et al. January 2008. "Chocolate Consumption and Bone Density in Older Women." *American Journal of Clinical Nutrition* 87(1): 175–180.

Kim, Min, Xiaofang Wu, Insun Song, et al. June 1, 2008. "Selective Cytotoxicity of Synthesized Procyanidin 3-o-Galloylepicatecthin-4b,8-3-o-Galloylcatechin to Human Cancer Cells." *Cell Cycle* 7(11): 1648–1657.

Miller, Kenneth B., William Jeffrey Hurst, Mark J. Payne, et al. September 24, 2008. "Impact of Alkalization on the Antioxidant and Flavanol Content of Commercial Cocoa Powders." *Journal of Agriculture and Food Chemistry* 56(18): 8527–8533.

Parker, Gordon and Joanna Crawford. October 2007. "Chocolate Craving When Depressed: A Personality Marker." *The British Journal of Psychiatry* 191: 351–352.

Savill, Peter. June 29, 2007. "Cardiovascular Disease: Chocolate Shown to Reduce Blood Pressure." *The Practitioner*: 11.

Serafini, Mauro, Rossana Bugianesi, Giuseppe Maiani, et al. August 28, 3003. "Plasma Antioxidants from Chocolate." *Nature* 424(6952): 1013.

Taubert, Dirk, Reinhard Berkels, Renate Roesen, et al. August 27, 2003. "Chocolate and Blood Pressure in Elderly Individuals with Isolated Systolic Hypertension." *JAMA, The Journal of the American Medical Association* 290(8): 1029–1030.

Website

All Chocolate. http://www.allchocolate.com.

CRANBERRIES

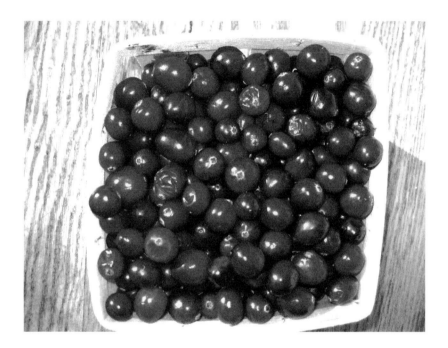

It is known that American Indians used cranberries to make poultices for wounds. In addition, they enjoyed cooked cranberries that were sweetened with maple syrup or honey. When the colonists arrived, they also developed a taste for sweetened versions of these tart-flavored red berries.

By the beginning of the 18th century, the colonists were exporting cranberries to England. But, the history of cranberry cultivation changed forever in 1840 when a Massachusetts man observed that cranberries grew in abundance when the winds and tides filled his bog with sand.[1] Bogs became the ideal medium for cranberry growth. It did not take long for cranberry cultivation to spread across the United States, especially in the states of Wisconsin, Massachusetts, New Jersey, Oregon, and Washington.[2]

Cranberries contain excellent amounts of vitamin C, and a very good amount of dietary fiber. They have good levels of manganese and vitamin K.[3]

Though probably best known for preventing and treating urinary tract infections, cranberries are thought to be useful for a number of other medical problems including cardiovascular disease and ulcers. There has been a good deal of research on cranberries. It is time to review some of what the researchers have learned.

URINARY TRACT INFECTIONS

In a study published in 2007 in *Phytomedicine*, researchers attempted to determine if treatment with cranberry extract could help 12 women, between the ages of 25 and 70, who had a history of a minimum of six urinary tract infections in the preceding year. For 12 weeks, the women took one 200-mg capsule of a concentrated cranberry extract standardized to 30 percent phenolics twice each day. During the study, none of the women had a urinary tract infection. Two years later, eight of the 12 women who continued to take cranberry remained free of urinary infections. The researchers noted that, "A cranberry preparation with a high phenolic content may completely prevent UTIs [urinary tract infections] in women who are subject to recurrent infections."[4]

In a study published in 2009 in the *Journal of Antimicrobial Chemotherapy*, Scottish researchers compared the effectiveness of cranberry extract to a low dose of the antibiotic trimethoprim for preventing recurrent urinary infections in older women. The subjects consisted of 137 women who had two or more antibiotic-treated urinary tract infections during the previous year. For six months, the women took either 500 mg of cranberry extract or 100 mg of trimethoprim. While more of the women taking cranberry extract developed a urinary tract infection, the amount of time before an infection occurred was about the same in the two groups—84.5 days for the women taking cranberry extract and 91 days for those on the antibiotic. But, while the cranberry extract had no side effects, people taking antibiotics for extended periods of time may experience side effects such as nausea, stomach upset, vomiting, sensitivity to sun, and/or a resistance to the medication.[5]

How do cranberries prevent these infections? Previously, it was thought that the levels of acidity in cranberries stopped the growth of bacteria. However, in a laboratory study published in 2009 in the *Journal of Medicinal Food*, researchers from Worcester Polytechnic Institute in Worcester, Massachusetts, determined that it was not the acidity of the cranberries but, rather, chemicals in cranberries. About 85 percent of all urinary tract infections are caused by the adhesion of *E. coli* bacteria to the cells lining the urinary tract. The researchers determined that the proanthocyanidins contained in cranberries change the surface properties of the bacteria so that they are unable to cling to the urinary tract epithelial cells. Moreover, the effect may be reversed—"because bacteria that were regrown in cranberry-free medium regained their ability to attach to uroepithelial cells and their adhesion forces reverted to the values observed in the control condition." Thus, when people stop their consumption of cranberries in food or supplementation, the urinary tract infections will likely return.[6]

CARDIOVASCULAR HEALTH

In a study published in 2006 in the *British Journal of Nutrition*, researchers from Quebec investigated the effect of increasing daily doses of low-calorie cranberry juice cocktail on the plasma lipid levels of 30 abdominally obese men, with a mean age of 51. During three periods of four weeks, the men drank 125 ml/day, 250 ml/day, or 500 ml/day. While no changes were noted in total and LDL (bad) cholesterol levels, the men's levels of HDL (good) cholesterol did rise. The researchers concluded that foods like cranberries that are filled with antioxidants such as flavonoids, may well be protective of cardiac health.[7]

In a Finnish study published in 2008 in *The American Journal of Clinical Nutrition*, researchers asked 72 middle-aged "unmedicated" subjects with cardiovascular risk factors to consume moderate amounts of berry products (such as cranberries), or a control product, for eight weeks. At the end of the study, the subjects with high baseline blood pressure showed a significant decrease in their systolic blood pressure. Furthermore, though the levels of total cholesterol remained the same, the concentrations of serum HDL cholesterol increased significantly more in the berry-eating group than in the control group. The researchers noted that the regular intake of berries "may play a role in the prevention of cardiovascular disease."[8]

ULCER TREATMENT AND PREVENTION OF STOMACH CANCER

In a study published in 2007 in *Molecular Nutrition & Food Research*, Israeli researchers treated 177 patients with the *H. pylori* bacteria, which causes ulcers and may be associated with stomach cancer, with the standard one-week triple therapy—omeprazole, amoxicillin, and clarithromycin (OAC). While taking this therapy, eighty-nine patients received cranberry juice twice daily and 88 received a placebo. At the end of the week, the patients stopped taking the OAC therapy but continued with the cranberry juice or placebo for another two weeks. Seven hundred twelve patients treated for *H. pylori* only with OAC served as an additional control group.

Initially, there did not appear to be a significant difference between the cranberry and placebo groups. Yet, when the data were analyzed according to gender, an important difference emerged. For females, the eradication rate was significantly higher in those drinking cranberry juice. No such differences were seen in males. The researchers concluded that, "the addition of cranberry to triple therapy improves the rate of *H. pylori* eradication in females."[9]

GUM HEALTH

In a study published in 2007 in the *Journal of Periodontal Research*, researchers from Quebec learned that cranberry extract inhibited the action of enzymes that have been associated with periodontal (gum) disease. The researchers noted that their results, "suggest that cranberry compounds offer promising perspectives for the development of novel host-modulating strategies for an adjunctive treatment of periodontitis."[10] (Periodontitis is a serious gum infection that kills soft tissue and bones that support teeth.)

HEALTHFUL FOR PEOPLE WITH TYPE 2 DIABETES

In a randomized, placebo-controlled, double-blind 12-week study published in 2008 in *Diabetic Medicine*, researchers enrolled 16 men and 14 women, with a mean age of about 65, who were taking oral glucose-lowering medication. The researchers, who wanted to examine the effect that cranberry supplements would have on their lipid profiles, determined that the people taking the cranberry supplements had reductions in total and LDL cholesterol levels. They also had improvements in their HDL (good) cholesterol ratios. At the same time, there was a "neutral effect on glycaemic control."

Should people eat cranberries, drink cranberry juice, and/or take supplements? For most people, they are a helpful addition to the diet. Be aware, cranberry products often contain fairly high amounts of sugar. It is best to select products with lower amounts or no added sugar.

NOTES

1. The George Mateljan Foundation Website. www.whfoods.com.

2. Sego, Sherril. February 2007. "Cranberry." *Clinical Advisor* 10(2): 163–164.

3. The George Mateljan Foundation Website.

4. Bailey, David T., Carol Dalton, F. Joseph Daugherty, and Michael S. Tempesta. April 10, 2007. "Can a Concentrated Cranberry Extract Prevent Recurrent Urinary Tract Infections in Women? A Pilot Study." *Phytomedicine* 14(4): 237–241.

5. McMurdo, Marion E. T., Ishbel Argo, Gabby Phillips, et al. 2009. "Cranberry or Trimethoprim for the Prevention of Recurrent Urinary Tract Infections? A Randomized Controlled Trial in Older Women." *Journal of Antimicrobial Chemotherapy* 63(2): 389–395.

6. Pinzón-Arango, Paola A., Yatao Liu, and Terri A. Camesano. 2009. "Role of Cranberry on Bacterial Adhesion Forces and Implications for *Escherichia coli*-Uroepithelial Cell Attachment." *Journal of Medicinal Food* 12(2): 259–270.

7. Ruel, Guillaume, Sonia Pomerleau, Patrick Couture, et al. 2006. "Favourable Impact of Low-Calorie Cranberry Juice Consumption on Plasma HDL-Cholesterol Concentrations in Men." *British Journal of Nutrition* 96: 357–364.

8. Erlund, Iris, Raika Koli, George Alfthan, et al. February 2008. "Favorable Effects of Berry Consumption on Platelet Function, Blood Pressure, and HDL Cholesterol." *The American Journal of Clinical Nutrition* 87(2): 323–331.

9. Shmuely, Haim, Jacob Yahav, Zmira Samra, et al. 2007. "Effect of Cranberry Juice on Eradication of *Helicobacter pylori* in Patients Treated with Antibiotics and a Proton Pump Inhibitor." *Molecular Nutrition & Food Research* 51(6): 746–751.

10. Bodet, C., F. Chandad, and D. Grenier. April 2007. "Inhibition of Host Extracellular Matrix Destructive Enzymes Production and Activity by a High-Molecular-Weight Cranberry Fraction." *Journal of Periodontal Research* 42(2): 159–168.

REFERENCES AND RESOURCES
Magazines, Journals, and Newspapers

Bailey, David T., Carol Dalton, F. Joseph Daugherty, and Michael S. Tempesta. April 10, 2007. "Can a Concentrated Cranberry Extract Prevent Recurrent Urinary Tract Infections in Women? A Pilot Study." *Phytomedicine* 14(4): 237–241.

Bodet, C., F. Chandad, and D. Grenier. April 2007. "Inhibition of Host Extracellular Matrix Destructive Enzyme Production and Activity by a High-Molecular-Weight Cranberry Fraction." *Journal of Periodontal Research* 42(2): 159–168.

Erlund, Iris, Raika Koli, Georg Alfthan, et al. February 2008. "Favorable Effects of Berry Consumption on Platelet Function, Blood Pressure, and HDL Cholesterol." *The American Journal of Clinical Nutrition* 87(2): 323–331.

Lee, I. T., Y. C. Chan, C. W. Lin, et al. December 2008. "Effect of Cranberry Extracts on Lipid Profiles in Subjects with Type 2 Diabetes." *Diabetic Medicine* 25(12): 1473–1477.

McMurdo, Marion E. T., Ishbel Argo, Gabby Phillips, et al. 2009. "Cranberry or Trimethoprim for the Prevention of Recurrent Urinary Tract Infections? A Randomized Controlled Trial in Older Women." *Journal of Antimicrobial Chemotherapy* 63(2): 389–395.

Pinzón-Arango, Paola A., Yatao Liu, and Terri A. Camesano. 2009. "Role of Cranberry on Bacterial Adhesion Forces and Implications for *Escherichia coli*-Uroepithelial Cell Attachment." *Journal of Medicinal Food* 12(2): 259–270.

Ruel, Guillaume, Sonia Pomerleau, Patrick Couture, et al. 2006. "Favourable Impact of Low-Calorie Cranberry Juice Consumption on Plasma HDL-Cholesterol Concentrations in Men." *British Journal of Nutrition* 96: 357–364.

Sego, Sherril. February 2007. "Cranberry." *Clinical Advisor* 10(2): 163–164.

Shmuely, Haim, Jacob Yahav, Zmira Samra, et al. 2007. "Effect of Cranberry Juice on Eradication of *Helicobacter pylori* in Patients Treated with Antibiotics and a Proton Pump Inhibitor." *Molecular Nutrition & Food Research* 51(6): 746–751.

Websites

Cranberry Institute. www.cranberryinstitute.org.

The George Mateljan Foundation. www.whfoods.com.

DRIED PLUMS

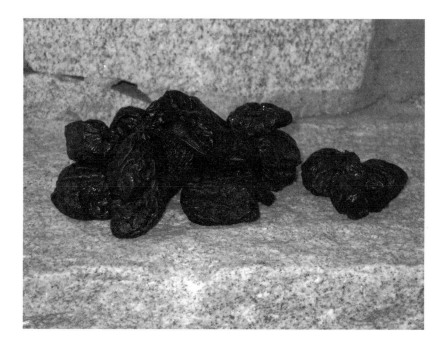

Plums are believed to have originated in areas near the Caspian Sea, which is an enclosed body of water between Russia, Azerbaijan, Iran, Turkmenistan, and Kazakhstan. The process of making dried plums, as prunes are now called, began in the same area thousands of years ago. Over time, dried plums (*Prunus domestica* L.) spread throughout Europe.

It was Louis Pellier who introduced plum trees to California in the mid-19th century. He planted plum tree cuttings from his native France, especially the Agen variety trees, which produce plums well-suited for drying. Today, California is the world's largest producer of dried plums.[1]

In the past, dried plums were often viewed more as a laxative—primarily for elderly people with sluggish digestive systems. Now, they are recognized as a food that has good amounts of vitamin A, dietary fiber, potassium, and copper, and some magnesium and boron. Dried plums have polyphenolic compounds that have antioxidant and anti-inflammatory properties, as well as beta-carotene, which lowers levels of free radicals.[2] Because they have a reduced water content, dried plums are a more concentrated source of nutrients than fresh plums. But, what have researchers learned?

OSTEOPOROSIS

As strange as it may sound, there is some good evidence that dried plums may be valuable for the millions of people throughout the world who are dealing with osteoporosis. In a study published in 2005 in *Menopause*, Oklahoma researchers sham-operated (conducted a placebo operation) or ovariectomized 90 Sprague-Dawley rats. Then, the rats were fed a standard diet with or without dried plum supplementation (5 percent, 15 percent, or 25 percent). After 60 days, the researchers analyzed blood and bone specimens. Their findings were dramatic. "Dried plum, as low as five percent, was effective in restoring femoral and tibial bone density. Dried plum increased lumbar bone density as well, with HD [high dose] achieving a statistical significance." Moreover, the researchers found improvements in bone quality and trabecular bone (tissue inside bone that resembles a sponge) not seen in the controls. This is of particular significance. Losses in trabecular connectivity were previously believed "to be an irreversible process."[3]

Oklahoma researchers also conducted a study published in 2006 in *Bone*. In this trial, researchers investigated feeding castrated rats (a procedure that triggers osteoporosis) either low, medium, or high amounts of dried plum extract. The researchers found that the rats fed medium and high amounts of dried plum extract experienced none of the castration-induced "decrease in whole body, femur, and lumbar vertebra bone mineral density (BMD)." Even the rats fed the low amount of dried plum had improvement in chemical markers of bone loss and bone strength.[4]

In an in vitro study published in 2009 in *The Journal of Nutritional Biochemistry*, researchers investigated the effects of different concentrations of dried plum polyphenols (ranging from zero to 20 micrograms per milliliter) on mouse cells. Twenty-four hours after mixing the cells with dried plum, the researchers introduced tumor necrosis factor-alpha (TNF-alpha), which inhibits the activity of the cells involved in bone formation. The researchers found that polyphenol doses of 5, 10, and 20 micrograms per milliliter aided the production of compounds associated with bone formation, even in the presence of TNF-alpha. They noted that, "It is possible that dietary consumption of dried plums could serve as a source of polyphenolic compounds that favorably modulate both bone formation and resorption, and provide a natural alternative for individuals at risk for osteoporosis."[5]

In an article published in 2009 in *Ageing Research Reviews*, Bahram H. Arjmandi, PhD, who has conducted extensive research on dried plums, and one of his graduate students, wrote "dried plum to our knowledge is the most effective natural compound in both preventing and reversing bone loss in male . . . and female animal models of osteoporosis . . . Based on our collective observations, the efficacy of dried plum surpasses that of other natural occurring compounds as well as functional foods."[6]

WEIGHT MANAGEMENT

In a study presented at the 2009 Experimental Biology meeting in New Orleans, San Diego State University researchers noted that on separate days, after fasting, nineteen adult women consumed either of two 238-calorie snacks (dried plums or low-fat cookies), 238-calorie white bread, or water. At the end of the two-hour test period, the subjects were "presented with a meal to be consumed until satisfied." The subjects completed questionnaires on hunger, and their blood was periodically analyzed. The researchers found that the women who ate dried plums were more satisfied than the women who ate the low-fat cookies. In addition, the dried plum eaters had lower levels of blood glucose and insulin than the low-fat cookies eaters. According to the researchers, "These results suggest that consuming dried plums as a snack suppresses appetite relative to commercially available low-fat cookies, perhaps by producing lower glucose and/or appetite-regulating hormone concentrations."[7] (There are no comments on the consumption of white bread or water.)

ATHEROSCLEROSIS

In a five-month animal study published in 2009 in the *British Journal of Nutrition*, University of Minnesota researchers fed a strain of mice that quickly develops atherosclerosis ("hardening of the arteries") different amounts of dried plum powder. A control group of mice consumed no dried plum powder. The researchers found that the mice that ate the human equivalent of 10 to 12 dried plums per day had a significant reduction in their atherosclerotic lesions. They concluded that, "consuming dried plums may help slow the development of atherosclerosis."[8]

CARDIOVASCULAR HEALTH

In a study published in 2003 in the *Archives of Internal Medicine*, researchers followed the fiber intake of almost 10,000 adults for an average of 19 years. At the beginning of the study, none of the adults had cardiovascular disease. During the follow-up years, there were 1,843 incident cases of coronary heart disease and 3,762 incident cases of cardiovascular disease. The subjects who ate the most fiber (21 grams per day), such as the fiber contained in dried plums, had 12 percent less coronary heart disease and 11 percent less cardiovascular disease than those who ate the least amount of fiber (five grams per day). The subjects who consumed the most water-soluble dietary fiber, such as found in dried plums, had even better results. They experienced a 15 percent reduction in risk of coronary heart disease and a 10 percent reduction in risk of cardiovascular disease. The researchers wrote that, "higher intake of dietary fiber, particularly water-soluble fiber, reduces the risk of CHD [coronary heart disease]."[9]

BREAST CANCER

In a study published in 2008 in the *International Journal of Cancer*, Scandinavian and Japanese researchers examined the role fiber-rich foods, such as dried plums, play in the risk of breast cancer. The cohort consisted of close to 52,000 postmenopausal women; they were followed for an average of 8.3 years. When compared to the women who ate the least amounts of fiber-rich foods, the women who ate the most fiber-rich foods had a 34 percent lower risk of breast cancer. The researchers noted that their findings "suggest that dietary fiber intake from fruit and cereal may play a role in reducing breast cancer risk."[10]

ANOTHER FEATURE OF DRIED PLUMS

Dried plums have been proven to suppress the growth of major food-borne pathogens in ground meat. In fact, combining as little as three percent extract effectively kills 90 percent of food-borne pathogens. Unlike spices, which tend to change the taste of meat, dried plums do not alter taste.

ONE CAVEAT

Because of their polyphenol content, juices that are dark in color reduce the absorption of iron. So, people who have a tendency to be anemic should be careful when they drink dried plum juice. It is best not to drink the juice with meals. Instead, drink it between meals.

Should dried plums be part of the diet? Certainly. But, to prevent gastrointestinal upset, it is wise to increase the intake gradually.

NOTES

1. The George Mateljan Foundation Website. www.whfoods.com.

2. The George Mateljan Foundation Website.

3. Deyhim, Farzad, Barbara J. Stoecker, Gerald H. Brusewitz, et al. November/December 2005. "Dried Plum Reverses Bone Loss in an Osteopenic Rat Model of Osteoporosis." *Menopause* 12(6): 755–762.

4. Franklin, M., S. Y. Bu, M. R. Lerner, et al. December 2006. "Dried Plum Prevents Bone Loss in a Male Osteoporosis Model via IGF-I and the RANK Pathway." *Bone* 39(6): 1331–1342.

5. Bu, So Young, Tamara S. Hunt, and Brenda J. Smith. January 2009. "Dried Plum Polyphenols Attenuate the Detrimental Effects of TNF-α on Osteoblast Function Coincident with Up-Regulation on Runx2, Osterix and IGF-I." *The Journal of Nutritional Biochemistry* 20(1): 35–44.

6. Hooshmand, Shirin and Bahram H. Arjmandi. April 2009. "Viewpoint: Dried Plum, An Emerging Functional Food That May Effectively Improve Bone Health." *Ageing Research Reviews* 8(2): 122–127.

7. Furchner-Evanson, Allison, Yumi Petrisko, Leslie S. Howarth, et al. 2009. "Snack Selection Influences Satiety Responses in Adult Women." *The FASEB Journal* 23: 545.11.

8. Gallaher, Cynthia M. and Daniel D. Gallaher. 2009. "Dried Plums (Prunes) Reduce Atherosclerosis Lesion Area in Apolipoprotein E-Deficient Mice." *British Journal of Nutrition* 101: 233–239.

9. Bazzano, Lydia A., Jiang He, Lorraine G. Ogden, et al. September 8, 2003. "Dietary Fiber Intake and Reduced Risk of Coronary Heart Disease in U.S. Men and Women." *Archives of Internal Medicine* 163(16): 1897–1904.

10. Suzuki, Reiko, Tove Rylander-Rudqvist, Weimin Ye, et al. January 15, 2008. "Dietary Fiber Intake and Risk of Postmenopausal Breast Cancer Defined by Estrogen and Progesterone Receptor Status—A Prospective Cohort Study Among Swedish Women." *International Journal of Cancer* 122(2): 403–412.

REFERENCES AND RESOURCES
Magazines, Journals, and Newspapers

Bazzano, Lydia A., Jiang He, Lorraine G. Ogden, et al. September 8, 2003. "Dietary Fiber Intake and Reduced Risk of Coronary Heart Disease in U.S. Men and Women." *Archives of Internal Medicine* 163(16): 1897–1904.

Bu, So Young, Tamara S. Hunt, and Brenda J. Smith. January 2009. "Dried Plum Polyphenols Attenuate the Detrimental Effects of TNF-Alpha on Osteoblast Function Coincident with Up-Regulation of Runx2, Osterix and IGF-I." *The Journal of Nutritional Biochemistry* 20(1): 35–44.

Deyhim, Farzad, Barbara J. Stoecker, Gerald H. Brusewitz, et al. November/December 2005. "Dried Plum Reverses Bone Loss in an Osteopenic Rat Model of Osteoporosis." *Menopause* 12(6): 755–762.

Franklin, M., S. Y. Bu, M. R. Lemer, et al. December 2006. "Dried Plum Prevents Bone Loss in a Male Osteoporosis Model via IGF-I and the RANK Pathway." *Bone* 39(6): 1331–1342.

Furchner-Evanson, Allison, Yumi Petrisko, Leslie S. Howarth, et al. 2009. "Snack Selection Influences Satiety Responses in Adult Women." *The FASEB Journal* 23: 545.11.

Gallaher, Cynthia M. and Daniel D. Gallaher. 2009. "Dried Plums (Prunes) Reduce Atherosclerosis Lesion Area in Apolipoprotein E-Deficient Mice." *British Journal of Nutrition* 101: 233–239.

Hooshmand, Shirin and Bahram H. Arjmandi. April 2009. "Viewpoint: Dried Plum, An Emerging Functional Food That May Effectively Improve Bone Health." *Ageing Research Reviews* 8(2): 122–127.

Suzuki, Reiko, Tove Rylander-Rudqvist, Weimin Ye, et al. January 15, 2008. "Dietary Fiber Intake and Risk of Postmenopausal Breast Cancer Defined by Estrogen and Progesterone Receptor Status—A Prospective Cohort Study Among Swedish Women." *International Journal of Cancer* 122(2): 403–412.

Website

The George Mateljan Foundation. www.whfoods.com.

EGGS

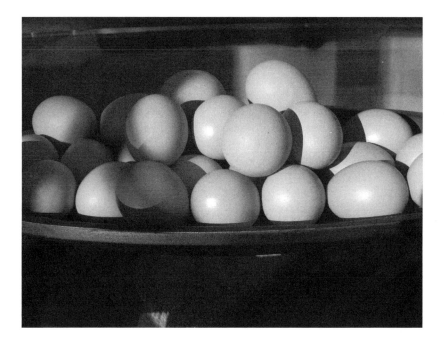

For years, eggs were truly vilified. The high cholesterol content of their yokes—about 213 milligrams (mg) per egg—was believed to raise human cholesterol levels. Concern about the large numbers of Americans with elevated levels of blood cholesterol, health professionals generally advised people to abstain from eating eggs and other high cholesterol foods. More recently, there has been research suggesting that eggs do not seem to be a problem for healthy adults who do not have a history of heart disease or high blood cholesterol. Moreover, a number of research studies have demonstrated some additional benefits derived from the consumption of eggs.

WEIGHT CONTROL

There is some evidence that eggs may be useful for weight management as well as the health problems associated with excess weight and obesity. A 2008 article in the *International Journal of Obesity* compared overweight people who ate two eggs for breakfast with overweight people who ate a bagel for breakfast. The calorie counts for both breakfasts were the same. After eight weeks, the people who ate the eggs breakfast lost 65 percent more weight and had a 61 percent greater reduction in body mass than the people who ate the bagel breakfast. They also reported having more energy. The researchers concluded that, "the inclusion of eggs in a weight management program may offer a nutritious supplement to enhance weight loss."[1]

In a study that appeared in 2008 in the online *British Journal of Nutrition*, researchers at Purdue University found that overweight or obese men who eat high-quality protein foods, such as eggs and Canadian bacon, with breakfast are more satisfied than when they eat protein with lunch or dinner. Since the men were not hungry, they were more likely to adhere to their dietary restrictions. "The initial and sustained feelings of fullness following protein consumption at breakfast suggest that the timing of protein intake differentially influences satiety."[2]

Commenting on this study, a 2008 article in *Natural Health* noted that people feel fuller after eating protein because it takes longer to digest than fat or carbohydrates. "Have you ever noticed that a dish made with eggs . . . keeps you satisfied all morning long? That's because eggs are loaded with protein plus an array of other nutrients. In a 75-calorie, 11-cent package, the egg is a versatile essential that is rapidly shedding its bad cholesterol rap."[3]

In a study published in 2008 in *The Journal of Nutrition* researchers placed overweight men, between the ages of 40 and 70, on carbohydrate-restricted diets that included the consumption of three eggs per day. More than half the men (a total of 18) had been diagnosed with metabolic syndrome, a disorder defined by high cholesterol, high blood pressure, and belly fat. The men remained on this diet for twelve weeks. By the end of the study, only three men were still considered to have metabolic syndrome. In addition, as a group, the men experienced significant decrease in body weight and improvement in triglycerides and HDL or "good cholesterol."[4] Considering that the dietary changes were relatively modest, these are truly dramatic results.

In an English study that was published in 2008 in the *European Journal of Nutrition*, two groups of people were placed on energy-restricted diets for twelve weeks. One group was told to eat two eggs every day; the other group excluded eggs from their diets. Both groups experienced moderate weight loss. Yet, participants in the egg-eating group did not have an increase in total or LDL cholesterol. "These findings suggest that cholesterol-rich foods should not be excluded from dietary advice to lose weight on account of an unfavorable influence on plasma LDL cholesterol."[5] While this may in fact be true, it is also possible that other foods or factors may be preventing increases in the cholesterol levels.

IMPROVED MEMORY

A Massachusetts Institute of Technology study investigated the cognitive results that occurred after adult gerbils were placed on different combinations of uridine, choline, and docosahexaenoic acid, compounds that normally circulate in the blood and are found in eggs. When tested separately, each of these compounds had previously been shown to improve cognitive function. The results of the study, which continued for four weeks, were published in 2008 in *The FASEB Journal*. Researchers found that the cognitive function of the gerbils was greatest among those that received all three compounds. Researchers concluded that these compounds improve brain synapse function—the passing of information between neurons.[6] As a result, there is at least the possibility that eggs may help prevent Alzheimer's disease and other forms of dementia.

A study in 2007 in *The American Journal of Clinical Nutrition* reported the results of a ten-year review of men and women age 65 or older. Those with low levels of vitamin B_{12}, which is found in eggs, were found to be at significantly higher risk for cognitive decline. In fact, the researchers noted that, "low vitamin B_{12} status was associated with more rapid cognitive decline."[7]

Commenting on this study and the importance of vitamin B_{12} in a 2008 issue of *Food and Fitness Advisor*, Elina Kaminsky, RPh, a nutritionist pharmacist, explained that vitamin B_{12} is instrumental in the production of acetylcholine, a neurotransmitter that helps memory and learning. Vitamin B_{12} is also needed for the proper development of nerve cells.[8]

Though neither the study nor Kaminsky suggest that eating eggs will prevent cognitive decline, the regular consumption of eggs most certainly helps to boost the amount of vitamin B_{12} in the body. And, in so doing, it may fight against cognitive decline. Often, however, as Kaminsky noted, as people age, in addition to the consumption of foods containing vitamin B_{12}, they require vitamin B_{12} supplementation.[9]

BREAST CANCER

Although very few people would probably associate the consumption of eggs with the prevalence of breast cancer, in a study conducted at Boston University and published in 2008 at *The FASEB Journal*, researchers fed varying amounts of choline, which is found in eggs, to pregnant rats. Some rats received a standard amount of choline, others received no choline, and still others received extra choline. All the rats were given a chemical that induces breast cancer. While rats in all three groups developed breast cancer, the daughters of the rats who had been given extra choline had tumors that grew more slowly than those of the daughters of the rats who had no choline. So, the consumption of choline during pregnancy seems to affect the breast cancer outcomes for the mother's children. If the results of this study proves to be true, then pregnant moms may be able to help prevent the incidence of breast cancer in their children even before they are born.[10]

Krzysztof Blusztajn, PhD, a professor of pathology at Boston University and the senior researcher of the study, noted in a December 2008 article in *Women's Health Weekly* that the "study provides additional support for the notion that choline is an important nutrient that has to be considered when dietary guidelines are developed. We hope it will be possible to develop nutritional guidelines for pregnant women that ensure the good health of their offspring well into old age."[11]

In addition to these results, the researcher observed that the slow growing tumors in the rats appeared to have a genetic pattern that is similar to breast cancer in women believed to have better outcomes; likewise, fast growing tumors in rats were genetically similar to those in women with more aggressive breast cancer. The researchers noted that there was some support for the belief that choline acts on the DNA of the mammary gland of the fetuses while they are still growing inside the womb.[12]

Though humble in appearance, eggs appear to pack a huge nutritional punch. And, for the average healthy person, who does not have symptoms of cardiovascular disease, they should probably be a frequent part of the diet. Those still concerned about the high cholesterol in the yolke may want to try omelets filled with egg whites and only a tiny drop of yolke.

NOTES

1. Wal, J. S. Vander, A. Gupta, P. Khosla, and N. V. Dhurandhar. 2008. "Egg Breakfast Enhances Weight Loss." *International Journal of Obesity* 32: 1545–1551.

2. *British Journal of Nutrition* Website. http://journalscambridge.org/action/search#.

3. Brugeman, Stacey. April 2008. "The Good Egg: Lose Weight, Get Energized, and Protect Your Heart—Three Simple Reasons to Eat More Eggs." *Natural Health* 38(4): 68–77.

4. Mutungi, Gisella, Joseph Ratliff, Michael Puglisi, et al. February 2008. "Dietary Cholesterol from Eggs Increases Plasma HDL Cholesterol in Overweight Men Consuming a Carbohydrate-Restricted Diet." *The Journal of Nutrition* 138: 272–276.

5. Harman, Nicola L., Anthony R. Leeds, and Bruce A. Griffin. September 2008. "Increased Dietary Cholesterol Does Not Increase Plasma Low Density Lipoprotein When Accompanied by an Energy-Restricted Diet and Weight Loss." *European Journal of Nutrition* 47(6): 287–293.

6. Holguin, Sarah, Joseph Martinez, Camille Chow, and Richard Wurtman. 2008. "Dietary Uridine Enhances the Improvement in Learning and Memory Processed by Administering DHA to Gerbils." *The FASEB Journal* 22: 3938–3946.

7. Clarke, Robert, Jacqueline Birks, Ebba Nexo, et al. November 2007. "Low Vitamin B$_{12}$ Status and Risk of Cognitive Decline in Older Adults." *The American Journal of Clinical Nutrition* 86(5): 1384–1391.

8. April 2008. "Vitamin B12 May Help Memory: Protein-Rich Foods and Supplements Can Provide the Recommended Daily Levels of This Essential Nutrient." *Food & Fitness Advisor* 11(4): 11.

9. "Vitamin B$_{12}$ May Help Memory: Protein-Rich Foods and Supplements Can Provide the Recommended Daily Levels of This Essential Nutrient." April 2008.

10. Kovacheva, Vesela P., Jessica M. Davison, Tiffany J. Mellott, et al. published online December 1, 2008. "Raising Gestational Choline Intake Alters Gene Expression in DMBA-Evoked Mammary Tumors and Prolongs Survival." *The FASEB Journal* 2009; 23: 1054–1063.

11. "Eating Eggs When Pregnant Affects Breast Cancer in Offspring." December 18, 2008. *Women's Health Weekly*: 434.

12. "Eating Eggs When Pregnant Affects Breast Cancer in Offspring," 434.

REFERENCES AND RESOURCES
Magazines, Journals, and Newspapers

Brugeman, Stacey. April 2008. "The Good Egg: Lose Weight, Get Energized, and Protect Your Heart—Three Simple Reasons to Eat More Eggs." *Natural Health* 38(4): 68–77.

Clarke, Robert, Jacqueline Birks, Ebba Nexo, et al. November 2007. "Low Vitamin B$_{12}$ Status and Risk of Cognitive Decline in Older Adults." *The American Journal of Clinical Nutrition* 86(5): 1384–1391.

"Eating Eggs When Pregnant Affects Breast Cancer in Offspring." December 18, 2008. *Women's Health Weekly*: 434.

Harman, Nicola, Anthony R. Leeds, and Bruce A. Griffin. September 2008. "Increased Dietary Cholesterol Does Not Increase Plasma Low Density Lipoprotein When Accompanied by an Energy-Restricted Diet and Weight Loss." *European Journal of Nutrition* 47(6): 287–293.

Holguin, Sarah, Joseph Martinez, Camille Chow, and Richard Wurtman. 2008. "Dietary Uridine Enhances the Improvement in Learning and Memory Produced by Administering DHA to Gerbils." *The FASEB Journal* 22: 3938–3946.

Kovacheva, Vasela P., Jessica M. Davison, Tiffany J. Mellot, et al. December 1, 2008. "Raising Gestational Choline Intake Alters Gene Expressions in DMBA-Evoked Mammary Tumors and Prolongs Survival." *The FASEB Journal* 2009; 23: 1054–1063.

Mutungi, Gisella, Joseph Ratliff, Michael J. Puglisi, et al. February 2008. "Dietary Cholesterol from Eggs Increases Plasma HDL Cholesterol in Overweight Men Consuming a Carbohydrate-Restricted Diet." *The Journal of Nutrition* 138: 272–276.

Smith, Rod. September 8, 2008. "Study Supports Eggs for Weight Loss." *Feedstuffs* 80(35): 9.

"Vitamin B$_{12}$ May Help Memory: Protein Rich Foods and Supplements Can Provide the Recommended Daily Levels of This Essential Nutrient." April 2008. *Food & Fitness Advisor* 11(4): 11.

Wal, J. S. Vander, A. Gupta, P. Khosla, and N.V. Dhurandhar. 2008. "Egg Breakfast Enhances Weight Loss." *International Journal of Obesity* 32: 1545–1551.

Websites

British Journal of Nutrition. http://journalscambridge.org/action/search
The FASEB Journal. www.fasebj.org.

FLAXSEEDS

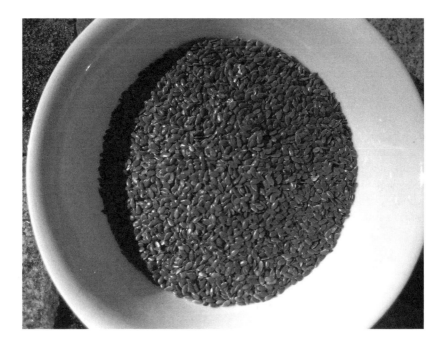

The flax plant has a truly ancient history. During the Stone Age, it grew in Mesopotamia, which is now the southern portion of Iraq. There are recordings of the use of flaxseeds in the preparation of food in ancient Greece. In both ancient Greece and ancient Rome, flaxseeds were believed to have a number of healthful benefits. But, after the decline of the Roman Empire, interest in flaxseeds waned.

That changed in the eighth and ninth centuries. The Emperor Charlemagne reintroduced flaxseeds to the European palate. Centuries later, the colonists planted flaxseeds in the United States. In the 17th century, flaxseeds arrived in Canada. Today, Canada is the world's largest producer of flaxseeds.[1] (Flaxseeds have also been used to make products such as rope, linen, linseed oil, and linoleum.)

Flaxseeds contain very good amounts of manganese and dietary fiber. They have good amounts of magnesium, folate, copper, phosphorus, and vitamin B_6.[2] Additionally, flaxseeds have alpha-linolenic acid (ALA), an omega fat that is a precursor to eicosapentaenoic acid (EPA), the type of omega-3 that is found in fish oil. Furthermore, they have lignans, phytochemicals (plant based substances) that have estrogenic and anti-cancer effects.[3] But, it is important to review the research.

CANCER

Breast Cancer

In a study published in 2004 in *The American Journal of Clinical Nutrition*, Canadian researchers supplemented the diet of 46 postmenopausal women with a daily muffin. For 16 weeks, the women ate muffins with a placebo or soy (25 grams of soy flour) or flaxseed (25 grams of ground flaxseed). At the end of the study, the researchers determined that the estrogen metabolism of those eating the flaxseed muffins, but not the soy or placebo muffins, had undergone a few changes. The levels of 2-hydroxyestrone, which is believed to be protective against breast cancer, had increased significantly. Second, the ratio of 2-hydroxyestrone to 16-alpha-hydroxyestrone (a metabolite that is thought to promote cancer) increased dramatically. This is also indicative of cancer prevention. So, flaxseeds appeared to have anti-cancer properties while the blood levels of the estrogen fractions (estradiol, estrone, and estrone sulfate) remained the same, which is important for bone health.[4]

Prostate Cancer

In a study published in 2008 in *Cancer Epidemiology, Biomarkers & Prevention*, researchers placed 161 men with prostate cancer on one of four diets at least 21 days before their scheduled prostatectomy: a flaxseed-supplemented diet (30 grams/day), a low-fat diet (<20 percent total energy), a flaxseed supplement low-fat diet, or a control (usual) diet. The men, who had a mean age of 59 years, remained on the diet for an average of 30 days.

Following surgery, the tumors were analyzed. Researchers found that tumors in the men who followed the diets that contained flaxseeds grew 40 to 50 percent more slowly than in the men who ate the low-fat or control diets. The researchers concluded that, "flaxseed is safe and associated with biological alterations that may be preventive for prostate cancer."[5]

HOT FLASHES

In a small study published in 2007 in the *Journal of the Society for Integrative Oncology*, Mayo Clinic researchers examined the use of flaxseeds to help women, who did not want to take hormonal therapy, manage their hot flashes. In order to be included in the study, women had to experience 14 hot flashes per week for at least one month.

For six weeks, everyday, the women took 40 grams (g) of crushed flax-seeds. At the conclusion of the study, the researchers found that the frequency of hot flashes had decreased by 50 percent—from 7.3 hot flashes to 3.6. However, a significant number of the women experienced gastrointestinal problems, a side effect that is not uncommon with flaxseed supplementation. Nevertheless, the researchers noted that flaxseed dietary therapy "decreases hot flash activity in women not taking estrogen therapy."[6]

On the other hand, a study published in 2006 in *Menopause* compared the effects of the 16-week consumption of daily muffins containing either 25 g of soy flour, 25 g of ground flaxseed, or wheat flour (control) on the frequency and severity of hot flashes in 99 postmenopausal women. Eighty-seven women completed the study. Of these, 31 ate the soy flour muffins; 28 ate the ground flaxseed muffins; and 28 ate wheat flour muffins. Although the researchers conducted extensive analysis of the results, they found that, "neither dietary flaxseed nor soy flour significantly affected menopause-specific quality of life or hot flash symptoms in this study."[7]

REDUCE SYMPTOMS OF ATTENTION DEFICIT HYPERACTIVITY DISORDER (ADHD)

In a study published in 2006 in *Prostaglandins, Leukotrienes and Essential Fatty Acids,* researchers reviewed the effect that flax oil had on 30 children with ADHD in Pune, India. The average age of the boys was seven years; the average age of the girls was 8.5 years. Boys outnumbered girls by three to one. The control group consisted of 30 healthy children without ADHD.

For three months, the children with ADHD were given daily flax oil supplementation "corresponding to 200 mg ALA [alpha-linolenic acid] content along with 25 mg vitamin C twice a day." All of the children completed the study; no one had any side effects.

The researchers observed dramatic improvements in the symptoms of children with ADHD. "All the symptoms like impulsivity, restlessness, inattention, self-control, psychosomatic problems and learning problems showed highly significant improvement."

Social and learning problems, so often seen with ADHD, also improved. The researchers noted that "flax oil-based emulsion could be a useful adjunct for effective therapy of ADHD."[8]

LOWER BLOOD PRESSURE

In a 12-week study published in 2007 in the *European Journal of Clinical Nutrition*, Greek researchers supplemented the diets of 59 middle-aged men who had dyslipoidemia (abnormal fats in the blood) with flaxseed oil. The diet of a control group of 28 men was supplemented with safflower oil. The goal was to determine the effect that flaxseed oil had on the blood pressure.

The researchers found that when compared to supplementation with safflower oil, supplementation with flaxseed oil resulted in significant reductions in both systolic and diastolic blood pressure levels. By lowering blood pressure levels, flaxseed oil helps to maintain cardiovascular health.[9]

IMPROVED COGNITION

In a study published in 2005 in *The Journal of Nutrition*, Dutch researchers examined the association between dietary intake of phytoestrogens, specifically lignans, such as those contained in flaxseeds, and cognitive function in 394 healthy postmenopausal women who consume a Western diet. The researchers found that the women who included higher amounts of lignans in their diets had significantly better cognitive performance. This was particularly apparent in the women who were 20 to 30 years postmenopausal. The researchers wrote, "From our results, we conclude that higher dietary intake of lignans is associated with better cognitive function in postmenopausal women." Even so, the researchers noted that the results are far from conclusive. "Data on the relation between phytoestrogens and cognitive function are still sparse and far from sufficient to become conclusive."[10]

TWO CAVEATS

Since the body is unable to break down whole flaxseeds, they must be ground before consumed or added to another food such as yogurt or oatmeal. The small grinding machines, such as those used to grind coffee, are useful for grinding flaxseed.

It is generally recommended that people add one to two tablespoons of flaxseeds to their daily diets. However, as has previously been noted, flaxseeds may cause gastrointestinal problems. So, it is best to begin with a relatively small amount of flaxseeds, and slowly increase the amount.

Should flaxseeds be part of the diet? For many people, they may well be an excellent addition.

NOTES

1. The George Mateljan Foundation Website. www.whfoods.com.

2. The George Mateljan Foundation Website.

3. Turner, Lisa. June 2009. "Just the Flax: Discover Delicious Flax Products—and Get the Most from Flaxseeds and Oils." *Better Nutrition* 71(6): 60.

4. Brooks, Jennifer D., Wendy E. Ward, Jacqueline E. Lewis, et al. February 2004. "Supplementation with Flaxseed Alters Estrogen Metabolism in Postmenopausal Women to a Greater Extent Than Does Supplementation with an Equal Amount of Soy." *The American Journal of Clinical Nutrition* 79(2): 318–325.

5. Demark-Wahnefried, Wendy, Thomas J. Polascik, Stephen L. George, et al. 2008. "Flaxseed Supplementation (Not Dietary Fat Restriction) Reduces Prostate Cancer Proliferation Rates in Men Presurgery." *Cancer Epidemiology, Biomarkers & Prevention* 17(12): 3577–3587.

6. Pruthi, S., S. L. Thompson, P. J. Novotny, et al. Summer 2007. "Pilot Evaluation of Flaxseed for the Management of Hot Flashes." *Journal of the Society for Integrative Oncology* 5(3): 106–112.

7. Lewis, Jacqueline E., Leslie A. Nickell, Lilian U. Thompson, et al. July–August 2006. "A Randomized Controlled Trial of the Effect of Dietary Soy and Flaxseed Muffins on Quality of Life and Hot Flashes During Menopause." *Menopause* 13(4): 631–642.

8. Joshi, Kalpana, Sagar Lad, Mrudula Kale, et al. January 2006. "Supplementation with Flax Oil and Vitamin C Improves the Outcome of Attention Deficit Hyperactivity Disorder (ADHD)." *Prostaglandins, Leukotrienes & Essential Fatty Acids* 74(1): 17–21.

9. Paschos, G. K., F. Magkos, D. B. Panagiotakos, et al. 2007. "Dietary Supplementation with Flaxseed Oil Lowers Blood Pressure in Dyslipidaemic Patients." *European Journal of Clinical Nutrition* 61: 1201–1206.

10. Franco, Oscar H., Huibert Burger, Corinne E. I. Lebrun, et al. May 2005. "Higher Dietary Intake of Lignans Is Associated with Better Cognitive Performance in Postmenopausal Women." *The Journal of Nutrition* 135: 1190–1195.

REFERENCES AND RESOURCES
Magazines, Journals, and Newspapers

Brooks, Jennifer D., Wendy E. Ward, Jacqueline E. Lewis, et al. February 2004. "Supplementation with Flaxseed Alters Estrogen Metabolism in Postmenopausal Women to a Greater Extent Than Does Supplementation with an Equal Amount of Soy." *The American Journal of Clinical Nutrition* 79(2): 318–325.

Demark-Wahnefried, Wendy, Thomas J. Polascik, Stephen I. George, et al. 2008. "Flaxseed Supplementation (Not Dietary Fat Restriction) Reduces Prostate Cancer Proliferation in Men Presurgery." *Cancer Epidemiology, Biomarkers & Prevention* 17(12): 3577–3587.

Franco, Oscar H., Huibert Burger, Corinne E. I. Lebrun, et al. May 2005. "Higher Dietary Intake of Lignans Is Associated with Better Cognitive Performance in Postmenopausal Women." *The Journal of Nutrition* 135: 1190–1195.

Joshi, Kalpana, Sagar Lad, Mrudula Kale, et al. January 2006. "Supplementation with Flax Oil and Vitamin C Improves the Outcome of Attention Deficit Hyperactivity Disorder (ADHA)." *Prostaglandins, Leukotrienes & Essential Fatty Acids* 74(1): 17–21.

Lewis, Jacqueline E., Leslie A. Nickell, Lilian U. Thompson, et al. July–August 2006. "A Randomized Controlled Trial of the Effect of Dietary Soy and Flaxseed Muffins on Quality of Life and Hot Flashes During Menopause." *Menopause* 13(4): 631–642.

Paschos, G. K., F. Magkos, D. B. Panagiotakos, et al. 2007. "Dietary Supplementation with Flaxseed Oil Lowers Blood Pressure in Dyslipidaemic Patients." *European Journal of Clinical Nutrition* 61: 1201–1206.

Pruthi, S., S. L. Thompson, P. J. Novotny, et al. Summer 2007. "Pilot Evaluation of Flaxseed for the Management of Hot Flashes." *Journal of the Society for Integrative Oncology* 5(3): 106–112.

Turner, Lisa. June 2009. "Just the Flax: Discover Delicious Flax Products—and Get the Most from Flaxseeds and Oils." *Better Nutrition* 71(6): 60.

Website

The George Mateljan Foundation. www.whfoods.com.

GARLIC

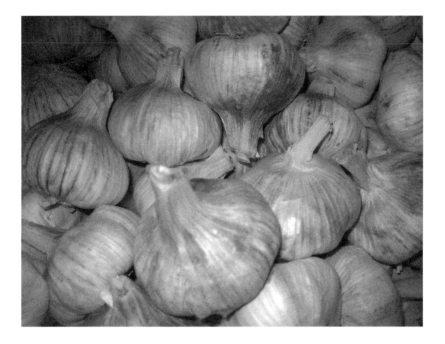

Garlic has long been acclaimed as one of the healthiest of all foods. The ancient Egyptians thought it made people stronger and was an excellent medicinal food. They fed it to the slaves who built the pyramids, and buried it with their pharaohs for their long journeys ahead.

Later, the ancient Greeks and Romans also revered garlic. To this day, many believe that garlic, which is a member of the onion family and is botanically known as *Allium sativum*, has an extraordinary ability to prevent cardiovascular disease, cancer, colds, and dementia disorders while fostering good health. One cannot help but wonder how much of this is hype and how much is backed by solid research.

CARDIOVASCULAR HEALTH

A 2007 study published the *Proceedings of the National Academy of Sciences of the United States* examined the association between the consumption of garlic and cardiovascular health. In the study conducted on rats, researchers from the University of Alabama at Birmingham found that when the compounds in garlic interacted with red blood cells, hydrogen sulfide was produced. The hydrogen sulfide relaxed blood vessels. Eating the equivalent of only two cloves of garlic may trigger a relaxation rate of up to 72 percent. And, that relaxation begins the process of lowering blood pressure.[1]

Another study on blood pressure was published in 2008 in *The Annals of Pharmacotherapy*. In order to determine the effect garlic had on people with and without elevated levels of systolic blood pressure, researchers conducted a meta-analysis of randomized controlled trials. The researchers found that garlic did indeed lower the systolic blood pressure in people with elevated levels of systolic blood pressure. But, the garlic did not lower either the systolic or diastolic blood pressure in people without elevated levels of systolic blood pressure.[2]

In an Iranian study published in 2007 in *Lipids in Health and Disease*, 150 patients with high levels of cholesterol were divided into three groups of 50. The members of the first group were given enteric-coated garlic powder tablets that were equal to 400 mg garlic, 1 mg allicin. They were told to take them twice daily. The members of the second group were given anethum (dill) tablets, 650 mg. They were also told to take them twice daily. The members of the last group were given placebos. Everyone was placed on a diet recommended by the National Cholesterol Education Program. (This diet advises people to obtain about 55 percent of their total calories from carbohydrates and no more than 30 percent of their total energy intake from dietary fat. Of this, polyunsaturated fats should be less than 10 percent and saturated fat and trans fat should be limited to less than 10 percent of calories. Protein intake should be about 0.6 g/kg desirable body weight per day.) The study continued for six weeks.

The people who ate the diets with garlic powder had significant reductions in total cholesterol and LDL (bad) cholesterol. Their levels of HDL (good) cholesterol increased. Though their triglycerides levels dropped, the drops were not statistically significant. The subjects who took anethum had small, statistically insignificant reductions in cholesterol and LDL cholesterol, and their levels of triglycerides increased. The people on placebos saw no improvement.[3]

But, markedly different results were obtained in a study published in 2007 in the *Archives of Internal Medicine*. Researchers assigned 192 adults with LDL levels between 130 and 190 (so they all had elevated levels of LDL) to one of four types of treatments: raw garlic, powdered garlic supplement, aged garlic extract, or placebo. For six months, six days per week, the subjects consumed the equivalent of a four-gram clove of garlic.

The researchers were surprised to find that none of the types of garlic had a statistically significant effect on the LDL levels of the participants.[4]

CANCER

An Australian study published in 2007 in *The Journal of Nutrition* reviewed scientific studies completed during the previous ten years that had examined the relationship between consumption of garlic and the incidence of colorectal cancer. After noting a number of studies in which consumption of garlic dramatically lowered the incidence of colorectal cancer, the researchers concluded that, "there is consistent scientific evidence derived from RCT [randomized controlled trials] of animal studies reporting protective effects of garlic on CRC [colorectal cancer] despite great heterogeneity of measures of intakes among human epidemiological studies."[5]

In an Italian and Swiss study published in 2006 in *The American Journal of Clinical Nutrition*, researchers used a number of case-control studies of south European populations to analyze the association between the frequency of consumption of onions and garlic and the incidence of several types of cancer, such as colorectal and ovarian cancer. The researchers found an inverse relationship between the consumption of garlic and onions and the incidence of cancer. So, the people who ate the highest amount of garlic and onions had the lowest rates of cancer.[6]

And, in a study conducted at the Medical University of South Carolina and published in 2007 in *Apoptosis—An International Journal of Programmed Cell Death*, researchers used garlic compounds to kill cancerous human brain cells. However, their research is very preliminary. It needs to be duplicated in animal tests. If, successful, it may be studied in humans.[7]

COLDS

In a study published in 2001 in *Advances in Therapy*, 146 subjects were randomly placed in one of two groups. For 12 winter weeks, one group took a daily garlic supplement; for the same period of time, the second group took a placebo. The subjects assessed their health in daily diaries. At the end of the study, the researchers determined that the people who took the garlic supplement had significantly fewer colds than the placebo group, and their colds lasted for shorter periods of time.[8]

MEMORY

Research conducted at the University of Illinois at Chicago and published in 2007 in *Phytotherapy Research* examined whether aged garlic extract could slow the progression of Alzheimer's disease and "prevent progressive behavioral impairment" in mice. The researchers, who have been studying the association between garlic and Alzheimer's disease for years, noted that the aged garlic extract reduced the amount of amyloid beta in the brains of the treated mice. Amyloid beta is found in the brains of people with Alzheimer's disease, and it is known to limit the creation of new neurons in the brain and to interfere with the brain's neuronal communications. The mice that were fed aged garlic extract had far less progression of the disease. The researchers suggest that "aged garlic extract has a potential for preventing AD [Alzheimer's disease] progression."[9]

SEVERAL CAVEATS

After cutting or crushing garlic, wait about 15 minutes before cooking it. When used too soon, garlic may lose the properties that enable it to fight cancer.

Cook garlic as briefly as possible. Browning garlic may destroy its protective effects.

Garlic has been known to cause indigestion and/or diarrhea.

Garlic may interfere with medications, such as the blood-thinning medication warfarin. People who eat a good deal of garlic or take regular garlic supplements should discuss this with their healthcare providers.[10]

Should garlic be part of the diet? For most people, yes.

NOTES

1. Benavides, Gloria A., Giuseppe L. Squadrito, Robert W. Mill, et al. November 13, 2007. "Hydrogen Sulfide Mediates the Vasoactivity of Garlic." *Proceedings of the National Academy of Sciences* 104(46): 17977–17982.

2. Reinhart, Kurt M., Craig I. Coleman, Colleen Teevan, et al. December 2008. "Effects of Garlic on Blood Pressure in Patients with and without Systolic Hypertension: A Meta-Analysis." *The Annals of Pharmacotherapy* 42(12): 1766–1771.

3. Kojuri, Javad, Amir R. Vosoughi, and Majid Akrami. March 1, 2007. "Effects of *Anethum graveolens* and Garlic on Lipid Profile in Hyperlipidemic Patients." *Lipids in Health and Disease* 6: 5.

4. Gardner, Christopher D., Larry D. Lawson, Eric Block, et al. 2007. "Effect of Raw Garlic vs. Commercial Garlic Supplements on Plasma Lipid Concentrations in Adults with Moderate Hypercholesterolemia." *Archives of Internal Medicine* 167(4): 346–353.

5. Ngo, Suong, Desmond B. Williams, Lynne Cobiac, and Richard J. Head. October 2007. "Does Garlic Reduce Risk of Colorectal Cancer? A Systematic Review." *The Journal of Nutrition* 137: 2264–2269.

6. Galeone, Carlotta, Claudio Pelucchi, Fabio Levi, et al. November 2006. "Onion and Garlic Use and Human Cancer." *The American Journal of Clinical Nutrition* 84(5): 1027–1032.

7. Karmakar, Surajit, Naren L. Banik, Sunil J. Patel, and Swapan K. Ray. April 2007. "Garlic Compounds Induced Calpain and Intrinsic Caspase Cascade for Apoptosis in Human Malignant Neuroblastoma SH-SY5Y Cells." *Apoptosis—An International Journal on Programmed Cell Death* 12(4): 671–684.

8. Josling, Peter. July–August 2001. "Preventing the Common Cold with a Garlic Supplement: A Double-Blind, Placebo-Controlled Survey." *Advances in Therapy* 18(4): 189–193.

9. Chauhan, N. B. and J. Sandoval. July 2007. "Amelioration of Early Cognitive Deficits by Aged Garlic Extract in Alzheimer's Transgenic Mice." *Phytotherapy Research* 21(7): 629–640.

10. "Another Role for Garlic: Colon Cancer Prevention: Garlic May Help Lower Cholesterol, but Studies Confirm Its Anti-Colorectal Cancer Properties as Well." January 2008. *Food & Fitness Advisor* 11(1): 8.

REFERENCES AND RESOURCES
Magazines, Journal, and Newspapers

"Another Role for Garlic: Colon Cancer Prevention: Garlic May Help Lower Cholesterol, but Studies Confirm Its Anti-Colorectal Cancer Properties as Well." January 2008. *Food & Fitness Advisor* 11(1): 8.

Benavides, Gloria A., Giuseppe L. Squadrito, Robert W. Mills, et al. November 13, 2007. "Hydrogen Sulfide Mediates the Vasoactivity of Garlic." *Proceedings of the National Academy of Sciences* 104(46): 17977–17982.

Chauhan, N. B., and J. Sandoval. July 2007. "Amelioration of Early Cognition Deficits by Aged Garlic Extract in Alzheimer's Disease." *Phytotherapy Research* 21(7): 629–640.

Galeone, Carlotta, Caludio Pelucchi, Fabio Levi, et al. November 2006. "Onions and Garlic Use and Human Cancer." *The American Journal of Clinical Nutrition* 84(5): 1027–1032.

Gardner, Christopher D., Larry D. Lawson, Eric Block, et al. 2007. "Effect on Raw Garlic vs. Commercial Garlic Supplements on Plasma Lipid Concentrations in Adults with Moderate Hypercholesterolemia." *Archives of Internal Medicine* 167(4): 346–353.

Josling, Peter. July-August 2001. "Preventing the Common Cold with a Garlic Supplement: A Double-Blind, Placebo-Controlled Survey." *Advances in Therapy* 18(4): 189–193.

Karmakar, Surajit, Naren L. Banik, Sunil J. Patel, and Swapan K. Ray. April 2007. "Garlic Compounds Induced Calpain and Intrinsic Caspase Cascade for Apoptosis in Human Malignant Neuroblastoma SH-SY5Y Cells." *Apoptosis—An International Journal on Programmed Cell Death* 12(4): 671–684.

Kojuri, Javad, Amir R. Vosoughi, and Majid Akrami. March 1, 2007. "Effects of *Anethum graveolens* and Garlic on Lipid Profile in Hyperlipidemic Patients." *Lipids in Health and Disease* 6: 5.

Ngo, Suong N. T., Desmond B. Williams, Lynne Cobiac, and Richard J. Head. October 2007. "Does Garlic Reduce Risk of Colorectal Cancer? A Systematic Review." *The Journal of Nutrition* 137: 2264–2269.

Reinhart, Kurt M., Craig I. Coleman, Colleen Teevan, et al. December 2008. "Effects of Garlic on Blood Pressure in Patients with and without Systolic Hypertension: A Meta-Analysis." *The Annals of Pharmacotherapy* 42(12): 1766–1771.

Website

The George Mateljan Foundation. http://www.whfoods.com.

GINGER

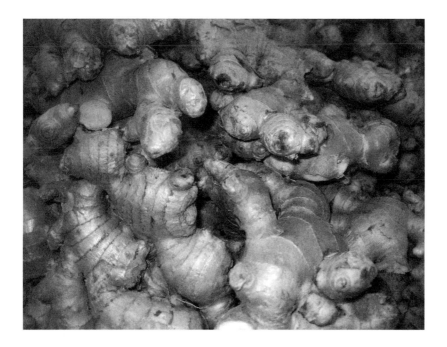

Ginger, which is mentioned in the ancient writings from China, India, and the Middle East, has long been praised for its aromatic and culinary qualities. However, it is probably best known for having a myriad of different medicinal properties. Of these, the first and foremost, is ginger's ability to bring relief from gastrointestinal problems such as nausea. Ginger is also thought to be useful for anti-inflammatory illnesses such as osteoarthritis. And, at least some people think that ginger may promote cardiovascular health.[1] Of course, it is important to review the research.

NAUSEA

An Australian study published in 2003 in the *Australian and New Zealand Journal of Obstetrics and Gynaecology* examined the effect ginger extract had on the morning sickness of 120 women, all of whom were less than 20 weeks pregnant. The study only included women who had daily bouts with morning sickness for at least one week and women for whom no relief was obtained from dietary modifications.

The women received either 125 mg of ginger extract (1.5 g of dried ginger) or a placebo four times per day for four days. After the first day of treatment, the women consuming ginger extract had significantly less nausea than the women taking the placebo. While there were no significant differences in vomiting, the women on ginger experienced less retching. The researchers concluded that, "Ginger can be considered a useful treatment for women suffering from morning sickness."[2]

A second study on the use of ginger for morning sickness in Australian women was published in 2004 in Obstetrics & Gynecology. For three weeks, 291 women, who were less than 16 weeks pregnant, were given either 1.05 g of ginger or 75 mg of vitamin B_6 every day. In both groups, more than half of the women improved; there were no significant differences in outcomes. The researchers concluded, that, for "women looking for relief from their nausea, dry retching, and vomiting, the use of ginger in early pregnancy will reduce their symptoms to an equivalent extent as vitamin B6."[3]

A third study, published in 2003 in the American Journal of Obstetrics and Gynecology, compared 187 pregnant women who took ginger for nausea and vomiting with a control group of 187 who did not take any treatments. The ginger appeared to "mildly" help the women with their nausea and vomiting, and it did not "appear to increase the rate of major malformations above the baseline rate."[4]

In a study conducted in Thailand and published in 2007 in Alternative Medicine Review, researchers attempted to determine if ginger could reduce or prevent the nausea and vomiting that often follows major gynecologic surgery. Researchers studied a total of 120 women undergoing major gynecologic surgery. Before surgery, 60 women received two capsules of ginger; another 60 women received a placebo. The researchers indicated that the women who had pre-surgery ginger had statistically significantly less nausea and vomiting that the women who took the placebo. The researchers noted that, "ginger has efficacy in prevention of nausea and vomiting after major gynecologic surgery."[5]

Another study from Thailand, published in 2006 in the American Journal of Obstetrics & Gynecology, reviewed five randomized, double-blinded, placebo-controlled trials including a total of 363 patients. All of the studies compared the use of a fixed dose of ginger to a placebo on 24-hour-post-operative nausea and vomiting in patients having gynecological or lower extremity surgery. The incidence of postoperative nausea and vomiting in those who received at least one gram of ginger was more than a third less than those who received placebos. Still, the study has some limitations. For example, the majority of the patients were Asian with an average weight of only 50 kg. Dosage requirements may need to be increased for people who are larger. Nevertheless, the researchers concluded that "use of ginger is an effective means for reducing postoperative nausea and vomiting."[6]

It is also well known that people receiving chemotherapy treatments frequently experience nausea. A study published in 2006 in *Neurogastroenterology & Motility* attempted to determine if high-protein meals combined with ginger could help control the post-chemotherapy nausea. For three days after chemotherapy treatments, 28 cancer patients were placed in one of three groups. The control group ate their normal diets. A second group ate a protein drink and one gram of ginger root twice each day. A third group ate a protein drink and additional protein power and one gram of ginger root twice a day. The researchers found that the "high protein meals with ginger reduced the delayed nausea of chemotherapy, and reduced the use of antiemetic [anti-nausea] medications. Anti-nausea effects of high protein meals with ginger were associated with enhancement of normal gastric myoeletrical [electricity generated by muscle] activity and decreased gastric dysrhythmias [abnormal stomach electrical activity]."[7]

CARDIOVASCULAR AND DIABETIC HEALTH

Researchers at Kuwait University studied the role that ginger may play in rats who have been treated to develop diabetes. In a study published in 2006 in the *British Journal of Nutrition*, researchers noted that rats that developed diabetes tended to have high blood sugar and weight loss. The researchers fed these rats raw ginger–500 mg per kg of body weight per day—for seven weeks. A separate group of rats, which did not receive any ginger, served as the control group. At the end of the study, the rats that were fed ginger had considerably lower levels of blood sugar, cholesterol, and triglycerides than the rats in the control group. Ginger also appeared to lessen some of the complications associated with diabetes such as protein in the urine, excessive urine output, and excess water intake. "Therefore, it can be concluded from these studies that raw ginger has significant potential in the treatment of diabetes."[8]

OSTEOARTHRITIS OF THE KNEE

In a study published in 2001 in *Arthritis & Rheumatism*, subjects with moderate to severe pain from osteoarthritis in their knees were divided into two groups. One group took 255 mg of concentrated ginger root twice daily for six weeks, while the other group had placebos. Following a washout period, the group who originally had ginger was given placebos, and the group who originally had placebos was given ginger. In the end, 247 patients were evaluated. The researchers found that the ginger markedly improved the pain from osteoarthritis. "A highly purified and standardized ginger extract had a statistically significant effect on reducing symptoms of OA [osteoarthritis] of the knee." But, some of the participants reported gastrointestinal side effects such as belching, gas, nausea, and mild heartburn.[9]

In an article published in 2005 in the *Journal of Medicinal Food*, researchers from the Department of Orthopedic Surgery at Johns Hopkins University School of Medicine noted that the anti-inflammatory properties of ginger have been known for centuries. More recently, many studies have been conducted on these properties, and it is now generally recognized that "ginger modulates biochemical pathways activated in chronic inflammation."[10] But, an article published in 2007 in *American Family Physician* appears to disagree. Commenting on the use of ginger for arthritis, Brett White, MD, wrote, "Mixed results have been found in limited studies of ginger for the treatment of arthritis symptoms."[11]

TWO CAVEATS

Though ginger allergies are uncommon, they are known to exist. And, people taking blood-thinning medications, such as warfarin, should check with their healthcare provider before consuming even moderate amounts of ginger.

Should ginger be part of the diet? For the vast majority of people, yes.

NOTES

1. Klotter, Jule. February–March 2009. "The Many Benefits of Ginger." *Townsend Letter*: 45–46.

2. Willetts, Karen E., Abie Ekangaki, and John A. Eden. March 2003. "Effect of a Ginger Extract on Pregnancy-Induced Nausea: A Randomised Controlled Trial." *Australian and New Zealand Journal of Obstetrics and Gynaecology* 43(2): 139–144.

3. Smith, C., C. Crowther, K. Willson, et al. April 2004. "A Randomized Controlled Trial of Ginger to Treat Nausea and Vomiting in Pregnancy." *Obstetrics and Gynecology* 103(4): 639–645.

4. Portnoi, G., L. A. Chng, L. Karimi-Tabesh, et al. November 2003. "Prospective Comparative Study of the Safety and Effectiveness of Ginger for the Treatment of Nausea and Vomiting in Pregnancy." *American Journal of Obstetrics and Gynecology* 189(5): 1374–1377.

5. Roxas, Mario. December 2007. "The Efficacy of Ginger in Prevention of Postoperative Nausea and Vomiting After Major Gynecologic Surgery." *Alternative Medicine Review* 12(4): 373.

6. Chaiyakunapruk, Nathorn, Nantawarn Kitikannakorn, Surakit Nathisuwan, et al. January 2006. "The Efficacy of Ginger for the Prevention of Postoperative Nausea and Vomiting: A Meta-Analysis." *American Journal of Obstetrics and Gynecology* 194(1): 95–99.

7. Levine, M. E., M. Gillis, S. Yanchis, et al. June 2006. "Protein and Ginger for the Treatment of Chemotherapy-Induced Delayed Nausea and Gastric Dysrhythmia." *Neurogastroenterology & Motility* 18(6): 488.

8. Al-Amin, Zainab M., Martha Thomson, Khaled K. Al-Qattan, et al. 2006. "Anti-Diabetic and Hypolipidaemic Properties of Ginger (*Zingiber officinale*) in Streptozotocin-Induced Diabetic Rats." *British Journal of Nutrition* 96: 660–666.

9. Altman, R. D. and K. C. Marcussen. 2001. "Effects of a Ginger Extract on Knee Pain in Patients with Osteoarthritis." *Arthritis & Rheumatism* 44: 2531–2538.

10. Grzanna, Reinhard, Lars Lindmark, and Carmelita G. Frondoza. 2005. "Ginger—An Herbal Medicinal Product with Broad Anti-Inflammatory Actions." *Journal of Medicinal Food* 8(2): 125–132.

11. White, Brett. 2007. "Ginger: An Overview." *American Family Physician* 75: 1689–1691.

REFERENCES AND RESOURCES
Magazine, Journals, and Newspapers

Al-Amin, Zainab M., Martha Thomson, Khaled K. Al-Qattan, et al. 2006. "Anti-Diabetic and Hypolipidaemic Properties of Ginger (*Zingiber officinale*) in Streptozotocin-Induced Diabetic Rates." *British Journal of Nutrition* 96: 660–666.

Altman, R. D. and K. C. Marcussen. 2001. "Effects of a Ginger Extract on Knee Pain in Patients with Osteoarthritis." *Arthritis & Rheumatism* 44: 2531–2538.

Chaiyakunapruk, Nathorn, Nantawarn Kitikannakorn, Surakit Nathisuwan, et al. January 2006. "The Efficacy of Ginger for the Prevention of Postoperative Nausea and Vomiting: A Meta-Analysis." *American Journal of Obstetrics and Gynecology* 194(1): 95–99.

Grzanna, Reinhard, Lars Lindmark, and Carmelita G. Frondoza. 2005. "Ginger—An Herbal Medicinal Product with Broad Anti-Inflammatory Actions." *Journal of Medicinal Food* 8(2): 125–132.

Klotter, Jule. February–March 2009. "The Many Benefits of Ginger." *Townsend Letter*: 45–46.

Levine, M. E., M. Gillis, S. Yanchis, et al. June 2006. "Protein and Ginger for the Treatment of Chemotherapy-Induced Delayed Nausea and Gastric Dysrhythmia. *Neurogastroenterology & Motility* 18(6): 488.

Portnoi, G., L. A. Chng, L. Karimi-Tabesh, et al. November 2003. "Prospective Comparative Study of the Safety and Effectiveness of Ginger for the Treatment of Nausea and Vomiting in Pregnancy." *American Journal of Obstetrics and Gynecology* 189(5): 1374–1377.

Roxas, Mario. December 2007. "The Efficacy of Ginger in Prevention of Postoperative Nausea and Vomiting After Major Gynecologic Surgery." *Alternative Medicine Review* 12(4): 373.

Smith, S., C. Crowther, K. Willson, et al. April 2004. "A Randomized Controlled Trial of Ginger to Treat Nausea and Vomiting in Pregnancy." *Obstetrics & Gynecology* 103(4): 639–645.

White, Brett. 2007. "Ginger: An Overview." *American Family Physician* 75: 1689–1691.

Willets, Karen E., Abie Ekangaki, and John A. Eden. March 2003. "Effect of a Ginger Extract on Pregnancy-Induced Nausea: A Randomised Controlled Trial." *Australian and New Zealand Journal of Obstetrics and Gynaecology*. 43(2): 139–144.

Website

The George Mateljan Foundation. www.whfoods.com.

GRAPEFRUIT

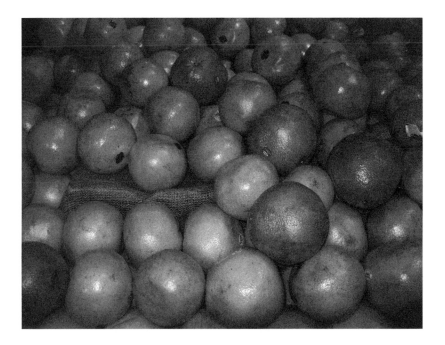

For generations, grapefruit has been considered one of the healthiest of foods. Throughout the world, millions of people begin each day with a breakfast that includes grapefruit or a glass of grapefruit juice. However, over the past few decades, some questions have arisen about this delicious food. Naturally, it is important to investigate the research.

CARDIOVASCULAR HEALTH

In a study that was published in 2006 in the *Journal of Agricultural and Food Chemistry*, fifty-seven men and women with high blood cholesterol and recent coronary bypass surgery were divided into three groups. For 30 days, each person was given a single serving of either fresh red grapefruit, fresh white grapefruit, or no grapefruit. The people who ate the grapefruit experienced reductions in blood lipid levels; the people who ate no grapefruit had no change in lipid levels. Reductions in lipid levels, especially blood triglycerides, were greatest in those who ate the red grapefruit. Red grapefruit also has higher levels of antioxidants than white grapefruit. The researchers concluded that, "The addition of fresh red grapefruit to generally accepted diets could be beneficial for hyperlipidemic, especially hypertriglyceridemic, patients suffering from coronary atherosclerosis."[1]

WEIGHT LOSS

In a 12-week study, published in 2006 in the *Journal of Medicinal Food*, researchers divided almost 100 obese people into four groups. One group received grapefruit extract; a second group drank grapefruit juice with each meal; a third group ate half of a grapefruit with each meal; and a fourth group took a placebo. By the end of the study, the fresh grapefruit group had lost the most weight—an average of 3.6 pounds per person. And, those who drank three glasses of grapefruit juice lost an average of 3.3 pounds. The researchers noted that the people who ate the grapefruit had lower levels of insulin in their blood, and they hypothesized that this might have caused the weight loss. How does that work? It is known that after eating, people who have lower amounts of insulin in their blood use more food for energy and store less fat. Also, because the people who ate grapefruit and drank grapefruit juice lost weight, the researchers suggested that the weight loss was the result of a natural plant compound in grapefruit, not the fiber.[2]

HEPATITIS C VIRUS (HCV)

In a study published in 2008 in *Hepatology*, researchers used naringenin, a common flavonoid found in grapefruit and other citrus fruits, to block the secretion of hepatitis C virus from infected cells. Without such secretion, a chronic state of hepatitis infection cannot be maintained. Still, since the gastrointestinal track does not absorb naringenin very well, if naringenin becomes part of the treatment for hepatitis C it will likely be delivered intravenously.[3] So, the consumption of grapefruit does not appear to be an effective treatment of hepatitis C.

PREMALIGNANT ORAL LESIONS

An article published in 2006 in the *American Journal of Epidemiology* describes a study in which researchers traced the diet of more than 42,000 men for 16 years. They found that the daily consumption of half a grapefruit or a whole orange (the equivalent of six ounces of orange or grapefruit juice) reduced the risk of oral cancer by up to 40 percent. The researchers noted, "The risk of oral premalignant lesions was significantly reduced with higher consumption of fruits, particularly citrus fruits and juices."[4]

BONE LOSS

An article published in 2008 in *Nutrition* describes a study conducted at Texas A & M University on 42 castrated male rats and a control group of 14 non-castrated male rats. (Castrating the rats increases the amount of oxidative stress and fosters the development of osteoporosis.) The castrated rats were divided into three groups. One group was fed a normal diet; the second group was fed the normal diet plus five percent grapefruit pulp; the third group was fed a normal diet plus 10 percent grapefruit pulp. At the end of 60 days, the researchers found that the more grapefruit the rats ate, the more protection they had against bone loss.[5]

BREAST CANCER

In 2007, a striking piece of research was published in the *British Journal of Cancer*. A study of more than 50,000 postmenopausal women from five racial or ethnic groups (African American, Japanese American, Hispanic/Latino, Native Hawaiian, and Caucasian) found that women who ate the most grapefruit—about one-quarter grapefruit per day or half a grapefruit every other day—had a 30 percent higher risk for breast cancer than women who ate no grapefruit. After the researchers, who were from California and Hawaii, controlled for risk factors for breast cancer (such as excess weight and family history of the disease), the association between breast cancer and grapefruit consumption remained high. The researchers noted that previous studies have found a molecule known as cytochrome P450 3A4 (CYP3A4) plays a role in metabolizing estrogen hormones. The researchers suggested that grapefruit may inhibit the actions of this molecule, thereby increasing the levels of estrogen in the blood.[6] Higher levels of estrogen in the blood are directly related with higher rates of breast cancer.

While the results of this study are clearly interesting, especially to those at increased risk for breast cancer or who have already dealt with estrogen-receptor positive breast cancer, it is also important to note that this is one epidemiologic study that deals only with postmenopausal women. Are younger women also at risk? Does the consumption of smaller amounts of grapefruit increase risk? Is it safe to have grapefruit even once a week? At present, the answers to these and other questions are not known. Worried citrus fruit lovers may wish to eat more oranges and fewer grapefruits.

GRAPEFRUIT, GRAPEFRUIT JUICE, AND MEDICATIONS

More than two decades ago, David G. Bailey, PhD, and his fellow researchers wanted to determine if it was necessary to stop drinking alcohol when taking felodipine (Plandil), a calcium channel blocker that lowers blood pressure. Dr. Bailey decided to test the felodipine/alcohol combination on himself. But, because he disliked the taste of alcohol, he added grapefruit juice. When he tested his own blood, he found that it contained rates of felodipine that were far higher than they should have been, a potentially very dangerous situation. The addition of the grapefruit juice made the felodipine more powerful. This came to be known as the "Grapefruit Juice Effect."[7] Grapefruit and grapefruit juice have "chemicals that interfere with the enzymes that normally break down drugs in the digestive system." When these enzymes are not working properly, medications enter the "bloodstream at higher-than-acceptable levels," which increases the risk of side effects.[8]

Since then, researchers have determined that the consumption of grapefruit and grapefruit juice may not only boost levels of many different types of medications, they may also lower the amounts of medications in the body. And, the effects of even a relatively small amount of grapefruit or grapefruit juice may remain in the body for quite some time.

In a small four-phase crossover Japanese study that appeared in 2005 in the *British Journal of Clinical Pharmacology*, eight healthy people ingested water or grapefruit juice three times a day for four days. On the fourth day, all eight people were given single doses of either atorvastatin (20 mg) or pitavastatin (4 mg), statin medications that lower blood cholesterol levels. Grapefruit juice was found to cause a substantial increase of the amount of atorvastatin in the blood but only a slight increase in the amount of pitavastatin.[9]

And, an article published in 2006 in *The American Journal of Clinical Nutrition* described the cause of these interactions—a family of plant toxins known as furanocoumarins. When these are removed from grapefruit juice, people may safely take their medications and drink grapefruit juice.[10]

Most often, grapefruit will interact with medications used for anxiety, depression, seizures, blood pressure, high cholesterol, impotence, and human immunodeficiency virus (HIV). But, there are reports for interactions with immunosuppressants (used to prevent organ rejection) and cardiovascular medications.

Should grapefruits be included in the diet? That is for people to discuss with their health providers.

NOTES

1. Gorinstein, Shela, Abraham Caspi, Imanuel Libman, et al. 2006. "Red Grapefruit Positively Influences Serum Triglyceride Level In Patients Suffering from Coronary Atherosclerosis: Studies in Vitro and in Humans." *Journal of Agricultural and Food Chemistry* 54(5): 1887–1892.

2. Fujioka, Ken, Frank Greenway, Judy Sheard, and Yu Ying. Spring 2006. "The Effects of Grapefruit on Weight and Insulin Resistance: Relationship to the Metabolic Syndrome." *Journal of Medicinal Food* 9(1): 49–54.

3. Nahmias, Yaakov, Jonathan Goldwasser, Monica Casali, et al. 2008. "Apolipoprotein B-Dependent Hepatitis C Virus Secretion Is Inhibited by the Grapefruit Flavonoid Naringenin." *Hepatology* 47(5): 1437–1445.

4. Maserejian, Nancy Nairi, Edward Giovannucci, Bernard Rosner, et al. 2006. "Prospective Study of Fruits and Vegetables and Risk of Oral Premalignant Lesions in Men." *American Journal of Epidemiology* 164(6): 556–566.

5. Deyhim, Farzad, Kranthi Mandadi, Bhimangouda S. Patil, and Bahram Faraji. 2008. "Grapefruit Pulp Increases Antioxidant Status and Improves Bone Quality in Orchidectomized Rats." *Nutrition* 24(10): 1039–1044.

6. Monroe, K. R., S. P. Murphy, L. N. Kolonel, and M. C. Pike. 2007. "Prospective Study of Grapefruit Intake and Risk of Breast Cancer in Postmenopausal Women: The Multiethnic Cohort Study." *British Journal of Cancer* 97: 440–445.

7. "Warning: These Health Drinks Can Make Your Blood Pressure Medications and Antibiotics Worthless." January 2009. *Women's Health Letter* 15(1): 3–5.

8. Dowd, Rachel. November 2007. "Ask the Experts." *Natural Health* 37(10): 102–104.

9. Ando, Hitoshi, Shuichi Tsuruoka, Hayato Yanagihara, et al. "Effects of Grapefruit Juice on the Pharmacokinetics of Pitavastatin and Atorvastatin." *British Journal of Clinical Pharmacology* 60(5): 494–497.

10. Paine, Mary F., Wilbur W. Widmer, Heather L. Hart, et al. May 2006. "A Furanocoumarin-Free Grapefruit Juice Establishes Furanocoumarins as the Mediators of the Grapefruit Juice-Felodipine Interaction." *The American Journal of Clinical Nutrition* 83(5): 1097–1105.

REFERENCES AND RESOURCES
Magazines, Journals, and Newspapers

Ando, Hitoshi, Shuichi Tsuruoka, Hayato Yanagihara, et al. 2005. "Effects of Grapefruit Juice on the Pharmacokinetics of Pitavastatin and Atorvastatin." *British Journal of Clinical Pharmacology* 60(5): 494–497.

Deyhim, Farzad, Kranthi Mandadi, Bhimanagouda S. Patil, and Bahram Faraji. October 2008. "Grapefruit Pulp Increases Antioxidant Status and Improves Bone Quality in Orchidectomized Rats." *Nutrition* 24(10): 1039–1044.

Dowd, Rachel. November 2007. "Ask the Experts." *Natural Health* 37(10): 102–104.

Fujioka, Ken, Frank Greenway, Judy Sheard, and Yu Ying. Spring 2006. "The Effects of Grapefruit on Weight and Insulin Resistance: Relationship to the Metabolic Syndrome." *Journal of Medicinal Food* 9(1): 49–54.

Gorinstein, Shela, Abraham Caspi, Imanuel Libman, et al. 2006. "Red Grapefruit Positively Influences Serum Triglyceride Level in Patients Suffering from Coronary Atherosclerosis: Studies In Vitro and in Humans." *Journal of Agricultural and Food Chemistry* 54(5): 1887–1892.

Maserejian, Nancy Nairi, Edward Giovannucci, Bernard Rosner, et al. 2006. "Prospective Study of Fruits and Vegetables and Risk of Oral Premalignant Lesions in Men." *American Journal of Epidemiology* 164(6): 556–566.

Monroe, K. R., S. P. Murphy, L. N. Kolonel, and M. C. Pike. 2007. "Prospective Study of Grapefruit Intake and Risk of Breast Cancer in Postmenopausal Women: The Multiethnic Cohort Study." *British Journal of Cancer* 97: 440–445.

Nahmias, Yaakov, Jonathan Goldwasser, Monica Casali, et al. 2008. "Apolipoprotein B-Dependent Hepatitis C Virus Secretion Is Inhibited by the Grapefruit Flavonoid Naringenin." *Hepatology* 47(5): 1437–1445.

Paine, Mary F., Wilbur W. Widmer, Heather L. Hart, et al. May 2006. "A Furanocoumarin-Free Grapefruit Juice Establishes Furanocoumarins as the Mediators of the Grapefruit Juice–Felodipine Interaction." *The American Journal of Clinical Nutrition* 83(5): 1097–1105.

"Warning: These Health Drinks Can Make Your Blood Pressure Medications and Antibiotics Worthless." January 2009. *Women's Health Letter* 15(1): 3–5.

Website

Medical News Today. www.medicalnewstoday.com.

GRAPES

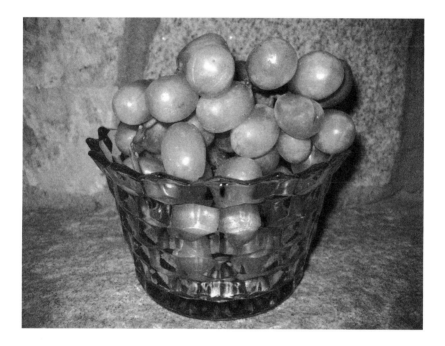

It is generally believed that grapes have been grown since prehistoric times. They are thought to have been cultivated in Asia as early as 5000 BCE. Grapes are also referenced in several biblical stories; in the Bible, they are referred to as the "fruit of the vine." Moreover, grapes are contained in the hieroglyphics in the tombs of ancient Egypt.

By the rise of the ancient Greek and Roman civilizations, grapes were used to make wine. But, it was not until the early 17th century that grapes were first planted in America—in a Spanish mission in what is now New Mexico.

Grapes are considered to be an excellent source for manganese and a good source of vitamins B_1, B_6, and C, and potassium. Furthermore, grapes contain flavonoids—phytochemicals that are antioxidant compounds, such as quercitin and resveratrol.[1] But what has the research determined?

CANCER
Breast Cancer

In a study that was published in 2008 in *Cancer Prevention Research*, researchers from Nebraska found that in laboratory studies, resveratrol slowed the abnormal cell formation that leads to the majority of cases of breast cancer. The researchers noted that estrogen reacts with DNA molecules to form adducts, also known as DNA adducts. A DNA adduct is a piece of DNA covalently bonded to a cancer-causing chemical. It is the very early stage of a cancer cell. The researchers determined that resveratrol is able to stop the formation of these DNA adducts.[2]

Colorectal Cancer

In a California study published in 2007 in *Nutrition and Cancer*, researchers investigated outcomes of 499 cases of colorectal cancer. Of these, 141 were familial and 358 were sporatic. The patients were placed in one of two categories: regular or infrequent wine consumers. The researchers found that among those patients with a family history of colorectal cancer, the people who drank a moderate amount of wine during the year before the cancer diagnosis had better survival outcomes. In a stunning finding, researchers learned that 75 percent of these familial patients were alive after ten years compared with only 47 percent among the familial patients who did not regularly drink wine.[3]

Prostate Cancer

A laboratory study published in 2007 in *Cancer Research* described how researchers were able to use an extract from the skin of muscadine grapes to inhibit the growth of different stages of prostate cancer. Yet, muscadine grape skin extract does not contain significant amounts of resveratrol. Instead, it is filled with anthocyanins, antioxidant flavonoids that have demonstrated anti-tumor activity. The researchers concluded that, "the unique properties of MSKE [muscadine grape skin extract] suggest that it may be an important source for further development of chemopreventive or therapeutic agents against prostate cancer."[4]

CARDIOVASCULAR HEALTH

In a study published in 2008 in *Journal of Gerontology: Biological Sciences*, researchers fed five groups of rats one of five types of diets: low salt, low salt, and grape powder; high salt, high salt, and grape powder; or high salt diet and the vasodilator hydralazine, a medication that lowers blood pressure. After 18 weeks, compared to the rats that ate the high-salt diet without grapes, the rats that ate the high-salt, grape-enriched diet had reduced levels of inflammation, lower blood pressure, better heart function, and fewer

signs of heart muscle damage. The rats that ate a salty diet and took medication had lower blood pressure, but they obtained no protection from heart
damage. The low-salt and grape powder diet reduced heart damage. The
researchers concluded that the grapes themselves support cardiovascular
health.[5]

In a study published in 2005 in *The Journal of Nutrition*, 24 pre-menopausal
women and 20 post-menopausal women were randomly asked to consume
water containing 1.26 ounces of freeze dried grapes or a control drink everyday for four weeks. After a three-week washout period, the subjects drank
the alternate drink for another four weeks. Both pre- and post-menopausal
women experienced improvements in cardiovascular health. "Through alterations in lipoprotein metabolism, oxidative stress, and inflammatory
markers, LGP [lyophilized grape powder] intake beneficially affects key
risk factors for coronary heart disease in both pre- and postmenopausal
women."[6]

HEALTH PROBLEMS ASSOCIATED WITH OBESITY

In a Spanish study published in 2008 in *Obesity*, researchers attempted to
determine if the quercetin found in grapes could assist obese rats with the
medical problems associated with obesity. For ten weeks, the rats received
either 2 or 10 mg/kg of body weight doses of quercetin. The obese rats who
received either of the doses had improvements in systolic blood pressure,
tryglycerides, total cholesterol, free fatty acids, and levels of insulin. Only
the high dose of quercetin was associated with a reduction in body weight
and anti-inflammatory effects in visceral adipose tissue.[7]

HEALTHIER AGING

In a study published in 2008 in *Cell Metabolism*, researchers compared mice
fed the following types of diets: standard diet, high-calorie diet, or an every-
other-day feeding regimen with or without high or low amounts of resveratrol. The findings indicated that the addition of resveratrol to the diet
resulted in a number of positive outcomes. Some of these were as follows:

- After ten months on resveratrol, the total cholesterol levels of 22-
  month-old non-obese mice were significantly reduced.
- When treated with resveratrol, the aortas of 18-month-old obese and
  non-obese mice functioned significantly better.
- Compared to the non-treated control group, mice taking resveratrol had
  better bone health.
- By the age of 30 months, mice taking resveratrol had reduced cataract
  formation.
- As they aged, mice taking resveratrol had better balance and motor
  coordination.

The mice on the high-calorie diets without resveratrol had the shortest lives; the mice that ate every other day lived the longest, whether or not they had resveratrol. While the resveratrol improved the quality of life for these mice, it did not actually extend their lifespan.[8]

In a study published in 2006 in *Nutrition*, Boston researchers investigated the effects of the consumption of two different concentrations (10 percent and 50 percent) of Concord grape juice by aged rats (versus rats fed a calorie-matched placebo). The rats fed the 10 percent juice experienced improvements in cognition, and the rats fed the 50 percent juice had better motor function. The researchers noted that their findings "suggest that, in addition to their known beneficial effects on cancer and heart disease, polyphenolics in foods may be beneficial in reversing the course of neuronal and behavioral aging, possibly through a multiplicity of direct and indirect effects that can affect a variety of neuronal parameters."[9]

MEMORY

In a study published in 2007 in *The Journal of Neuroscience*, researchers compared mice that were fed a standard diet to those given a diet supplemented with epicatechin, a flavonol found in grapes. Half of the mice devoted two daily hours to running on a wheel. At the end of a month, the researchers taught mice to locate a platform contained in some water. The mice that had consumed epicatechin and exercised had a better memory of the location of the platform. When the researchers examined the brains of the dead mice, they found more blood vessel growth in the dentate gyrus, the area of the brain dedicated to the formation of learning and memory as well as more mature nerve cells, which indicates enhanced communication.[10]

ONE CAVEAT

Non-organic imported grapes are generally grown with large amounts of pesticides. So, organic grapes are preferable.

Should grapes be part of the diet? Of course.

NOTES

1. The George Mateljan Foundation Website. www.whfoods.com.

2. Lu, Fang, Muhammad Zahid, Cheng Wang, et al. July 1, 2008. "Resveratrol Prevents Estrogen-DNA Adduct Formation and Neoplastic Transformation in MCF-10F Cells." *Cancer Prevention Research* 1(2): 135–145.

3. Zell, Jason A., Archana J. McEligot, Argyrios Ziogas, et al. September 1, 2007. "Differential Effects of Wine Consumption on Colorectal Cancer Outcomes Based on Family History of the Disease." *Nutrition and Cancer* 59(1): 36–45.

4. Hudson, Tamaro S., Diane K. Hartle, Stephen D. Hursting, et al. September 1. 2007. "Inhibition of Prostate Cancer Growth by Muscadine Grape Skin Extract and Resveratrol Through Distinct Mechanisms." *Cancer Research* 67(17): 8396–8405.

5. Seymour, E. M., Andrew A. M. Singer, Maurice R. Bennink, et al. October 2008. "Chronic Intake of Phytochemical-Enriched Diet Reduces Cardiac Fibrosis and Diastolic Dysfunction Caused by Prolonged Salt-Sensitive Hypertension." *Journal of Gerontology: Biological Sciences* 63A(10): 1034–1042.

6. Zern, Tosca L., Richard J. Wood, Christine Greene, et al. August 2005. "Grape Polyphenols Exert a Cardioprotective Effect in Pre- and Postmenopausal Women by Lowering Plasma Lipids and Reducing Oxidative Stress." *The Journal of Nutrition* 135: 1911–1917.

7. Rivera, Leonor, Rocío Morón, Manuel Sánchez, et al. 2008. "Quercetin Ameliorates Metabolic Syndrome and Improves the Inflammatory Status in Obese Zucker Rats." *Obesity* 16(9): 2081–2087.

8. Pearson, Keven J., Joseph A. Baur, Kaitlyn N. Lewis, et al. August 6, 2008. "Resveratrol Delays Age-Related Deterioration and Mimics Transcriptional Aspects of Dietary Restriction Without Extending Life Span." *Cell Metabolism* 8(2): 157–168.

9. Shukitt-Hale, B., A. Carey, L. Simon, et al. March 2006. "Effects of Concord Grape Juice on Cognition and Motor Deficits in Aging." *Nutrition* 22(3): 295–302.

10. van Praag, Henriette, Melanie J. Lucero, Gene W. Yeo, et al. May 30, 2007. "Plant-Derived Flavanol (−)Epicatechin Enhances Angiogenesis and Retention of Spatial Memory in Mice." *The Journal of Neuroscience* 27(22): 5869–5878.

REFERENCES AND RESOURCES
Magazines, Journals, and Newspapers

Hudson, Tamaro S., Diane K. Hartle, Stephen D. Hursting, et al. September 1, 2007. "Inhibition of Prostate Cancer Growth by Muscadine Grape Skin Extract and Resveratrol Through Distinct Mechanisms." *Cancer Research* 67(17): 8396–8405.

Lu, Fang, Muhammad Zahid, Cheng Wang, et al. July 1, 2008. "Resveratrol Prevents Estrogen-DNA Adduct Formation and Neoplastic Transformation in MCF-10F Cells." *Cancer Prevention Research* 1(2): 135–145.

Pearson, Kevin J., Joseph A. Baur, Kaitlyn N. Lewis, et al. August 6, 2008. "Resveratrol Delays Age-Related Deterioration and Mimics Transcriptional Aspects of Dietary Restriction without Extending Life Span." *Cell Metabolism* 8(2): 157–168.

Rivera, Leonor, Rocío Morón, Manuel Sánchez, et al. 2008. "Quercetin Ameliorates Metabolic Syndrome and Improves the Inflammatory in Obese Zucker Rats." *Obesity* 16(9): 2081–2087.

Seymour, E. M., Andrew A. M. Singer, Maurice R. Bennink, et al. October 2008. "Chronic Intake of a Phytochemical-Enriched Diet Reduces Cardiac Fibrosis and Diastolic Dysfunction Caused by Prolonged Salt-Sensitive Hypertension." *Journal of Gerontology: Biological Sciences* 63A(10): 1034–1042.

Shukitt-Hale, B., A. Carey, L. Simon, et al. March 2006. "Effects of Concord Grape Juice on Cognitive and Motor Deficits in Aging." *Nutrition* 22(3): 295–302.

van Praag, Henriette, Melanie J. Lucero, Gene W. Yeo, et al. May 30, 2007. "Plant-Derived Flavanol (−)Epicatechin Enhances Angiogenesis and Retention of Spatial Memory in Mice." *The Journal of Neuroscience* 27(22): 5869–5878.

Zell, Jason A., Archana J. McEligot, Argyrios Ziogas, et al. September 1, 2007. "Differential Effects of Wine Consumption on Colorectal Cancer Outcomes Based on Family History of the Disease." *Nutrition and Cancer* 59(1): 36–45.

Zern, Tosca L., Richard J. Wood, Christine Greene, et al. August 2005. "Grape Polyphenols Exert a Cardioprotective Effect in Pre- and Postmenopausal Women by Lowering Plasma Lipids and Reducing Oxidative Stress." *The Journal of Nutrition* 135: 1911–1917.

Website

The George Mateljan Foundation. www.whfoods.com.

KALE

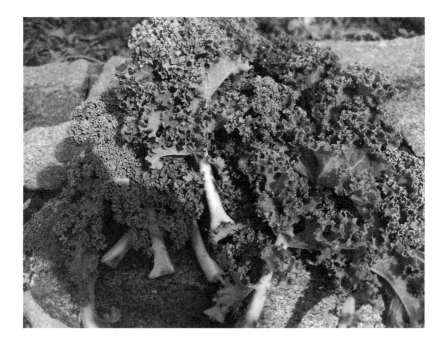

Kale is believed to have originated in Asia Minor, the most western section of the continent of Asia. Around 600 BCE, Celtic wanderers brought it to Europe. It is known that during ancient Roman times, curly kale was a significant crop. With the English settlers, kale made its way to America in the 17th century.

Kale is filled with a wide variety of vitamins and nutrients. It has excellent amounts of manganese and vitamins A, C, and K. It has very good quantities of dietary fiber, copper, tryptophan, calcium, vitamin B_6, and potassium. And, kale contains a good amount of iron, magnesium, omega-3 fatty acids, protein, folate, phosphorus, and vitamins E, B_1, B_2, and B_3.[1] Kale also has carotenoids, especially lutein and zeaxanthin. To many, kale may well be considered a "superfood." But, what have the researchers learned?

CANCER

In a laboratory study published in 2009 in *Food Chemistry*, Canadian researchers evaluated whether 34 different vegetable extracts inhibited the growth of cancer cells from the stomach, lung, breast, kidney, skin, pancreas, prostate, and brain. In addition to vegetables from the genus *Allium*, such as garlic, the best results were obtained from cruciferous vegetables, such as kale. The researchers noted that their findings "indicate that vegetables have very different inhibitory activities toward cancer cells and that the inclusion of cruciferous and *Allium* vegetables in the diet is essential for effective dietary-based chemopreventive strategies."[2]

In a study published in 2006 in *Carcinogenesis*, researchers attempted to determine if sulforaphane, a strong glucosinolate (sulfur-containing compound) polynutrient which is formed when kale and other cruciferous vegetables are chewed or chopped, could slow genetically-related cancers. To accomplish this goal, the researchers used mice that were bred to develop intestinal polyps. (Left intact, intestinal polyps may grow into colorectal cancer.) For three weeks, the mice were fed diets that were supplemented with two different doses of sulforaphane. The researchers found that the mice that were fed sulforaphane had a lower risk of tumors. When the tumors did appear, they were smaller and grew more slowly. In addition, more of the cancerous cells experienced cell death (apoptosis).[3]

Ovarian Cancer

In a European study published in 2008 in the *International Journal of Cancer*, researchers reviewed the association between six classes of flavonoids, such as those found in kale, and the risk of ovarian cancer. The study consisted of 1,031 women with confirmed epithelial ovarian cancer and 2,411 controls. The researchers found an inverse relationship between consumption of flavonoids and risk of ovarian cancer; the women who ate the higher amounts of flavonoids reduced their risk by 49 percent.[4]

Prostate Cancer

In a study published in 2007 in the *Journal of the National Cancer Institute*, Canadian researchers investigated the association between the risk of prostate cancer and intake of fruits and vegetables in 1,338 men with prostate cancer. Five hundred twenty of these men had aggressive disease. While the researchers found no association between risk of prostate cancer and intake of fruits and vegetables, the men who ate higher amounts of vegetables, especially cruciferous vegetables such as kale, had a reduced risk of the prostate cancer spreading beyond the prostate gland.[5]

TYPE 2 DIABETES

In a study published in 2008 in *Diabetes Care*, researchers reviewed the association between intake of fruit, vegetables, and fruit juice and the development of type 2 diabetes. Researchers analyzed 18 years of diet and health data from 71,346 nurses, between the ages of 38 and 63, who participated in the Nurses' Health Study from 1984 to 2002. During the follow-up years, there were 4,529 cases of diabetes. The researchers found that an increase of one serving per day of a green leafy vegetable, such as kale, was associated with a "modest" reduction in risk of type 2 diabetes. The researchers noted that the study did not prove causality and that it was limited by the reliance on self-reported data.[6] Still, with rates of type 2 diabetes rising rapidly in the United States, it may well be wise to incorporate more green leafy vegetables into the diet.

CARDIOVASCULAR HEALTH

In a study published in 2009 in the *American Journal of Clinical Nutrition,* researchers attempted to determine if a higher intake of fruit, vegetables, and dark fish would have a positive effect on cardiovascular health. As part of the Normative Aging Study, from November 2000 to June 2007, the researchers measured heart rate variability factors among 586 older men–a total of 928 observations. Researchers found a significant relationship between the consumption of green leafy vegetables, such as kale. They noted that a "higher intake of green leafy vegetables may reduce the risk of cardiovascular disease through favorable changes in cardiac autonomic function."[7]

COGNITIVE FUNCTIONING

In a study published in 2006 in *Neurology,* Chicago researchers examined the association between consumption of fruits and vegetables and rates of cognitive change in 3,718 subjects (62 percent female, 60 percent African American) who were at least 65 years old. (The average age was 74.) The researchers observed that when compared to the people who ate an average of less than one vegetable serving per day, the subjects who ate an average of 2.8 servings each day had a 40 percent decrease in cognitive decline. And, the least cognitive decline in older people was associated with intake of green leafy vegetables, such as kale.[8]

RHEUMATOID ARTHRITIS

In a prospective, population-based, case-control study published in 2004 in the *Annals of the Rheumatic Diseases,* British researchers examined the association between the consumption of fruits and vegetables and dietary antioxidants and the risk of developing rheumatoid arthritis. The cohort consisted of men and women, residents of Norfolk, UK, between the ages of 45 and 74. The researchers found that the people who developed rheumatoid arthritis had lower intakes of fruits and vegetables and vitamin C.[9] As has previously been noted, since kale is an excellent source of vitamin C, eating higher amounts of kale may well help prevent rheumatoid arthritis.

AGE-RELATED MACULAR DEGENERATION

In a study published in 2006 in the *Archives of Ophthalmology*, researchers reviewed the relationship between intake of dietary lutein and zeaxanthin, which is found in abundance in kale, and risk of intermediate age-related macular degeneration (AMD). The cohort consisted of women, between the ages of 50 and 79, who lived in Iowa, Wisconsin, and Oregon. At first, the researchers did not find any difference between the women with high and low intakes of lutein and zeaxanthin. However, when they limited the analysis to women younger than 75 years, "with stable intake of lutein plus zeaxanthin, without a history of chronic diseases that are often associated with diet changes," the lutein and zeaxanthin appeared to offer some benefit. The researchers concluded that, "Diets rich in lutein plus zeaxanthin may protect against intermediate AMD in healthy women younger than 75 years."[10]

TWO CAVEATS

The carotenoids, flavonoids, and vitamin K contained in kale are fat-soluble nutrients. That means that in order to be absorbed, they must be eaten with some form of dietary fat.[11]

Also, farmers who grow kale conventionally tend to use a good deal of pesticides. When purchasing kale, it is best to buy organically grown.

Should kale be part of the diet? Certainly.

NOTES

1. The George Mateljan Foundation Website. www.whfoods.com.

2. Boivin, Dominique, Sylvie Lamy, Simon Lord-Dufour, et al. January 15, 2009. "Antiproliferative and Antioxidant Activities of Common Vegetables: A Comparative Study." *Food Chemistry* 112(2): 374–380.

3. Hu, Rong, Tin Oo Khor, Guoxiang Shen, et al. 2006. "Cancer Chemoprevention of Intestinal Polyposis in ApcMin/+ Mice by Sulforaphane, a Natural Product Derived from Cruciferous Vegetable." *Carcinogenesis* 27(10): 2038–2046.

4. Rossi, Marta, Eva Negri, Pagona Lagiou, et al. August 15, 2008. "Flavonoids and Ovarian Cancer Risk: A Case-Control Study in Italy." *International Journal of Cancer* 123(4): 895–898.

5. Kirsh, V. A., U. Peters, S. T. Mayne, et al. August 1, 2007. "Prospective Study of Fruit and Vegetables and Risk of Prostate Cancer." *Journal of the National Cancer Institute* 99(15): 1200–1209.

6. Bazzano, Lydia A., Tricia Y. Li, Kamudi J. Joshipura, and Frank B. Hu. July 2008. "Intake of Fruit, Vegetables, and Fruit Juices and Risk of Diabetes in Women." *Diabetes Care* 31: 1311–1317.

7. Park, Sung Kyun, Katherine L. Tucker, Marie S. O'Neill, et al. March 2009. "Fruit, Vegetable, and Fish Consumption and Heart Rate Variability: the Veterans Administration Normative Aging Study." *American Journal of Clinical Nutrition* 89(3): 778–786.

8. Morris, M. C., D. A. Evans, C. C. Tangney, et al. 2006. "Association of Vegetable and Fruit Consumption with Age-Related Cognitive Change." *Neurology* 67: 1370–1376.

9. Pattison, D. J., A. J. Silman, N. J. Goodson, et al. 2004. "Vitamin C and the Risk of Developing Inflammatory Polyarthritis: Prospective Nested Case-Control Study." *Annals of Rheumatic Diseases* 63: 843–847.

10. Moeller, Suzen M., Niyati Parekh, Lesley Tinker, et al. August 2006. "Association Between Intermediate Age-Related Macular Degeneration and Lutein and Zeaxanthin in the Carotenoids in Age-Related Eye Disease Study (CAREDS)." *Archives of Ophthalmology* 124(8): 1151–1162.

11. Kohlstadt, Ingrid. May 2009. "Optimizing Metabolism: Preventing Age-Related Macular Degeneration with Leafy Greens." *Townsend Letter* 310: 109–110.

REFERENCES AND RESOURCES
Magazines, Journals, and Newspapers

Bazzano, Lydia A., Tricia Y. Li, Kamudi J. Joshipura, and Frank B. Hu. July 2008. "Intake of Fruit, Vegetables, and Fruit Juices and Risk of Diabetes in Women." *Diabetes Care* 31: 1311–1217.

Boivin, Dominique, Sylvie Lamy, Simon Lord-Dufour, et al. January 15, 2009. "Antiproliferative and Antioxidant Activities of Common Vegetables: A Comparative Study." *Food Chemistry* 112(2): 374–380.

Hu, Rong, Tin Oo Khor, Guoxiang Shen, et al. 2006. "Cancer Chemoprevention of Intestinal Polyposis in ApcMin/+ Mice by Sulforaphane, A Natural Product Derived from Cruciferous Vegetable." *Carcinogenesis* 27(10): 2038–2046.

Kirsh, V. A., U. Peters, S. T. Mayne, et al. August 1, 2007. "Prospective Study of Fruit and Vegetable Intake and Risk of Prostate Cancer." *Journal of the National Cancer Institute* 99(15): 1200–1209.

Kohlstadt, Ingrid. May 2009. "Optimizing Metabolism: Preventing Age-Related Macular Degeneration with Leafy Greens." *Townsend Letter* 310: 109–110.

Moeller, Suzen M., Niyati Parekh, Lesley Tinker, et al. August 2006. "Associations Between Intermediate Age-Related Macular Degeneration and Lutein and Zeaxanthin in the Carotenoids in Age-Related Eye Disease Study (CAREDS)." *Archives of Ophthalmology* 124(8): 1151–1162.

Morris, M. C., D. A. Evans, C. C. Tangney, et al. 2006. "Associations of Vegetable and Fruit Consumption with Age-Related Cognitive Change." *Neurology* 67: 1370–1376.

Park, Sung Kyun, Katherine L. Tucker, Marie S. O'Neill, et al. March 2009. "Fruit, Vegetable, and Fish Consumption and Heart Rate Variability: the Veterans Administration Normative Aging Study." *American Journal of Clinical Nutrition* 89(3): 778–786.

Pattison, D. J., A. J. Silman, N. J. Goodson, et al. 2004. "Vitamin C and the Risk of Developing Inflammatory Polyarthritis: Prospective Nested Case-Control Study." *Annals of Rheumatic Diseases* 63: 843–847.

Rossi, Marta, Eva Negri, Pagona Lagiou, et al. August 15, 2008. "Flavonoids and Ovarian Cancer Risk: A Case-Control Study in Italy." *International Journal of Cancer* 123(4): 895–898.

Website

The George Mateljan Foundation. www.whfoods.com.

KIWIS

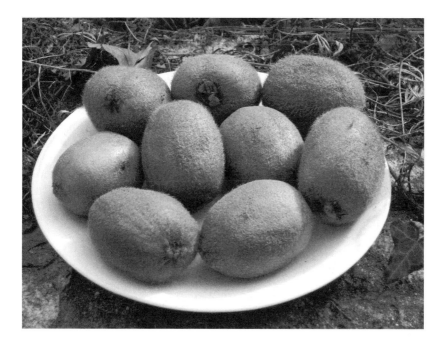

Kiwis, which are also known as kiwifruit, are fuzzy brown or gold fruits that are actually berries. They are the fruit of a vine. Named by the New Zealand Marketing Board after New Zealand's flightless bird, kiwifruit pack an enormous nutritional punch in a relatively small piece of produce.

While most people think of bananas as the fruit with high levels of potassium and oranges as an excellent source of vitamin C, two kiwis have more potassium—505 milligrams—than a banana and twice as much vitamin C—114 milligrams—as an orange. They also contain folate, magnesium, vitamins A and E, soluble and insoluble fiber, lutein, and copper. "By one scientific measure, kiwifruit has been dubbed the most nutrient dense fruit."[1] Moreover, there have been a number of intriguing research studies on these berries.

SUPPORTS HEALTH BY FIGHTING DAMAGING EFFECTS OF FREE RADICALS

Kiwis are filled with antioxidants, which neutralize the assaults of free radicals. A study that appeared in the 2007 in the *Journal of the American College of Nutrition* examined how several fruits, all known to contain high amounts of antioxidants, influenced the amount of antioxidants in the blood of volunteers. Of the fruits that they tested, the best results were obtained from grapes, kiwis, and wild blueberries. The researchers noted that the increased amounts of antioxidants in the blood were associated with a decreased risk for chronic illness. They advised people to eat high antioxidant foods with each meal.[2]

CANCER PREVENTION

Because kiwifruit is so rich in antioxidants and because it neutralizes free radicals, it may well play a role in cancer prevention. In a European study published in 2003 in *Carcinogenesis*, healthy, non-smoking volunteers, who did not take antioxidant supplement or medication, ate varying amounts of kiwis for three-week periods of time. The study times were followed by two-week washout periods. Researchers measured the ability to repair DNA oxidation with an in vitro test; concentrations of dietary antioxidants were measured in blood plasma. They found that the daily consumption of kiwis provides protection against the DNA damage that may cause cancer. "The magnitude of these effects was generally not related to the number of kiwifruits consumed per day. Kiwifruit provides a duel protection against oxidative DNA damage, enhancing antioxidant levels and stimulating DNA repair. It is probably that together these effects would decrease the risk of mutagenic changes leading to cancer."[3]

Similar findings were obtained in a study published in 2006 in *Nutrition Research*. A small group of only 12 healthy volunteers was further divided into two groups of six each. One group consumed kiwis every day; the other group ate no kiwis. As in the previous study, researchers found that the volunteers who ate kiwis had a much greater ability to repair the DNA breakage caused by free radicals. According to the researchers, eating a daily kiwi "may provide a sustainable population intervention that could reduce some of the risk factors associated with cancer."[4]

CARDIOVASCULAR HEALTH

In a study published in 2004 in *Platelets*, researchers from the University of Oslo in Norway found that eating two or three kiwifruits each day both thinned the blood, reducing the risk of blood clots, and lowered the amount of circulating fat in the blood. In the study, subjects ate two to three kiwis a day for 28 days. By the end of the study, the level of blood clotting was 18 percent lower and the amount of plasma triglyceride (fat in the blood) was reduced by 15 percent.[5] This effect was similar to taking a daily thera-peutic aspirin, but without the side effects of inflammation and gastrointes-tinal problems so often seen with the frequent use of aspirin. After the study ended, the subjects were told to remove all kiwifruit from their diets. Two weeks later, "their blood levels returned to pre-supplement period base line."[6]

Another study, published in 2009 in the *Journal of Food Sciences and Nutrition*, investigated 43 subjects who had hyperlipidemia or high levels of blood fat. Everyone ate two kiwifruits each day for eight weeks. "After eight weeks of consumption of kiwifruit, the HDL-C concentration was signifi-cantly increased and the LDL cholesterol/HDL-C ratio and total cholesterol/HDL-C ratio were significantly decreased. Vitamin C and vitamin E also increased significantly."[7] In other words, people dealing with high levels of blood fat obtain significant cardiovascular benefits from including kiwifruit in their diets.

RELIEVES CONSTIPATION

In a study conducted at the University of Hong Kong and published in 2007 in the *World Journal of Gastroenterology*, researchers recruited 33 peo-ple who suffered from constipation as well as 20 healthy volunteers. For four weeks, everyone ate a kiwifruit twice daily. The researchers noted that there was improvement not only in the constipation symptoms, "but also in terms of colonic transit times and rectal sensation." Moreover, none of the subjects reported problems with gas or bloating.[8]

In a study from New Zealand published in 2002 in the *Asia Pacific Jour-nal of Clinical Nutrition*, 38 people over the age of 60 consumed their normal diet with or without one kiwifruit for each 30 kg (each kg is equiva-lent to 2.2 pounds) of body weight. After three weeks, the subjects crossed over and consumed what they hadn't consumed during the first part of the study. Daily records chronicled the frequency of defecation and characteris-tics of the stool. The researchers noted that, "the regular use of kiwifruit appeared to lead to a bulkier and softer stool, as well as more frequent stool production."[9]

POSSIBLE RELIEF FROM BENIGN PROSTATIC HYPERPLASIA

While it is not a serious condition, benign prostatic hyperplasia (BPH), the enlargement of the prostate gland (only found in men) that often occurs as men age, may be very uncomfortable and challenging to everyday life. Men may experience urinary frequency that often disrupts sleep. A 2007 article in *Life Extension* magazine notes that members of the Life Extension Foun-dation have been reporting that eating a kiwi before bedtime has helped with their nighttime symptoms. Though there appears to be no research on the association between kiwi consumption and symptoms of BPH, men dealing with this medical problem may wish to try eating kiwi for several nights in a row.[10]

TWO CAVEATS
When Possible, Select Organic Kiwis

A study published in 2007 in the *Journal of the Science of Food and Agriculture* examined organic and conventional kiwifruits grown on the same farm in California. Researchers found that the organic fruit contained higher levels of the health-promoting factors found in kiwis such as antioxidants and vitamin C.[11]

Kiwi May Be an Allergen

In a 2004 article in *Clinical & Experimental Allergy*, researchers in South-ampton, England, maintained that allergic reactions to kiwifruit are fairly common. They note that, "kiwi fruit should be considered a significant food allergen, capable of causing severe reactions, particularly in young children."[12] Yet, this is a poorly studied field. It is known that people who tend to be allergic are more likely to be allergic to kiwi.

Should kiwis be part of the diet? Unless someone has a known allergy, absolutely.

NOTES

1. "Vibrant Green (and Gold) Kiwifruit Boasts Key Nutrients." August 2003. *Environmental Nutrition* 26(8): 8.

2. Prior, Ronald L., Liwei Gu, Xianli Wu, et al. April 2007. "Plasma Antioxidant Capacity Changes Following a Meal as a Measure of the Ability of a Food to Alter In Vivo Antioxidant Status." *Journal of the American College of Nutrition* 26(2): 170–181.

3. Collins, Andrew R., Vikki Harrington, Janice Drew, and Rachel Melvin. March 2003. "Nutritional Modulation of DNA Repair in a Human Intervention Study." *Carcinogenesis* 24(3): 511–515.

4. Rush, Elaine, Lynnette R. Ferguson, Michelle Cumin, et al. May 2006. "Kiwifruit Consumption Reduces DNA Fragility: A Randomized Controlled Pilot Study in Volunteers." *Nutrition Research* 26(5): 197–201.

5. Duttaroy, Asim K. and Aud Jørgensen. August 2004. "Effects of Kiwi Fruit Consumption on Platelet Aggregation and Plasma Lipids in Health Human Volunteers." *Platelets* 15(5): 287–292.

6. "Kiwifruit and Aspirin Have Similar Effects for Heart Health, Study Shows." October 20, 2004. *Heart Disease Weekly*: 68.

7. Chang, W. H. and J. F. Liu. February 2009. "Effects of Kiwifruit Consumption on Serum Lipid Profiles and Antioxidative Status in Hyperlipidemic Subjects." *Journal of Food Sciences and Nutrition* 19: 1–8.

8. On On Chan, Annie, Gigi Leung, Teresa Tong, and Nina YH Wong. September 21, 2007. "Increasing Dietary Fiber Intake in Terms of Kiwifruit Improves

Constipation in Chinese Patients." *World Journal of Gastroenterology* 13(35): 4771–4775.

9. Rush, Elaine C., Meena Patel, Lindsay D. Plank, and Lynnette R. Ferguson. 2002. "Kiwifruit Promotes Laxation in the Elderly." *Asia Pacific Journal of Clinical Nutrition* 11(2): 164–168.

10. Weinmann, Ed. September 2007. "Does Kiwi Relieve Prostate Symptoms?" *Life Extension*: NA.

11. Amodio, Maria L., Giancarlo Colelli, Janine K. Hasey, and Adel A. Kader. 2007. "A Comparative Study of Composition and Postharvest Performance of Organically and Conventionally Grown Kiwifruits." *Journal of the Science of Food and Agriculture* 87(7): 1228–1236.

12. Lucas, J. S. A., K. E. C. Grimshaw, K. Collins, et al. 2004. "Kiwi Fruit is a Significant Allergen and Is Associated with Differing Patterns of Reactivity in Children and Adults." *Clinical & Experimental Allergy* 34(7): 1115–1121.

REFERENCES AND RESOURCES
Magazine, Journals, and Newspapers

Amodio, Maria L., Giancarlo Colelli, Janine K. Hasey, and Adel A. Kader. 2007. "A Comparative Study of Composition and Postharvest Performance of Organically and Conventionally Grown Kiwifruits." *Journal of the Science of Food and Agriculture* 87(7): 1228–1236.

Chang, W. H. and J. F. Liu. February 2009. "Effects of Kiwifruit Consumption on Serum Lipid Profiles and Antioxidative Status in Hyperlipidemic Subjects." *Journal of Food Sciences and Nutrition* 19: 1–8.

Collins, Andrew R., Vikki Harrington, Janice Drew, and Rachel Melvin. March 2003. "Nutritional Modulation of DNA Repair in a Human Intervention Study." *Carcinogenesis* 24(3): 511–515.

Duttaroy, Asim K. and Aud Jørgensen. August 2005. "Effects of Kiwi Fruit Consumption on Platelet Aggregation and Plasma Lipids in Health Human Volunteers." *Platelets* 15(5): 287–292.

"Kiwifruit and Aspirin Have Similar Effects for Heart Health, Study Shows." October 10, 2004. *Heart Disease Weekly*: 68.

Lucas, J. S. A., K. E. C. Grimshaw, K. Collins, et al. 2004. "Kiwi Fruit is a Significant Allergen and Is Associated with Differing Patterns of Reactivity in Children and Adults." *Clinical & Experimental Allergy* 34(7): 1115–1121.

On On Chan, Annie, Gigi Leung, Teresa Tong, and Nina YH Wong. September 21, 2007. "Increasing Dietary Fiber Intake in Terms of Kiwifruit Improves Constipation in Chinese Patients." *World Journal of Gastroenterology* 13(35): 4771–4775.

Prior, Ronald L. March 2008. "A Daily Dose of Antioxidants?" *Agricultural Research* 56(3): 4–5.

Prior, Ronald L., Liwei Gu, Xianli Wu, et al. April 2007. "Plasma Antioxidant Capacity Changes Following a Meal as a Measure of the Ability of a Food to Alter In Vivo Antioxidant Status." *Journal of the American College of Nutrition* 26(2): 170–181.

Rush, Elaine, Lynnette R. Ferguson, Michelle Cumin, et al. May 2006. "Kiwifruit Consumption Reduces DNA Fragility: A Randomized Controlled Pilot Study in Volunteers." *Nutrition Research* 26(5): 197–201.

Rush, Elaine C., Meena Patel, Lindsay D. Plank, and Lynnette R. Ferguson. 2002. "Kiwifruit Promotes Laxation in the Elderly." *Asia Pacific Journal of Clinical Nutrition* 11(2): 164–168.

"Vibrant Green (and Gold) Kiwifruit Boost Key Nutrients." August 2003. *Environmental Nutrition* 26(8): 8.

Weinmann, Ed. September 2007. "Does Kiwi Relieve Prostate Symptoms?" *Life Extension*: NA.

Website

Biotechnology Learning Hub. www.biotechlearn.org.

LEMONS AND LIMES

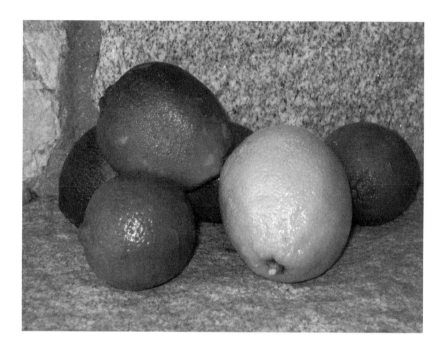

Though often used interchangeably, lemons and limes actually have separate histories. And, of course, they look quite different. Lemons are larger and yellow in color; limes are considerably smaller and green.

A cross between limes and citrons, lemons are thought to have originated in China or India about 2,500 years ago. Around the 11th century, Arabs brought lemons to Europe and North America. After finding lemons in Palestine, the crusaders traveled with them to still other European countries. And, it was in 1493, during his second voyage to the "New World," that Christopher Columbus took along lemons. By the 16th century, they were growing in what is now Florida. Today, the major commercial growers of lemons are the United States, Italy, Spain, Greece, Israel, and Turkey.[1]

Meanwhile, limes are believed to have originated in Southeast Asia. It is thought that around the 10th century, Arabs who traveled to Asia brought limes back to Egypt and Northern Africa. In the 13th century, Arab Moors introduced them to Spain. From there, limes spread throughout southern Europe. As with lemons, limes traveled on Christopher Columbus' second voyage to America. And, it was Columbus and his fellow explorers who introduced them to Caribbean countries. By the 16th century, they were growing in the United States. In addition to the United States, limes are now primarily grown in Brazil and Mexico.[2]

Both lemons and limes are excellent sources of vitamin C. Because the human body is unable to store vitamin C, it is needed in the daily diet. A 2009 article in *Environmental Nutrition* noted that lemons have twice the amount of vitamin C as limes; but, a single lemon contains about half the daily requirement for vitamin C. Furthermore, "both of these citrus cousins also contain potassium, as well as cancer-protecting antioxidants and bioflavonoids.[3] But, what have the researchers learned?

CARDIOVASCULAR HEALTH

In a study published in 2008 in *The American Journal of Clinical Nutrition*, British researchers examined the association between the amount of vitamin C, such as the vitamin C contained in lemons and limes, in blood plasma and the risk of incident stroke in the British population. The researchers reviewed data on 20,649 men and women between the ages of 40 and 70. At the time the data were collected, none of the subjects had suffered a stroke.

Over the course of 196,713 total person years (the average follow-up was 9.5 years), there were 448 incident strokes. The subjects in the top quartiles of baseline plasma vitamin C concentrations had a 42 percent lower risk of stroke than those in the bottom quartile. The researchers noted that, "Plasma vitamin C concentrations may serve as a biological marker of lifestyle or other factors associated with reduced stroke risk and may be useful in identifying those at high risk of stroke."[4]

In a similar study published in 2002 in *Stroke*, Finnish researchers attempted to determine if the amount of vitamin C in blood plasma could reduce the risk of strokes in hypertensive and overweight men from eastern Finland. The 10.4-year prospective population-based cohort study included 2,419 randomly selected men between the ages of 42 and 60. At baseline, no one had a history of a stroke. During the study, 120 had strokes. Of these, 96 were ischemic and 24 hemorrhagic.

The researchers found that the men with the lowest levels of plasma vitamin C had a 2.4 fold risk of any stroke compared with the men with the highest levels of vitamin C. They noted that, "Low plasma vitamin C was associated with increased risk of stroke, especially among hypertensive and overweight men."[5]

In a cross-sectional study published in 2006 in *The American Journal of Clinical Nutrition*, British researchers reviewed whether high dietary intake and high circulating concentrations of vitamin C could protect against ischemic heart disease, a medical problem in which there is an insufficient amount of blood and oxygen reaching the heart muscle. The study included 3,258 men, between the ages of 60 and 79 years, with no physician diagnosis of myocardial infarction, stroke, or diabetes. All the men were drawn from general practices in 24 British towns.

The researchers found that a diet rich in sources of vitamin C, such as lemons and limes, was associated with a 45 percent reduced risk of inflammation (with respect to levels of C-reactive protein). And, a high fruit intake was related to a 25 percent reduced risk of inflammation. The researchers concluded that, "vitamin C has anti-inflammatory effects and is associated with lower endothelial dysfunction in men with no history of cardiovascular disease or diabetes."[6]

KIDNEY STONE RECURRENCES

In a study published in 2007 in *The Journal of Urology*, researchers at the Duke University Medical Center in Durham, North Carolina, attempted to determine if lemonade therapy was useful for people with hypocitraturia, a medical condition in which low levels of urinary citrate are excreted, placing people at increased risk for kidney stone formation. The study included four males and seven females, with a mean age of 52.7 years. The subjects were treated with lemonade therapy for a mean of 44.4 months. The lemonade therapy consisted of 120 ml per day of concentrated lemon juice containing 5.9 g of citric acid. It was mixed with two liters of water and consumed throughout the day. The control group also had four males and seven females, with a mean age of 54.5 years. They were treated with potassium citrate for a mean of 42.5 months.

The researchers found that of the eleven people on lemonade therapy, ten had increases in their levels of urinary citrate; all the people in the control group had increases in urinary citrate levels. Moreover, during lemonade therapy, the stone formation rate dropped from 1.00 per person per year at baseline to 0.13 per year. The researchers noted that, "Due to its significant citraturic effect, lemonade therapy appears to be a reasonable alternative for patients with hypocitraturia who cannot tolerate first line therapy."[7]

GASTRIC CANCER

In a study published in 2008 in *Gastric Cancer*, Korean and Canadian researchers investigated the association between the dietary intake of citrus fruit and the risk of gastric (stomach) cancer. After searching the electronic databases and reference lists of publications, the researchers located 14 articles that dealt with the topic. The articles included six hospital-based case-control studies, six community-based case control studies, and two cohort studies. The researchers found that a high intake of citrus, such as contained in lemons and limes, was associated with a 28 percent reduction in the risk of stomach cancer. They noted that the, "pooled results from observational studies support a protective effect of high citrus fruit intake in the risk of stomach cancer."[8]

ONE CAVEAT—LEMON AND LIME JUICE—ARE ACIDIC

In a 20-week laboratory study published in 2009 in *General Dentistry*, Mohammed A. Bassiouny, DMD, MSc, PhD, of the Kornberg School of Dentistry, Temple University in Philadelphia, Pennsylvania, exposed teeth to two types of soda, green and black tea, and three juices, including lemon juice. Vinegar and water served as the controls. Dr. Bassiouny found that the lemon juice "demonstrated the highest erosive damage to enamel topography and morphology within the first four weeks." Additionally, "Among lemon juice specimens, the majority of enamel caps were lost by the four-week assessment. By week eight, the exposed coronal dentin core and root trunk displayed a leathery consistency that flaked easily upon exploration, although no volume change of dentin was noticeable."[9] Though these results may sound startling, they should not cause people to avoid lemons and limes. People should remember that saliva and the consumption of fluids reduce some of the erosion. Also, after exposure to acidic foods, it may be useful to rinse or brush the teeth.

Should lemons and limes be included in the diet? Absolutely.

NOTES

1. The George Mateljan Foundation Website. www.whfoods.com.

2. The George Mateljan Foundation Website.

3. Schepers, Anastasia. June 2009. "Pucker Up for Lemons and Limes: Tart, Refreshing and Healthful." *Environmental Nutrition* 32(6): 8.

4. Myint, P. K., R. N. Luben, A. A. Welch, et al. January 2008. "Plasma Vitamin C Concentrations Predict Risk of Incident Stroke Over 10 Years in 20,649 Participants in European Prospective Investigation into Cancer Norfolk Prospective Population Study." *The American Journal of Clinical Nutrition* 87(1): 5–7.

5. Kurl, S., T. P. Tuomainen, J. A. Laukkanen, et al. June 2002. "Plasma Vitamin C Modifies the Association Between Hypertension and Risk of Stroke." *Stroke* 33(6): 1568–1573.

6. Wannamethee, S. Goya, Gordon D. O. Lowe, Ann Rumley, et al. March 2006. "Association of Vitamin C Status, Fruit and Vegetable Intakes, and Markers of Inflammation and Hemostasis." *The American Journal of Clinical Nutrition* 83(3): 567–574.

7. Kang, David E., Roger L. Sur, George E. Haleblian, et al. April 2007. "Long-Term Lemonade Based Dietary Manipulation in Patients with Hypocitraturic Nephrolithiasis." *The Journal of Urology* 177(4): 1358–1362.

8. Bae, Jong-Myon, Eun Ja Lee, and Gordon Guyatt. March 2008. "Citrus Fruit Intake and Stomach Cancer Risk." *Gastric Cancer* 11(1): 23–32.

9. Bassiouny, Mohammed A. June 2009. "Effects of Common Beverages on the Development of Cervical Erosion Lesions." *General Dentistry* 57(3): 212–223.

REFERENCES AND RESOURCES
Magazines, Journals, and Newspapers

Bae, Jong-Myon, Eun Ja Lee, and Gordon Guyatt. March 2008. "Citrus Fruit Intake and Stomach Cancer Risk." *Gastric Cancer* 11(1): 23–32.

Bassiouny, Mohammed A. June 2009. "Effects of Common Beverage on the Development of Cervical Erosion Lesions." *General Dentistry* 57(3): 212–223.

Kang, David E., Roger L. Sur, George E. Haleblian, et al. April 2007. "Long-Term Lemonade Based Dietary Manipulation in Patients with Hypocitraturic Nephrolithiasis." *The Journal of Urology* 177(4): 1358–1362.

Kurl, S., T. P. Tuomainen, J. A. Laukkanen, et al. June 2002. "Plasma Vitamin C Modifies the Association Between Hypertension and Risk of Stroke." *Stroke* 33(6): 1568–1573.

Myint, P. K., R. N. Luben, A. A. Welch, et al. January 2008. "Plasma Vitamin C Concentrations Predict Risk of Incident Stroke Over 10 Years in 20,649 Participants in European Prospective Investigation into Cancer Norfolk Prospective Population Study." *The American Journal of Clinical Nutrition* 87(1): 5–7.

Schepers, Anastasia. June 2009. "Pucker Up for Lemons and Limes: Tart, Refreshing and Healthful." *Environmental Nutrition* 32(6): 8.

Wannamethee, S. Goya, Gordon D. O. Lowe, Ann Rumley, et al. March 2006. "Association of Vitamin C Status, Fruit and Vegetable Intakes, and Markers of Inflammation and Hemostasis." *The American Journal of Clinical Nutrition* 83(3): 567–574.

Website

The George Mateljan Foundation. www.whfoods.com.

LENTILS

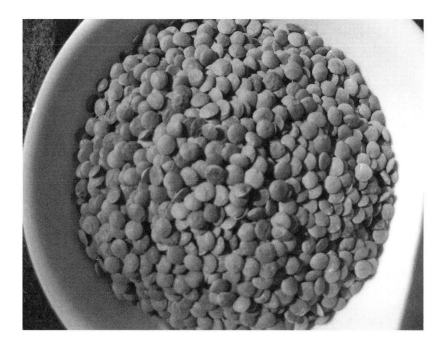

Consumed since prehistoric times, lentils (*Lens culinaris*) are thought to have originated in central Asia. These members of the legume family, which also includes peas, beans, soybeans, and peanuts, were one of the first foods to be cultivated. In fact, lentil seeds have been found in Middle East archeological sites that are 8,000 years old, and lentils are mentioned in the Bible.

For years, lentils have been considered a very healthful food. While they have almost no fat, they are thought to be high in minerals, two B vitamins and protein. At the same time, lentils have high amounts of soluble and insoluble fiber and are believed to be good sources for iron, copper, thiamin, magnesium, potassium, and phosphorus.[1] But, what does the research show?

CARDIOVASCULAR HEALTH

A study published in 2001 in the *Archives of Internal Medicine* examined the association between consumption of legumes, such as lentils, and the risk of coronary heart disease in men and women in the United States. Over an average of 19 years of follow-up, researchers evaluated almost 10,000 people who participated in the first National Health and Nutrition Examination Survey (NHANES) Epidemiologic Follow-Up Study (NHEFS). In the beginning of the study, everyone was free of cardiovascular disease. During the study, there were 1,802 cases of coronary heart disease and 3,880 cases of cardiovascular disease. People who ate legumes four or more times per week had a 22 percent lower risk of coronary heart disease and an 11 percent lower risk of cardiovascular disease when compared to those who ate legumes less than once a week.[2]

In 2002, another study of the same cohort was published in the journal *Stroke*. This time, the researchers reviewed the association between the dietary intake of folate and the risk of stroke and cardiovascular disease. Lentils are known to contain high amounts of folate, a water-soluble B vitamin that occurs naturally in food. (The synthetic version is folic acid.) The researchers found that the subjects who consumed the most folate (an average of 405 micrograms per day) had a 21 percent lower risk for stroke and a 14 percent lower risk for cardiovascular disease than those who consumed the least folate (an average of 99 micrograms per day).[3]

Two years later, *Stroke* reported on a Boston-area study of folate intake and the risk of stroke among women. Using data from the Nurses' Health Study, which included 83,272 females nurses between the ages of 34 and 59 who were followed for up to 18 years, the researchers identified 1,140 cases of stroke. Yet, they were unable to find any "appreciable association between the intake of folate and total incidence of stroke."[4]

Then, in 2005, *Stroke* published the work of Swedish researchers who studied the relationship between folate, B_{12}, and ischemic (caused by blockage of artery in the brain) and hemorrhagic (caused by burst vessel inside the brain) strokes. The researchers examined the blood and dietary levels of folate in 334 people who had an ischemic stroke and 62 people who had a hemorrhagic stroke. While no relationship was found between folate and ischemic stroke, folate appeared to have a protective role against hemorrhagic stroke.[5]

DIABETES

In a study published in 2008 in *The American Journal of Clinical Nutrition*, researchers from Vanderbilt University Medical Center in Nashville, Tennessee, joined with researchers from Shanghai, China, to determine if a higher intake of legumes, such as lentils, and soy foods reduced the risk of developing type 2 diabetes in 64,227 middle-aged Chinese women. At the beginning of the study, none of the subjects had a history of type 2 diabetes, cancer, or cardiovascular disease. The subjects were followed for an average of 4.6 years. Researchers found that the consumption of legumes and soy foods was inversely associated with the risk of type 2 diabetes in premenopausal and postmenopausal women. According to the study, a higher intake of legumes was associated with a reduced risk of type 2 diabetes.[6]

In another study published in 2008 in *JAMA, The Journal of the American Medical Association*, Canadian researchers investigated whether people with type 2 diabetes did better if they ate a diet high in low-glycemic foods (that release energy slowly), such as lentils, or ate a diet that placed more emphasis on high-cereal fiber foods. The 210 participants in the study were randomly assigned to receive one of the two diets for a period of six months. In addition to lentils, in the low-glycemic diet participants ate beans, peas, nuts, pasta, and rice that was briefly boiled; in the high-cereal fiber diet, the participants ate whole grain breakfast cereals, brown rice, potatoes with skins, and whole wheat bread, crackers, and breakfast cereals. The researchers found that people with type 2 diabetes experienced more improvement in glycemic control on the low-glycemic diet than on the high-cereal fiber diet.[7]

BREAST CANCER

A study published in 2005 in the *International Journal of Cancer* used information provided on 90,630 nurses in the Nurses' Health Study II to evaluate an association between the consumption of a type of flavonol found in legumes, such as lentils and beans, and the incidence of breast cancer. The researchers noted that animal studies have linked diets high in flavonols with a reduced risk of breast cancer. During the eight years of follow-up, there were 710 reported cases of breast cancer. While the researchers found no relationship between breast cancer and overall flavonol intake or consumption of flavonol-rich foods, they did observe that the women who consumed lentils (or beans) at least twice a week were 24 percent less likely to develop breast cancer than the women who consumed these foods less than one time per month.[8]

In a study published in 2009 in *The American Journal of Clinical Nutrition*, researchers investigated the association between dietary patterns and breast cancer risk in Asian Americans. The study, which was conducted in Los Angeles County, included 1,248 Asian American women with breast cancer and 1,148 controls who were matched by age, ethnicity, and neighborhoods. Researchers found that the women who ate more meat and starch had the highest rates of breast cancer; those who ate more legumes, such as lentils and soy foods, had the lowest risk.[9]

WEIGHT LOSS

In research that was published in *Cochrane Database of Systemic Reviews 2007*, Australian researchers studied the effects of eating foods that release energy slowly (low glycemic index) to foods that rapidly release sugar into the bloodstream (high glycemic index). In total, they examined six randomized control trials that included 202 subjects. The trials lasted from five weeks to six months. The researchers found that people who consumed foods, like lentils, with a low glycemic index instead of foods, like white bread, with a high glycemic index, were more likely to lose weight. According to Dr. Diana Thomas, the lead author of the study, a low-glycemic diet seems to be particularly useful for those who are obese. Moreover, she said that, "it may be easier to adhere to a low glycemic diet than a conventional weight loss diet, since there is less need to restrict the intake of food so long as the carbohydrates consumed have a low glycemic index."[10]

Should lentils be included in the diet? Unless one is allergic to them or experiences digestive problems when they are eaten, people should most definitely eat more lentil-rich foods.

NOTES

1. The George Mateljan Foundation Website. http://whfoods.com.

2. Bazzano, Lydia A., Jiang He, Lorraine G. Ogden, et al. November 21, 2001. "Legume Consumption and Risk of Coronary Heart Disease in US Men and Women." *Archives of Internal Medicine* 161(21): 2573–2578.

3. Bazzano, Lydia A., Jiang He, Lorraine G. Ogden, et al. May 2002. "Dietary Intake of Folate and Risk of Stroke in US Men and Women." *Stroke* 33(5): 1183–1189.

4. Al-Delaimy, Wael K., Kathryn M. Rexrode, Frank B. Hu, et al. June 2004. "Folate Intake and Risk of Stroke Among Women." *Stroke* 35(6): 1259–1263.

5. Van Guelpen, Bethany, Johan Hultdin, Ingegerd Johansson, et al. July 2005. "Folate, Vitamin B_{12}, and Risk of Ischemic and Hemorrhagic Stroke." *Stroke* 36(7): 1426–1431.

6. Villegas, Raquel, Yu-Tang Gao, Gong Yang, et al. January 2008. "Legume and Soy Food Intake and the Incidence of Type 2 Diabetes in the Shanghai Women's Health Study." *The American Journal of Clinical Nutrition* 87(1): 162–167.

7. Jenkins, David J. A., Cyril W. C. Kendall, Gail McKeown-Eyssen, et al. December 17, 2008. "Effect of a Low-Glycemic Index or a High-Cereal Fiber Diet on Type 2 Diabetes: A Randomized Trial." *JAMA, The Journal of the American Medical Association* 300(23): 2742–2753.

8. Adebamowo, Clement A., Eunyoung Cho, Laura Sampson, et al. April 20, 2005. "Dietary Flavonols and Flavonol-Rich Foods Intake and the Risk of Breast Cancer." *International Journal of Cancer* 114(4): 628–633.

9. Wu, Anna H., Mimi C. Yu, Chiu-Chen Tseng, et al. April 2009. "Dietary Patterns and Breast Cancer Risk in Asian American Women." *The American Journal of Clinical Nutrition* 89(4): 1145–1154.

10. Thomas, D. E., E. J. Elliott, and L. Baur. 2007. "Low Glycaemic Index or Low Glycaemic Load Diets for Overweight and Obesity." *Cochrane Database of Systematic Reviews 2007*. On website of The Cochrane Collaboration. http://www.cochrane.org.

RESOURCES AND REFERENCES
Magazines, Journals, and Newspapers

Adebamowo, Clement A., Eunyoung Cho, Laura Simpson, et al. April 20, 2005. "Dietary Flavonols and Flavonol-Rich Foods Intake and the Risk of Breast Cancer." *International Journal of Cancer* 114(4): 628–633.

Al-Delaimy, Wael K., Kathryn M. Rexrode, Frank Hu, et al. June, 2004. "Folate Intake and Risk of Stroke Among Women." *Stroke* 35(6): 1259–1263.

Bazzano, Lydia A., Jiang He, Lorraine G. Ogden, et al. November 26, 2001. "Legume Consumption and Risk of Coronary Heart Disease in US Men and Women." *Archives of Internal Medicine* 161(21): 2573–2578.

Bazzano, Lydia A., Jiang He, Lorraine G. Ogden, et al. May 2002. "Dietary Intake of Folate and Risk of Stroke in US Men and Women." *Stroke* 33(5): 1183–1189.

Jenkins, David J. A., Cyril W. C. Kendall, Gail McKeown-Eyssen, et al. December 17, 2008. "Effect of a Low-Glycemic Index or a High-Cereal Diet on Type 2 Diabetes: A Randomized Trial." *JAMA, The Journal of the American Medical Association* 300(23): 2742–2753.

Thomas, D. E., E. J. Elliott, and L. Baur. 2007. "Low Glycaemic Index or Low Glycaemic Load Diets for Overweight and Obesity." *Cochrane Database of Systemic Reviews 2007* Issue 3. On website for The Cochrane Collaboration, http://www.cochrane.org.

Van Guelpen, Bethany, Johan Hultdin, Ingegerd Johnsson, et al. July 2005. "Folate, Vitamin B_{12}, and Risk of Oschemic and Hemorrhagic Stroke." *Stroke* 36(7): 1426–1431.

Villegas, Raquel, Yu-Tang Gao, Gong Yang, et al. January 2008. "Legume and Soy Food Intake and the Incidence of Type 2 Diabetes in the Shanghai Women's Health Study." *The American Journal of Clinical Nutrition* 87(1): 162–167.

Wu, Anna H., Mimi C. Yu, Chiu-Chen Tseng, et al. April 2009. "Dietary Patterns and Breast Cancer Risk in Asian American Women." *The American Journal of Clinical Nutrition* 89(4): 1145–1154.

Websites

The Cochrane Collaboration. http://www.cochrane.org.
The George Mateljan Foundation. http://whfoods.com.

MACADAMIA NUTS

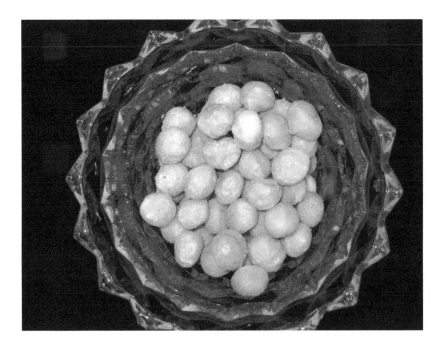

Even though the indigenous people of Australia were well aware of macadamia nuts, which they called "kindal kindal," it was not until the mid-nineteenth century that two European botanists discovered them growing in the rain forests of the eastern part of the country. The botanists named their finding after their friend Dr. John Macadam.[1]

Initially, macadamia nut trees were considered to be ornamental. But, in the 1890s, after the trees arrived on the shores of Hawaii, people began growing the nuts for human consumption. Still, it is important to note that macadamia nuts may be grown only in certain environments. They require tropical temperatures and abundant amounts of rain. While Australia and South Africa are the two top producing countries, macadamia nuts are also grown in the United States (Hawaii, California, and Florida), Guatemala, Brazil, Costa Rica, Malawi, Zimbabwe, and Kenya.[2]

Macadamia nuts are filled with fats. In fact, each 100 g of raw macadamia nuts consists of 74 g of fat. However, of the 74 g of fat, 60 g is monounsaturated (primarily oleic and palmitoleic acids), which is generally believed to be extremely healthful. Another 4 g is polyunsaturated fat, and 10 g is saturated. Macadamia nuts are high in potassium and phosphorus, and they have good amounts of protein, carbohydrates, dietary fiber, magnesium, and calcium. Furthermore, the nuts have small amounts of zinc, iron, selenium, manganese, copper, folate, niacin, and vitamins B_1, B_2, B_5, B_6, and E. They have polyphenols, which are antioxidant phytochemicals, and phytosterols, which are plant sterols.[3]

For years, people who were fearful of the high fat content of macadamia nuts avoided them. During the past decade or so, that seems to have changed. Still, the research on macadamia nuts is somewhat limited and has focused on cardiovascular health.

CARDIOVASCULAR HEALTH

In a study published in 2000 in the *Archives of Internal Medicine*, 30 volunteers between the ages of 18 and 53 were evaluated in a randomized crossover trial of three different 30-day diets: the "typical American" diet that is high in saturated fat, with 37 percent energy from fat; the American Heart Association Step 1 diet, which has 30 percent of energy from fat; and a macadamia nut-based monounsaturated fat diet, with 37 percent energy from fat. The researchers found that when compared with the typical American diet, the subjects eating the American Heart Association diet and the macadamia nut diets had significant reductions in total cholesterol and LDL ("bad") cholesterol. The subjects eating the macadamia nut based diet also experienced more reduction in their triglyceride values than the subjects eating the other two diets. The researchers concluded that the consumption of a diet with higher amounts of macadamia nuts seemed to lower levels of cholesterol "when total energy balance and percentage of energy from fat are maintained." As a result, "physicians can recommend the consumption of these and other nuts as part of a satisfying and healthy diet."[4]

A few years later, in 2003, Australian researchers reported on a similar study in *The Journal of Nutrition*. Their investigation included 17 men (mean age of 54 years) with elevated levels of cholesterol. For four weeks, the men ate 40 to 90 g/day of macadamia nuts; the amount of nuts was equivalent to a 15 percent energy intake. At the end of the study, the researchers determined that the total and LDL cholesterol levels in the men had been reduced by up to 5.3 percent. Levels of HDL ("good") cholesterol increased by 7.9 percent. The researchers noted, "This study demonstrated that macadamia nut consumption as part of a healthy diet favorably modifies the plasma lipid profile in hypercholesterolemic men despite their diet being high in fat."[5]

The next year, in 2004, Japanese researchers reported on their investigation of macadamia nut consumption in healthy, young Japanese women in *Clinical and Experimental Pharmacology and Physiology*. For three weeks, the women were placed on diets containing larger amounts of macadamia nuts, coconuts, or butter. At the end of the study, the researchers found that the women eating extra macadamia nuts and coconuts had significantly lowered levels of total cholesterol and LDL cholesterol. The group eating the macadamia nuts had a lowered body weight and body mass index. There were no statistically significant changes in the group who ate additional amounts of butter.[6]

Meanwhile, researchers from South Africa decided to conduct a systematic review of published research studies that have examined the effects of nuts on lipids. Their results were published in 2005 in *The Journal of Nutrition*. Twenty-three studies on almonds, peanuts, walnuts, and macadamia nuts were included. There was also one study on pecans. Except for macadamia nuts, all the studies showed that the consumption of nuts resulted in decreases of total cholesterol between 2 and 16 percent and decreases in LDL cholesterol between 2 and 19 percent. Commenting on the results from the macadamia nuts, the researchers noted that the "consumption of macadamia nuts (50–100 g/day) produced less convincing results."[7]

In a study published in 2007 in *Lipids*, the previously noted Australian researchers (plus one additional researcher) reviewed the information they had gathered on 17 men with elevated levels of cholesterol to determine if the consumption of macadamia nuts could have other cardiovascular benefits. The researchers found that the consumption of macadamia nuts did indeed have favorable effects on the "biomarkers of oxidative stress, thrombosis and inflammation, the risk factors for coronary artery disease." And, this occurred despite the increased intake of dietary fat, from the nuts. The researchers wrote "that regular consumption of macadamia nuts may play a role in the prevention of coronary artery disease."[8]

In a study published in 2008 in *The Journal of Nutrition*, researchers from Pennsylvania State University assigned 25 men and women with mildly elevated levels of cholesterol to one of two groups. One group added 1.5 ounces per day of macadamia nuts to their diets; the second group ate an average American diet. While the amount of fat in both diets remained essentially the same, the percentages of saturated and monounsaturated fats differed. The macadamia nut diet contained seven percent saturated fat, 18 percent monounsaturated fat, and five percent polyunsaturated fat. The standard American diet had 13 percent saturated fat, 11 percent monounsaturated fat, and five percent polyunsaturated fat. After five weeks, the subjects ate the alternate diet for another five weeks. The researchers determined that the subjects who ate macadamia nuts experienced a 9.4 percent reduction in total cholesterol and an 8.9 percent reduction in LDL cholesterol. The researchers concluded that, "macadamia nuts can be included in a heart-healthy dietary pattern that reduces lipid/lipoprotein CVD [cardiovascular]-risk factors. Nuts as an isocaloric [having similar caloric value] substitute for SFA [saturated fatty acid] foods increase the proportion of unsaturated fatty acids and decrease SFA, thereby lowering CVD risk."[9]

In a 12- to 18-week study conducted at the Human Nutrition Research Center on Aging at Tufts University and published in *The Journal of Nutrition* in 2009, researchers investigated the effects of diets enriched in canola, safflower, macadamia, or palm/coconut oils on the liprotein profiles and atherosclerosis of hamsters. (Some of the hamsters initially fed palm oil were later fed coconut oil.) When compared to the hamsters fed the palm/coconut diet, the hamsters fed the macadamia oil diet had lower non-HDL cholesterol and triglyceride values. When compared to the hamsters fed the coconut, canola, and safflower oil, the hamsters fed the macadamia nut oil had higher HDL cholesterol.[10]

Should macadamia nuts be included in the diet? Unless there is an allergy or intolerance to tree nuts, there is no reason to exclude them. And, there is a good chance that they are quite beneficial.

NOTES

1. Macadamia Advice Center Website. www.macadamias.org.uk.

2. Macadamia Advice Center Website.

3. Macadamia Advice Center Website.

4. Curb, J. David, Gilbert Wergowske, Joan C. Dobbs, et al. April 24, 2000. "Serum Lipid Effects of a High-Monounsaturated Fat Diet Based on Macadamia Nuts." *Archives of Internal Medicine* 160: 1154–1158.

5. Garg, Manohar L., Robert J. Blake, and Ron B. H. Wills. April 2003. "Macadamia Nut Consumption Lowers Plasma Total and LDL Cholesterol Levels in Hypercholesterolemic Men." *The Journal of Nutrition* 133(4): 1060–1063.

6. Hiraoka-Yamamoto J., K. Ikeda, H. Negishi, et al. December 2004. "Serum Lipid Effects of a Monounsaturated (Palmitoleic) Fatty Acid-Rich Diet Based on Macadamia Nuts in Healthy, Young Japanese Women." *Clinical and Experimental Pharmacology and Physiology* 31 Supplement 2: S37–S38.

7. Mukudden-Petersen, Janine, Welma Oosthuizen, and Johann C. Jerling. September 2005. "A Systematic Review of the Effects of Nuts on Blood Lipid Profiles in Humans." *The Journal of Nutrition* 135(9): 2082–2089.

8. Garg, Manohar L., Robert J. Blake, Ron B. H. Wills, and Edward H. Clayton. June 2007. "Macadamia Nut Consumption Modulates Favourably Risk Factors for Coronary Artery Disease in Hypercholesterolemic Subjects." *Lipids* 42(6): 583–587.

9. Griel, Amy E., Yumei Cao, Deborah D. Bagshaw, et al. April 2008. "A Macadamia Nut-Rich Diet Reduces Total and LDL-Cholesterol in Mildly Hypercholesterolemic Men and Women." *The Journal of Nutrition* 138: 761–767.

10. Matthan. Nirupa R., Alice Dillard, Jaime L. Lecker, et al. February 2009. "Effects of Dietary Palmitoleic Acid on Plasma Lipoprotein Profile and Aortic Cholesterol Accumulation Are Similar to Those of Other Unsaturated Fatty Acids in the F1B Golden Syrian Hamster." *The Journal of Nutrition* 139(2): 215–221.

REFERENCES AND RESOURCES
Magazines, Journals, and Newspapers

Curb, J. David, Gilbert Wergowske, Joan C. Dobbs, et al. April 24, 2000. "Serum Lipid Effects on a High-Monounsaturated Fat Diet Based on Macadamia Nuts." *Archives of Internal Medicine* 160: 1154–1158.

Garg, Manohar L., Robert J. Blake, and Ron B. H. Wills. April 2003. "Macadamia Nut Consumption Lowers Plasma Total and LDL Cholesterol Levels in Hypercholesterolemic Men." *The Journal of Nutrition* 133(4): 1060–1063.

Garg, Manohar L., Robert Blake, Ron B. H. Wills, and Edward H. Clayton. June 2007. "Macadamia Nut Consumption Modulates Favourably Risk Factors for Coronary Artery Disease in Hypercholesterolemic Subjects." *Lipids* 42(6): 583–587.

Griel, Amy E., Yumei Cao, Deborah D. Bagshaw, et al. April 2008. "A Macadamia Nut-Rich Diet Reduces Total and LDL-Cholesterol in Mildly Hypercholesterolemic Men and Women." *The Journal of Nutrition* 138: 761–767.

Hiraoka-Yamamoto, J., K. Ikeda, H. Negishi, et al. December 2004. "Serum Lipid Effects of Monounsaturated (Palmitoleic) Fatty Acid-Rich Diet Based on Macadamia Nuts in Healthy, Young Japanese Women." *Clinical Experimental Pharmacology and Physiology* 31 Supplement 2: S37–S38.

Matthan, Nirupa R., Alice Dillard, Jaime L. Lecker, et al. February 2009. "Effects of Dietary Palmitoleic Acid on Plasma Lipoprotein Profile and Aortic Cholesterol Accumulation Are Similar to Those of Other Unsaturated Fatty Acids in the F1B Golden Syrian Hamster." *The Journal of Nutrition* 139(2): 215–221.

Mukuddem-Petersen, Janine, Welma Oosthuizen, and Johann C. Jerling. September 2005. "A Systematic Review of the Effects of Nuts on Blood Lipid Profiles in Humans." *The Journal of Nutrition* 135(9): 2082–2089.

Website

Macadamia Advice Center. www.macadamias.org.uk.

MUSHROOMS

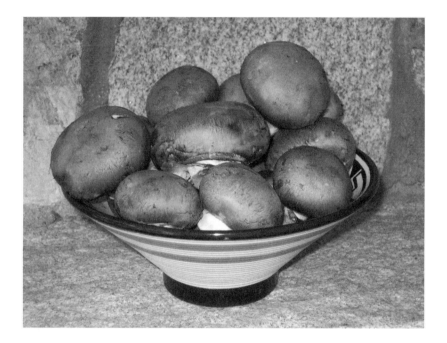

According to mushroom folklore, the ancient Egyptians believed that mushrooms were a plant of immortality. That is exactly what they indicated in their writings, known as hieroglyphics, 4,600 years ago. In fact, it has been said that the pharaohs, or Egyptian royal leaders, decreed that mushrooms could be consumed only by members of the royal family. Commoners could not even touch them.[1] Of course, since it is assumed that commoners prepared the food the royals ate, the folklore fails to explain exactly how this was accomplished.

Nevertheless, in recent years, many different types of mushrooms have grown in popularity. And, every year, hundred of millions of pounds are sold in the United States. The American Mushroom Institute notes that for the 2007 to 2008 sales year, the United States mushroom crop was 809 million pounds. Of these, the best selling mushroom is the white button (*Agaricus bisporus*). The majority of all mushrooms are grown in Pennsylvania.[2]

For years, it has been well established that mushrooms, which are fungi, are a very low calorie food that has lots of fiber and no fat. More recently, it has been learned that they contain vitamins as well as the minerals potassium, selenium, and copper. Mushrooms even have a little-known antioxidant ergothioneine and a high amount of the amino acid glutamate.[3] So, it should surprise no one that many researchers have found the study of mushrooms to be intriguing. Although they may have their research results published in a vast array of publications, mushroom researchers even have their own research journal—*International Journal of Medicinal Mushrooms*. In addition, the American Mushroom Institute publishes *Mushroom News*.

CANCER

A large portion of the research on mushrooms appears to focus on using mushrooms as part of the ongoing effort to prevent and treat different types of cancer. For example, a study published in 2008 in the *British Journal of Cancer* describes research at the Methodist Research Institute in Indianapolis, Indiana, in which an extract of the ancient Asian mushroom, *Phellinus linteus* (PL), was added to aggressive breast cancer cells. Researchers found that when exposed to *Phellinus linteus*, the breast cancer cells grew at a slower rate and were less aggressive. Moreover, the exposed cells had a lowered ability to form the blood vessels needed for tumor growth, and they stopped the action of an enzyme, AKT, necessary for the formation of blood vessels and cell growth. Commenting on the study, the researchers wrote, "Taken together, our study suggests potential therapeutic effects of PL against invasive breast cancer."[4]

In a 2008 article in *Current Medical Chemistry*, researchers at Beth Israel Deaconess Medical Center in Boston made a more sweeping claim for PL. They noted that there has been increasing evidence that PL causes cell death in many different types of cancer "without causing any measurable toxic effects to their normal counterparts." It also seems to have the "ability to enhance some conventional chemotherapeutic drugs." As a result, "PL [may well be] a promising candidate as an alternative anticancer agent or synergizer for existing antitumor drugs."[5]

But, it is not only exotic types of mushrooms that are been associated with preventing and/or treating cancer. Researchers at the Beckman Research Institute of the City of Hope in Duarte, California, have been studying white button mushrooms. They all contain the phytochemical conjugated linoleic acid, which is known to have anti-cancer properties. Using laboratory and mouse studies, the researchers determined that mice that ate mushrooms had a 58-percent reduction in growth of breast cancer. "The studies showed that mushroom extract decreased both tumor cell proliferation and tumor weight with no effect on rate of apoptosis [cell death]."[6] In a 2008 article that appeared in *Mushroom News*, the lead researcher, Shiuan Chen, PhD, said,

"Eating mushrooms would be an easy intervention. It could provide a cost-effective, whole-food option for cancer risk reduction."[7]

A 2007 article in *Urology Times* describes research by Jackilen Shannon, PhD, MPH, of the Oregon Health & Science University Cancer Institute, that was presented to an American Association of Cancer Research meeting held in Boston. Dr. Shannon examined the consumption of folate-rich foods, such as mushrooms, and alcohol among two groups of veterans. One group included 137 men who had received a diagnosis of prostate cancer; the second group included 238 men who had normal PSA levels. (PSA is a blood test used to detect prostate cancer.)

Dr. Shannon found that the men with the highest consumption of folate-rich foods were 52 percent less likely to have prostate cancer. As a result, she theorized that folate-rich foods give a level of protection against prostate cancer.[8]

And, the previously noted *P. linteus* mushrooms appear to be useful for prostate cancer as well. Researchers at Boston University School of Medicine found that the ancient mushroom increased the effects of chemotherapy in killing prostate cancer cells.[9]

There is also good evidence that mushrooms may be a tool in preventing and/or treating other types of cancer. In a 2002 study published in *The Journal of Alternative and Complementary Medicine*, researchers at the National University of Singapore studied the use of lentinan (from shiitake mushrooms) for colon cancer in mice. The researchers found that lentinan did "retard the development of tumors in these mice."[10]

And, in truly stunning research at New York Medical College, Sensuke Konno, PhD, examined the effects of eight natural agents on bladder cancer cells. While there were no effects from six of the agents, two agents, an active ingredient in maitake mushroom and an extract of *meshimakobu* (the Japanese name for *P. linteus*) reduced the growth, over a 72-hour period, more than 90 percent. Similar results were obtained when lower concentrations of the agents were used in conjunction with low levels of vitamin C. Dr. Konno concluded that, "It is thus possible that these substances could be used, solely or combined with conventional modalities, for the treatment of superficial bladder cancer."[11]

BONE HEALTH

It has been well documented that Americans tend to have very low levels of vitamin D in their blood. Most often, Americans receive too little sun to allow their bodies to make vitamin D. And, without adequate levels of vitamin D, the body is unable to maintain calcium absorption and bone health. This may lead to osteopenia or, the more serious, osteoporosis. Although vitamin D may be added to many foods, only a small number of foods actually contain vitamin D. Mushrooms have small amounts of vitamin D. However, when mushrooms are exposed to ultraviolet light, they become a rich source of this vitamin. A 2008 article in *Business Wire* and a 2009 issue of *Tufts University Health & Nutrition Letter* explain that researchers at the USDA's Agricultural Research Service joined with Monterey Mushroom, a California mushroom grower to create mushrooms with high levels of vitamin D. So, three ounces of Sun Bella mushrooms exposed to UV-B rays have 100 percent of the recommended daily intake of vitamin D.[12]

WEIGHT LOSS

In a study published in *Appetite* in 2008, Johns Hopkins University researchers recruited 54 men and women. Over four days, some received a lunch with beef; the others received a lunch with an equal amount of mushrooms. On the following week, the subjects ate the opposite lunches for four days. The meat meals averaged 420 more calories and 30 more fat grams per day than the mushroom meals. Both groups had similar ratings for after-eating fullness, the appeal of the food, and general satiety. The researchers found it intriguing that the subjects appeared to accept the mushrooms as a substitute for beef, and they didn't attempt to compensate for their lower calorie meal by eating more later in the day.[13]

Are mushrooms a good food choice? Absolutely. And, more people should make them an integral part of the diet.

NOTES

1. Mushroom Council Website. http://mushroomcouncil.com.

2. American Mushroom Institute Website. www.americanmushroom.org.

3. Schepers, Anastasia. February 2006. "Mushrooms Sprout Unique Flavor and Nutrients." *Environmental Nutrition* 29(2): 8.

4. Sliva, D., A. Jedinak, J. Kawasaki, et al. 2008. "*Phellinus linteus* Suppresses Growth, Angiogenesis and Invasive Behaviour of Breast Cancer Cells Through the Inhibition of AKT Signalling." *British Journal of Cancer* 98(8): 1348–1356.

5. Zhu, T., S. H. Kim, and C. Y. Chen. 2008. "A Medicinal Mushroom: *Phellinus linteus*." *Current Medical Chemistry* 15(13): 1330–1335.

6. Chen, Shiuan, Sei-Ryang Oh, Sheryl Phung, et al. December 15, 2006. "Anti-Aromatase Activity of Phytochemicals in White Button Mushrooms (*Agaricus bisporus*)." *Cancer Research* 66: 12026–12034.

7. Di Rado, Alicia. September 2008. "Researchers Study Mushrooms' Cancer Fighting Potential." *Mushroom News* 56(9): 26–27.

8. "Food Nutrients May Reduce Risk of Prostate Cancer." February 2007. *Urology Times* 35(2): 44.

9. Collins, L., T. Zhu, J. Guo, et al. 2006. "*Phellinus linteus* Sensitises Apoptosis Induced by Doxorubicin in Prostate Cancer." *British Journal of Cancer* 95: 282–288.

10. Ng, Mah-Lee and Ann-Teck Yap. October 1, 2002. "Inhibition of Human Colon Carcinoma Development by Lentinan from Shiitake Mushrooms (*Lentinus edodes*)." *The Journal of Alternative and Complementary Medicine* 8(5): 581–589.

11. Konno, Sensuke. November 1, 2007. "Effect of Various Natural Products on Growth of Bladder Cancer Cells: Two Promising Mushroom Extracts." *Alternative Medicine Review* 12(1): 63–68.

12. "UV-B Light Makes Mushrooms a Vitamin D Powerhouse." January 2009. *Tufts University Health & Nutrition Letter* 26(11): 3; "Monterey Mushrooms Help Combat National Vitamin D Deficiency with a New Year's Resolution." December 18, 2008. *Business Wire*: NA.

13. Cheskin, L. J., L. M. Davis, L. M. Lipsky, et al. July 2008. "Lack of Energy Consumption over 4 Days When White Button Mushrooms Are Substituted for Beef." *Appetite* 51(1): 50–57.

REFERENCES AND RESOURCES
Magazines, Journals, and Newspapers

Chen, Shiuan, Sei-Ryang Oh, Sheryl Phung, et al. December 15, 2006. "Anti-Aromatase Activity of Phytochemicals in White Button Mushrooms *(Agaricus bisporus)*." *Cancer Research* 66: 12026–12034.

Cheskin, L. J., L. M. Davis, L. M. Lipsky, et al. July 2008. "Lack of Energy Compensation over 4 Days When White Button Mushrooms Are Substituted for Beef." *Appetite* 51(1): 50–57.

Collins, L., T. Zhu, J. Guo, et al. 2006. "*Phellinus linteus* Sensitises Apoptosis Induced by Doxorubicin in Prostate Cancer." *British Journal of Cancer* 95: 282–288.

Di Rado, Alicia. September 2008. "Researchers Study Mushrooms' Cancer Fighting Potential." *Mushroom News* 56(9): 26–27.

Feeney, Mary Jo. January 2008. "Vitamin D$_2$ Enhanced Mushrooms—Coming Soon to Consumers Near You?" *Mushroom News* 56(1): 10–13.

"Food Nutrients May Reduce Risk of Prostate Cancer." February 2007. *Urology Times* 35(2): 44.

Konno, Senuke. November 1, 2007. "Effect of Various Natural Products on Growth of Bladder Cancer Cells: Two Promising Mushroom Extracts." *Alternative Medicine Review* 12(1): 63–68.

"Monterey Mushrooms Help Combat National Vitamin D Deficiency with a New Year's Resolution." December 18, 2008. *Business Wire*: NA.

Ng, Mah-Lee and Ann-Teck Yap. October 1, 2002. "Inhibition of Human Colon Carcinoma Developed by Lentinan from Shiitake Mushrooms *(Lentinus edodes)*." *The Journal of Alternative and Complementary Medicine* 8(5): 581–589.

Schepers, Anastasia. February 2006. "Mushrooms Sprout Unique Flavor and Nutrients." *Environmental Nutrition* 29(2): 8.

Sliva, D., A. Jedinak, J. Kawasaki, et al. 2008. "*Phellinus linteus* Suppresses Growth, Angiogenesis and Invasive Behaviour of Breast Cancer Cells Through the Inhibition of AKT Signalling." *British Journal of Cancer* 98(8): 1348–1356.

"UV-B Light Makes Mushrooms a Vitamin D Powerhouse." January 9, 2009. *Tufts University Health & Nutrition Letter* 26(11): 3.

Zhu, T., S. H. Kim, and C. Y. Chen. 2008. "A Medicinal Mushroom: Phellinus linteus." *Current Medical Chemistry* 15(13): 1330–1335.

Websites

American Mushroom Institute. www.americanmushroom.org.
Mushroom Council. http://mushroomcouncil.com.

OATS

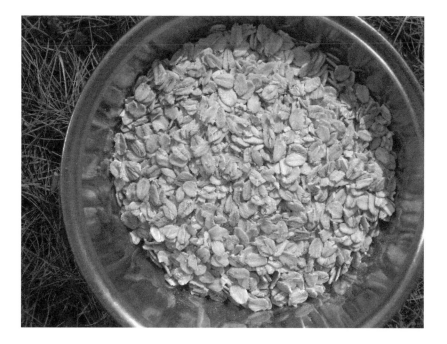

For about two thousand years, oats have been cultivated in various parts of the world. Initially, oats were used for medicinal purposes. Later, people began to consume them as food.

Over the past several decades, many people have viewed oats as a type of superfood. These people consider oats to be especially useful for those hoping to prevent or delay cardiovascular problems. Many are convinced that if they eat sufficient amounts of oats, they will lower both their cholesterol and blood pressure.

And, eating oats is so easy. What better way to start the day than with a steaming bowl of cooked whole-grain oats? A cup of such oats has just under 146 calories. Even if a little milk is added, the amount of calories remains low. Of course, there are also various types of oat breads. But, the amount of oats actually contained in these breads varies widely.

Oats are filled with manganese and selenium, and they have good amounts of vitamin B_1, magnesium, protein, tryptophan, and phosphorus. Do they really live up to all the hype?

CARDIOVASCULAR HEALTH
Cholesterol

In a study published in 2007 in *Nutrition Journal*, 75 men and women with high levels of cholesterol were randomly given either six grams/day of concentrated oat beta-glucan or six grams/day of dextrose (control). After six weeks, the researchers found that the subjects taking the oat beta-glucan had significant reductions in total cholesterol and LDL (bad) cholesterol.[1]

In a Colorado State University study, which was published in 2002 in *The American Journal of Clinical Nutrition*, 36 overweight men between the ages of 50 and 75 ate either an oat or wheat cereal providing 14 g of dietary fiber per day for 12 weeks. At the end of the study, researchers found that the men derived no lipoprotein benefit from the wheat cereal. However, the oat cereal group had a 17 percent reduction in their quantity of small LDL cholesterol.[2]

In a German study published in 2003 in the *Annals of Nutrition & Metabolism*, researchers at Wehrawald Hospital placed overweight subjects who had high cholesterol levels on one of three diets. Ninety-nine subjects consumed a fat modified diet with caloric restriction and a daily intake of 35 to 50 g of oat bran. One hundred thirty-six subjects ate a fat-modified oat bran-free diet with caloric restrictions. Fifty-three overweight men with normal cholesterol levels comprised the control group. At the end of four weeks, the most significant improvement in total cholesterol and LDL cholesterol was seen among the subjects who had a fat-modified diet that included oat bran.[3]

A study published in 2005 in the *Journal of the American Dietetic Association* describes research on 152 Hispanic men between the ages of 30 and 70 who had LDL cholesterol levels between 120 and 190 mg/dl. After they all ate a National Cholesterol Education Program Step 1 diet for five weeks, the subjects were randomly assigned to eat either corn or oat cereal for the next six weeks. While those who ate the corn cereal achieved no significant reduction in cholesterol, the subjects who ate the oat cereal had significant reductions in both total cholesterol and LDL cholesterol.[4]

On the other hand, a Swedish study published in 2008 in the *Annals of Nutrition & Metabolism* investigated whether the consumption of a daily meal that contains 4 g of oat beta-glucans would lower total and LDL cholesterol in subjects with elevated levels of cholesterol. For the first three weeks of the study, 43 healthy men and women with elevated levels of cholesterol consumed a daily soup that was high in fiber but low in energy and fat and without any oat beta-glucans. Then, the subjects were randomly assigned to either continue the same soup or consume a similar soup that contained oat beta-glucans for five more weeks. Though the total and LDL cholesterol levels of the subjects who consumed the oat soup with beta-glucans dropped, the decreases were not statistically significant.[5]

Blood Pressure

A small six-week study published in 2002 in the *Journal of Family Practice* divided a group of 18 men and women with mild to borderline high blood pressure into one of two groups. One group ate oat cereal (standardized to 5.52 g/day beta-glucan) and the other group ate a low-fiber cereal with less than 1.0 g/day total fiber. While the group eating the low-fiber cereal experienced essentially no change in blood pressure readings, the group eating the oat cereal had significant reductions in both systolic and diastolic blood pressure. The researchers concluded that, "soluble fiber-rich whole oats may be an effective dietary therapy in the prevention and adjunct treatment of hypertension."[6]

In a study conducted at the Jean Mayer U.S. Department of Agriculture Human Nutrition Research Center on Aging at Tufts University and published in 2001 in *The Journal of Nutrition*, researchers asked 43 overweight adults to consume their regular "control" diets for two weeks. Then, for the next six weeks, they ate one of two diets: the control diet or a diet containing 45 g/day of oats. Although the diastolic pressure of the members of the two groups remained similar, the members of the group who ate oats had significant decreases in systolic blood pressure.[7]

In a study published in 2007 in the *European Journal of Clinical Nutrition*, 97 men and women with resting systolic blood pressure of 130–179 mm Hg and/or diastolic blood pressure of 85–109 mm Hg (mildly elevated to profoundly elevated) were randomly assigned to eat either foods containing beta-glucan or control foods for 12 weeks. Although blood pressure tended to remain about the same in both groups, the subjects who had a mean body mass index above the median (in this case that meant they were obese) and who ate the oat beta-glucan foods experienced a lowering of the both systolic and diastolic blood pressure.[8]

BREAST CANCER

In a Swedish study that was published in 2008 in the *International Journal of Cancer*, researchers examined the association between the intake of fiber, such as oats, in 51,823 postmenopausal women who comprise the Swedish Mammography Screening Cohort and the incidence of breast cancer. Fiber intake was initially measured in a questionnaire that was collected between 1987 and 1997. During the follow-up, which continued for an average of 8.3 years, close to 1,200 cases of breast cancer were diagnosed. The findings were important. Among women who had ever used postmenopausal hormones, "total fiber intake and especially cereal fiber [such as oatmeal] were statistically significantly associated with approximately 50 percent reduced risk for overall and ER [estrogen receptor] and PR [progesterone receptor] tumors when comparing the highest to the lowest quartile, but no association was observed among PMH [postmenopausal] never users."[9]

While oats may or may not be a superfood, for most people, they are probably a useful addition to the diet. Still, unless one is absolutely certain that no cross-contamination occurred, people who have celiac disease or gluten intolerance should not consume oats in any form.

NOTES

1. Queenan, Katie M., Maria L. Stewart, Kristen N. Smith, et al. 2007. "Concentrated Oat beta-Glucan, a Fermentable Fiber, Lowers Serum Cholesterol in Hypercholesterolemic Adults in a Randomized Controlled Trial." *Nutrition Journal* 6: 6.

2. Davy, Brenda M., Kevin P. Davy, Richard C. Ho, et al. August 2002. "High-Fiber Oat Cereal Compared with Wheat Cereal Consumption Favorably Alters LDL-Cholesterol Subclass and Particle Numbers in Middle-Aged and Older Men." *The American Journal of Clinical Nutrition* 76(2): 351–358.

3. Berg, Aloys, Daniel König, Peter Deibert, et al. 2003. "Effect of an Oat Bran Enriched Diet on the Atherogenic Lipid Profile in Patients with an Increased Coronary Heart Disease Risk: A Controlled Randomized Lifestyle Intervention Study." *Annals of Nutrition & Metabolism* 47(6): 306–311.

4. Karmally, Wahida, Maria G. Montez, Walter Palmas, et al. June 2005. "Cholesterol-Lowering Benefits of Oat-Containing Cereal in Hispanic Americans." *Journal of the American Dietetic Association* 105(6): 967–970.

5. Biörklund, M., J. Holm, and G. Önning. 2008. "Serum Lipids and Postprandial Glucose and Insulin Levels in Hyperlipidemic Subjects After Consumption of an Oat beta-Glucan Containing Ready Meal." *Annals of Nutrition & Metabolism* 52(2): 83–90.

6. Keenan, J. M., J. J. Pins, C. Frazel, et al. April 2002. "Oat Ingestion Reduces Systolic and Diastolic Blood Pressure in Patients with Mild or Borderline Hypertension: A Pilot Trial." *Journal of Family Practice* 51(4): 369+.

7. Saltzman, Edward, Sai Krupa Das, Alice H. Lichtenstein, et al. 2001. "An Oat-Containing Hypocaloric Diet Reduces Systolic Blood Pressure and Improves Lipid Profile Beyond Effects of Weight Loss in Men and Women." *The Journal of Nutrition* 131: 1465–1470.

8. Maki, K. C., R. Galant, P. Samuel, et al. 2007. "Effects of Consuming Foods Containing Oat beta-Glucan on Blood Pressure, Carbohydrate Metabolism and Biomarkers of Oxidative Stress in Men and Women with Elevated Blood Pressure." *European Journal of Clinical Nutrition* 61: 786–795.

9. Suzuki, R., T. Rylander-Rudqvist, W. Ye, et al. January 15, 2008. "Dietary Fiber Intake and Risk of Postmenopausal Breast Cancer Defined by Estrogen and Progesterone Receptor Status—A Prospective Cohort Study Among Swedish Women." *International Journal of Cancer* 122(2): 403–412.

REFERENCES AND RESOURCES
Magazines, Journals, and Newspapers

Berg, Aloys, Daniel König, Peter Deibert, et al. 2003. "Effect of Oat Bran Enriched Diet on the Atherogenic Lipid Profile in Patients with an Increased Coronary

Heart Disease Risk: A Controlled Randomized Lifestyle Intervention Study." *Annals of Nutrition & Metabolism* 47(6): 306–311.

Biörklund, M., J. Holm, and G. Önning, G. 2008. "Serum Lipids and Postprandial Glucose and Insulin Levels in Hyperlipidemic Subjects After Consumption of an Oat beta-Glucan-Containing Ready Made Meal." *Annals of Nutrition & Metabolism* 52(2): 83–90.

Davy, Brenda M., Kevin P. Davy, Richard C. Ho, et al. August 2002. "High-Fiber Oat Cereal Compared with Wheat Cereal Consumption Favorably Alters LDL-Cholesterol Subclass and Particle Numbers in Middle-Aged and Older Men." *The American Journal of Clinical Nutrition* 76(2): 352–358.

Karmally, Wahida, Maria G. Montez, Walter Palmas, et al. June 2005. "Cholesterol-Lowering Benefits of Oat-Containing Cereal in Hispanic Americans." *Journal of the American Dietetic Association* 105(6): 967–970.

Keenan, J. M., J. J. Pins, C. Frazel, et al. April 2002. "Oat Ingestion Reduces Systolic and Diastolic Blood Pressure in Patients with Mild or Borderline Hypertension: A Pilot Trial." *Journal of Family Practice* 51(4): 369+.

Maki, K. C., R. Galant, P. Samuel, et al. 2007. "Effects of Consuming Foods Containing Oat beta-Glucan on Blood Pressure, Carbohydrate Metabolism and Biomarkers of Oxidative Stress in Men and Women with Elevated Blood Pressure." *European Journal of Clinical Nutrition* 61: 786–795.

Queenan, Katie M., Maria L. Stewart, Kristen N. Smith, et al. 2007. "Concentrated Oat beta-Glucan, a Fermentable Fiber, Lowers Serum Cholesterol in Hyper-cholesterolemic Adults in a Randomized Controlled Trial." *Nutritional Journal* 6: 6.

Saltzman, Edward, Sai Krupa Das, Alice H. Lichtenstein, et al. 2001. "An Oat-Containing Hypocaloric Diet Reduces Systolic Blood Pressure and Improves Lipid Profile Beyond Effects of Weight Loss in Men and Women." *The Journal of Nutrition* 131: 1465–1470.

Suzuki, R., T. Rylander-Rudqvist, W. Ye, et al. January 15, 2008. "Dietary Fiber Intake and Risk of Postmenopausal Breast Cancer Defined by Estrogen and Progesterone Receptor Status—A Prospective Cohort Study Among Swedish Women." *International Journal of Cancer* 122(2): 403–412.

Website

The George Mateljan Foundation. http://whfoods.com.

OLIVE OIL

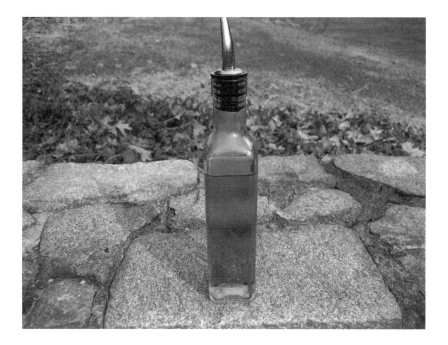

All olive oils contain 119 calories per tablespoon. Of these, 119 calories come from fat. Each tablespoon has 14 grams of fat: 9.8 grams of mono-unsaturated fat, 1.9 grams of saturated fat, and 1.4 grams of polyunsaturated fat. So, when someone refers to "light olive oil," it is a function of the color of the oil, not the fat content.

But, olive oils do differ in other ways. Green olive oils tend to be more bitter or pungent; yellow olive oils are generally milder. Olive oils may be fruity or buttery. Some are considered "well-rounded" or "full."[1]

Furthermore, there are different types of olive oil. Extra virgin olive oil is derived from the first pressing of the olives. It has the best flavor and the lowest acidity (0.8 percent). People may drizzle it on vegetables, or use it in a salad. Virgin oil is from the second pressing of the olives. With an acidity of less than two percent, it may be used for sautéing. Pure olive oil is a mixture of virgin oil and refined oil. It has an acidity of up to one percent. Though it is relatively inexpensive, it lacks flavor.[2]

There have been a number of studies on olive oil. Some have been focused only on the oil. More often, the studies investigate the Mediterranean diet, of which olive oil is a key component. So what have they determined?

WEIGHT LOSS

In a study published in 2008 in *Cell Metabolism*, researchers infused oleic acid, an omega-9 fatty acid found in olive oil, into the intestines of laboratory rats. There it was converted into oleoylethanolamide (OEA). Apparently, OEA stimulates brain cells that the stomach is full—that it is time to stop eating. The rats with infused oleic acid ate less. The researchers also infused oleic acid into rats that were unable to make OEA. Those rats continued to eat the usual amount of food. "The results suggest that activation of small-intestinal OEA mobilization . . . serves as a molecular sensor linking fat ingestion to satiety."[3]

A study published in 2004 in *The Journal of Nutrition* examined the relationship between body mass index (BMI) and obesity and the level of adherence to the traditional Mediterranean diet. The study, which was conducted in Spain, included 1,547 men and 1,615 women between the ages of 24 and 74. The researchers found that both men and women who most closely followed the Mediterranean diet were least likely to be obese. "The traditional Mediterranean dietary pattern is inversely associated with BMI and obesity."[4]

CARDIOVASCULAR HEALTH

An article published in 2005 in *Nature* explained that newly pressed extra virgin olive oil contains oleocanthal, which is similar in many ways to ibuprofen. Both oleocanthal and ibuprofen inhibit activity of cyclooxygenase (COX) enzymes, which means they have anti-inflammatory properties. The researchers suggest that since regular low doses of aspirin (which is also a COX inhibitor), confer cardiovascular benefits, then there is a good chance that comparable results may be obtained from olive oil.[5]

In a study published in 2007 in *The Journal of Nutrition*, researchers reviewed the association between olive oil consumption and blood pressure in 110 men from non-Mediterranean countries and 45 men from the Mediterranean countries of Spain and Italy. The crossover trial included three three-week interventions separated by two two-week wash out periods. At the end of the study, the systolic blood pressure of the non-Mediterranean men decreased by three percent. "The results of this study suggest that a moderate consumption of olive oil may be used as an effective tool to reduce SBP [systolic blood pressure] of healthy men who do not typically consume a Mediterranean diet."[6]

But, as has been previously noted, not all olive oils are alike. In a study published in 2006 in the *Annals of Internal Medicine*, researchers administered three different types of olive oil combinations to 200 healthy male volunteers. For two weeks, each man ate a daily tablespoon of either virgin olive oil, refined olive oil, or a combination of the two.

After a two-week washout period, the volunteers were retested with one of the other types of oil for two weeks. The researchers determined that the virgin olive oil, which contains higher amounts of polyphenols, raised the rates of high-density lipoprotein (HDL) cholesterol in the volunteers more than the other two types of olive oil. Moreover, the virgin olive oil increased the levels of substances that prevent the oxidation of low-density liproprotein (LDL) cholesterol, which has been associated with clot formation in blood vessels. The researchers noted that "olive oil is more than a monounsaturated fat. Its phenolic content can also provide benefits for plasma lipid levels and oxidative damage."[7]

CANCER

In a study that appeared in *BMC Cancer* in 2008, Spanish researchers attempted to determine the parts of olive oil that act against cancer cells. After separating extra virgin olive oil into fractions, the different fractions were tested against breast cancer cells. The researchers found that all the fractions that contained polyphenols (lignans and secoiridoids) were useful against the breast cancer gene HER2. Nevertheless, the researchers cautioned that, "The phenolics that were active (i.e. lignans and secoiridoids) exhibited tumor effects against cultured breast cancer cells at concentrations that are unlikely to be achieved in vivo [in real life by consuming olive oil]." Still, "these findings, together with the fact that humans have safely been ingesting significant amounts of lignans and secoiridoids as long as they have been consuming olives and extra virgin olive oil, strongly suggest that these polyphenols might provide an excellent and safe platform for the design of new anti breast cancer drugs."[8]

A study published in 2008 in the *British Journal of Cancer* reviewed the food intake and medical records of close to 26,000 people living in Greece. During a follow-up of 7.9 years, there were 851 medically confirmed cases of cancer. The people who most strictly adhered to the Mediterranean diet had the lowest incidence of the disease. The researchers noted that they "found evidence that adherence to the traditional MD [Mediterranean diet] is associated with markedly and significantly reduced incidence of cancer, which is apparently larger than predicted from examining individual MD components."[9]

MORTALITY

In a 2003 study that was published in *The New England Journal of Medicine*, researchers examined the association between mortality rates and adherence to the Mediterranean diet in population of 22,043 Greek adults between the ages of 20 and 80. During the 44 months of the study, there were 275 deaths. However, the death rate among those who ate a Mediterranean diet was significantly lower than those who did not follow this diet.[10]

An Italian study published in 2008 in the *British Medical Journal* reviewed findings from twelve different studies, which included a total of about 1.6 million people. The researchers hoped to determine the association between following a Mediterranean diet and the incidence of chronic diseases and mortality. Their findings were quite dramatic. "Greater adherence to a Mediterranean diet is associated with a significant improvement in health status, as seen by a significant reduction in overall mortality (9 percent), mortality from cardiovascular disease (9 percent), incidence of or mortality from cancer (6 percent), and incidence of Parkinson's disease and Alzheimer's disease (13 percent)."[11]

ONE CAVEAT

Are olives as healthful as olive oil? Unfortunately, the vast majority of olives are bottled in brine, which contains huge amounts of sodium. Unless one is able to purchase olives bottled in water, olives should comprise a limited part of the diet.

What about olive oil? Yes, it should be part of the diet. But, as with all high calorie foods, in moderation.

NOTES

1. Webb, Robyn. April 2008. "Ingredients in Depth: Olive Oil." *Diabetes Forecast* 61(4): 43.

2. Webb, Robyn: 43.

3. Schwartz, Gary J., Jin Fu, Giuseppe Astarita, et al. October 8, 2008. *Cell Metabolism* 8(4): 281–288.

4. Schröder, Helmut, Jaume Marrugat, Juan Vila, et al. December 2004. "Adherence to the Traditional Mediterranean Diet Is Inversely Associated with Body Mass Index and Obesity in a Spanish Population." *The Journal of Nutrition* 143: 3355–3361.

5. Beauchamp, Gary K., Russell S. J. Keast, Diane Morel, et al. September 2005. "Ibuprofen-Like Activity in Extra-Virgin Olive Oil. *Nature* 437: 45–46.

6. Bondia-Pons, Isabel, Helmut Schröder, Maria-Isabel Covas, et al. January 2007. "Moderate Consumption of Olive Oil by Healthy European Men Reduces Systolic Blood Pressure in Non-Mediterranean Participants." *The Journal of Nutrition* 137: 84–87.

7. Covas, Maria-Isabel, Kristina Nyyssönen, Henrik E. Poulsen, et al. September 5, 2006. "The Effect of Polyphenols on Olive Oil on Heart Disease Risk Factors." *Annals of Internal Medicine* 145(5): 333–341.

8. Menendez, Javier A., Alejandro Vazquez-Martin, Rocio Garcia-Villalba, et al. December 18, 2008. "tabAnti-HER2 (*erb*–2) Oncogene Effects of Phenolic Compounds Directly Isolated from Commercial Extra Virgin Olive Oil (EVOO)." *BMC Cancer* 8: 377.

9. Benetou, V., A. Trichopoulou, P. Orfanos, et al. 2008. "Conformity to Traditional Mediterranean Diet and Cancer Incidence: The Greek EPIC Cohort." *British Journal of Cancer* 99: 191–195.

10. Trichopoulos, Antonia, Tina Costacou, Christina Bamia, and Dimitrios Trichopoulos. June 26, 2003. "Adherence to a Mediterranean Diet and Survival in a Greek Population." *The New England Journal of Medicine* 348: 2599–2608.

11. Sofi, Francesco, Francesca Cesari, Rosanna Abbate, et al. September 11, 2008. "Adherence to Mediterranean Diet and Health Status: Meta-Analysis." *British Medical* Journal 337: a1344.

REFERENCES AND RESOURCES
Magazines, Journals, and Newspapers

Beauchamp, Gary K., Russell S. J. Keast, Diane Morel, et al. September 2005. "Ibuprofen-Like Activity in Extra-Virgin Olive Oil." *Nature* 437: 45–46.

Benetou, V., A. Trichopoulou, P. Orfanos, et al. 2008. "Conformity to Traditional Mediterranean Diet and Cancer Incidence: The Greek EPIC Cohort." *British Journal of Cancer* 99: 191–195.

Bondia-Pons, Isabel, Helmut Schröder, Maria-Isabel Covas, et al. January 2007. "Moderate Consumption of Olive Oil by Health European Men Reduces Systolic Blood Pressure in Non-Mediterranean Participants." *The Journal of Nutrition* 137: 84–87.

Covas, Maria-Isabel, Kristina Nyyssönen, Henrik E. Poulsen, et al. September 5, 2006. "The Effects of Polyphenols in Olive Oil on Heart Disease Risk Factors." *Annals of Internal Medicine* 145(5): 333–341.

Menendez, Javier A., Alejandro Vazquez-Martin, Rocio Garcia-Villalba, et al. December 18, 2008. "tabAnti-HER2 (*erb*B-2) Oncogene Effects of Phenolic Compounds Directly Isolated from Commercial Extra-Virgin Olive Oil (EVOO)." *BMC Cancer* 8: 377.

Schröder, Helmut, Jaume Marrugat, Juan Vila, et al. December 2004. "Adherence to the Traditional Mediterranean Diet Is Inversely Association with Body Mass Index and Obesity in a Spanish Population." *The Journal of Nutrition* 134: 3355–3361.

Schwartz, Gary J., Jin Fu, Giuseppe Astarita, et al. October 8, 2008. "The Lipid Messenger OEA Links Dietary Fat Intake to Satiety." *Cell Metabolism* 8(4): 281–288.

Sofi, Francesco, Francesca Cesari, Rosanna Abbate, et al. September 11, 2008. "Adherence to Mediterranean Diet and Health Status: Meta-Analysis." *British Medical Journal* 337: a1344.

Trichopoulou, Antonia, Tina Costacou, Christina Bamia, and Dimitrios Trichopoulos. June 26, 2003. "Adherence to a Mediterranean Diet and Survival in a Greek Population." *The New England Journal of Medicine* 348: 2599–2608.

Webb, Robyn. April 2008. "The Ingredients in Depth: Olive Oil." *Diabetes Forecast* 61(4): 43.

Website

North American Olive Oil Association. http://naooa.mytradeassociation.org.

ONIONS

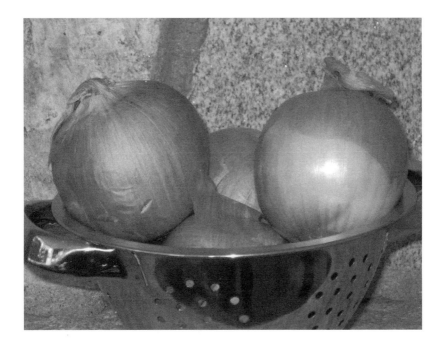

For at least 5,000 years, since onions were first cultivated, many people have believed that onions have medicinal powers. In fact, the ancient Egyptians considered onions to be an object of worship, and Dioscorides, a first-century Greek physician, advised athletes who participated in the Olympic Games to consume large amounts of onions. In addition, he told them to drink onion juice and rub it on their bodies. During the Middle Ages, onions were a commonly eaten food. They were also used for headaches, snakebites, and hair loss. Even the Pilgrims brought onions along when they traveled to the shores of America.[1]

Today, onions, which average only 45 calories per serving, are recognized as a fat- and cholesterol-free food that contains fiber and vitamin C but is very low in sodium. They also have a good deal of quercetin, a flavonoid, which is believed to provide protection from cancer and cardio-vascular disease. So, what does the research show?

CANCER
Colorectal Cancer

In a study published in 2008 in *Cancer Epidemiology, Biomarkers & Prevention*, adults (average age of 61) with precancerous colorectal polyps (adenomas) were assigned either to a group who would receive dietary intervention or a control group. During the study, researchers evaluated the participants' intake of 29 different flavonoids and the regrowth of colorectal adenomas. The researchers found that the high intake of flavonols, a subgroup of flavonoids, such as those found in onions, was associated with a decreased risk for the recurrence of advanced adenomas. When compared to those with the lowest intake of flavonols, those with the highest intake of flavonols had a 76 percent lower risk of adenoma recurrence.[2]

Ovarian Cancer

An Italian study, published in 2008 in the *International Journal of Cancer*, examined the relationship between ovarian cancer and the consumption of foods with large amounts of flavonoids. The study included 1,031 women with confirmed cases of ovarian cancer and 2,411 women in the control group. The researchers found that those who ate diets with generous amounts of flavonoids could reduce their risk of ovarian cancer by almost 50 percent.[3]

Pancreatic Cancer

Using data from the Multiethnic Cohort Study, which contains dietary and other data on 183,518 people between the ages of 45 and 75, researchers reviewed the association between intake of three flavonols (quercetin, kaempferol, and myricetin) and reduced risk for pancreatic cancer. The findings, which were published in 2007 in the *American Journal of Epidemiology*, indicated that the consumption of flavonols significantly lowered the risk of pancreatic cancer. Of the foods tested, onions appeared to offer some benefits to nonsmokers and even more benefits to current smokers.[4]

Prostate Cancer

In a study published in 2002 in the *Journal of the National Cancer Institute*, researchers from the National Cancer Institute and the Shanghai Cancer Institute in Shanghai, China, recruited 238 men with prostate cancer and 471 healthy men to serve as the control group. All the participants completed questionnaires that described their intake of allium vegetables, such as onions, over the past five years. (Other allium vegetables include garlic, scallions, leeks, and chives.) These vegetables, which contain flavonoids and sulfur-containing compounds, have repeatedly been shown in laboratory studies to reduce tumor growth.

The researchers found that the men who ate ten grams or more of these vegetables each day were far less likely to develop prostate cancer than those who ate less than 2.2 grams each day. (Ten grams is a relatively modest amount of food. For example, 3.5 cloves of garlic weigh about 10 grams.) The researchers concluded that, "The reduced risk of prostate cancer associated with allium vegetables was independent of body size, intake of other foods, and total calorie intake and was more pronounced for men with localized than with advanced prostate cancer."[5]

In another study, published in 2004 in *European Urology*, an independent health researcher, William B. Grant, PhD, investigated the relationship between varying national diets and rates of death from prostate cancer. Dr. Grant began with the knowledge that the rates of death from prostate cancer in northern Europe are about five times the rates in Hong Kong, Iran, Japan, and Turkey. Whatever the country, the consumption of animal products proved to be the strongest risk factor for prostate cancer mortality; the consumption of complex carbohydrates and antioxidants played the most significant role in reducing risk. Of all the risk-reducing foods, onions were at the top of the list.[6]

CARDIOVASCULAR HEALTH

The millions of Americans dealing with cardiovascular problems should heed this information. A study published in 2007 in *The Journal of Nutrition* found that quercetin, which is contained in abundance in onions, has the potential to help those dealing with high blood pressure (hypertension) and coronary artery disease. It is also useful in the prevention of stroke. During the study, men and women with either prehypertension or stage 1 hypertension were given either quercetin or a placebo. Although quercetin failed to alter the blood pressure in the men and women who have yet to develop high blood pressure, it did lower the blood pressure of those with stage 1 hypertension. The researchers noted that, "These data are the first to our knowledge to show that quercetin supplementation reduces blood pressure in hypertensive subjects."[7]

IMMUNITY

In a study published in 2007 in the *Journal of Applied Physiology*, researchers at Appalachian State University and the University of South Carolina gave 40 trained cyclists either quercetin or a placebo for five weeks. After three weeks, the participants rode their bicycles three hours a day for three days, until they were exhausted. Following the exercise, 45 percent of the placebo group became ill; only 5 percent of those who took quercetin developed an illness.[8]

Another study, published in 2008 in the *American Journal of Physiology: Regulatory, Integrative and Comparative Physiology*, tested the use of quercetin in mice. Mice were randomly assigned to one of four groups: exercise-placebo, exercise-quercetin, control-placebo, or control-quercetin. The two groups that exercised ran to exhaustion three days in a row. Then, all four groups were exposed to flu virus. The researchers found that the mice that exercised to exhaustion were more at risk for developing the flu than the mice that did not exercise. Mice that exercised and took quercetin developed the flu at about the same rate as those that did not exercise; mice that did not exercise or who exercised and took the quercetin had about the same severity of symptoms. The researchers concluded that the "data suggest that short-term quercetin feedings may prove to be an effective strategy to lessen the impact of stressful exercise on susceptibility to respiratory infection."[9]

ONE CAVEAT

One would think that just about all types of onions have similar cancer-inhibiting abilities. But, according to researchers at Cornell University, that is not true. In a study published in 2004 in the *Journal of Agricultural and Food Chemistry*, researchers found that the strongest onions have more antioxidant activity than the milder varieties, and, as a result, have a greater ability to destroy free radicals. Free radicals are thought to play an important role in a number of illnesses, particularly cancer. The strongest cancer-fighting onions were the New York Bold variety and the Western Yellow. Unfortunately, at least in this study, the much loved, sweet-tasting Vidalia was found to have little ability to fight cancer. The researchers noted that, "These results may influence consumers toward purchasing onion varieties exhibiting greater potential health benefits and may significantly affect future breeding efforts to enhance onion nutritional qualities."[10]

Should onions be included in the diet? Of course.

NOTES

1. National Onion Association Website. www.onions-usa.org.

2. Bobe, Gerd, Leah B. Sansbury, Paul S. Albert, et al. June 1, 2008. "Dietary Flavonoids and Colorectal Adenoma Recurrence in the Polyp Prevention Trial." *Cancer Epidemiology, Biomarkers & Prevention* 17(6): 1344–1353.

3. Rossi, Marta, Eva Negri, Pagona Lagiou, et. al. 2008. "Flavonoids and Ovarian Cancer Risk: A Case-Control Study in Italy." *International Journal of Cancer* 123(4): 895–898.

4. Nöthlings, Ute, Suzanne P. Murphy, Lynne R. Wilkens, et al. October 15, 2007. "Flavonols and Pancreatic Cancer Risk." *American Journal of Epidemiology* 166(8): 924–931.

5. Hsing, Ann W., Anand P. Chokkalingam, Yu-Tang Gao, et al. November 6, 2002. "Allium Vegetables and Risk of Prostate Cancer: A Population-Based Study. *Journal of the National Cancer Institute* 94(21): 1648–1651.

6. Grant, William B. March 2004. "A Multicountry Ecologic Study of Risk and Risk Reduction Factors for Prostate Cancer Mortality." *European Urology* 45(3): 271–279.

7. Edwards, Randi, Tiffany Lyon, Sheldon E. Litwin, et al. November 2007. "Quercetin Reduces Blood Pressure in Hypertensive Subjects." *The Journal of Nutrition* 137: 2405–2411.

8. Nieman, David C., Dru A. Henson, J. Mark Davis, et al. 2007. "Quercetin's Influence on Exercise-Induced Changes in Plasma Cytokines and Muscle and Leukocyte mRNA." *Journal of Applied Physiology* 103: 1728–1735.

9. Davis, J. M., E. A. Murphy, J. L. McClellan, et al. 2008. "Quercetin Reduces Susceptibility to Influenza Infection Following Stressful Exercise." *American Journal of Physiology–Regulatory, Integrative and Comparative Physiology* 295: R505–R509.

10. Yang, Jun, Katherine J. Meyers, Jan van der Heide, and Rui Hai Liu. 2004. "Varietal Differences in Phenolic Content and Antioxidant and Antiproliferative Activities of Onions." *Journal of Agricultural and Food Chemistry* 52(22): 6787–6793.

REFERENCES AND RESOURCES
Magazines, Journals, and Newspapers

Bobe, Gerd, Leah B. Sansbury, Paul S. Albert, et al. June 1, 2008. "Dietary Flavonoids and Colorectal Adenoma Recurrence in the Polyp Prevention Trial." *Cancer Epidemiology, Biomarkers & Prevention* 17(6): 1344–1353.

Davis, J. M., E. A. Murphy, J. L. McClellan, et. al. August 2008. "Quercetin Reduces Susceptibility to Influenza Infection Following Stressful Exercise." *American Journal of Physiology-Regulatory, Integrative and Comparative Physiology* 295: R505–R509.

Edwards, Randi L., Tiffany Lyon, Sheldon E. Litwin, et al. November 2007. "Quercetin Reduces Blood Pressure in Hypertensive Subjects." *The Journal of Nutrition* 137: 2405–2411.

Grant, William B. March 2004. "A Multicountry Ecologic Study of Risk and Risk Reduction Factors for Prostate Cancer Mortality." *European Urology* 45(3): 271–279.

Hsing, Ann W., Anand P. Chokkalingam, Yu-Tang Gao, et al. November 6, 2002. "Allium Vegetables and Risk of Prostate Cancer: A Population-Based Study." *Journal of the National Cancer Institute* 94(21): 1648–1651.

Nieman, David C., Dru A. Henson, J. Mark Davis, et al. 2007. "Quercetin's Influence on Exercise-Induced Changes in Plasma Cytokines and Muscle and Leukocyte Cytokine mRNA." *Journal of Applied Physiology* 103: 1728–1735.

Nöthlings, Ute, Suzanne P. Murphy, Lynne R. Wilkens, et al. October 15, 2007. "Flavonols and Pancreatic Cancer Risk." *American Journal of Epidemiology* 166(8): 924–931.

Rossi, Marta, Eva Negri, Pagona Lagiou, et al. 2008. "Flavonoids and Ovarian Cancer Risk: A Case-Control Study in Italy." *International Journal of Cancer* 123(4): 895–898.

Yang, Jun, Katherine J. Meyers, Jan van der Heide, and Rui Hai Liu. 2004. "Varietal Differences in Phenolic Content and Antioxidant and Antiproliferative Activities of Onions." *Journal of Agricultural and Food Chemistry* 52(22): 6787–6793.

Website

National Onion Association. www.onions-usa.org.

ORANGES

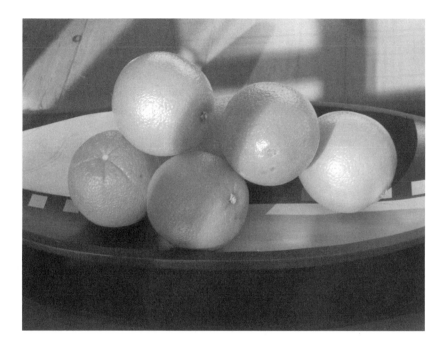

Oranges originated thousands of years ago in the area that spans from southern China to Indonesia. From there, they spread to India. By the 15th century, explorers and traders had brought oranges to Europe. It was in the late 15th century, on the second voyage that Christopher Columbus made to the "New World," that orange seeds arrived in the Caribbean. During the 16th century, Spanish explorers brought oranges to Florida, and, in the 18th century, they arrived in California with the Spanish missionaries. Today, the largest commercial growers of oranges are the United States, Brazil, Mexico, Spain, China, and Israel.[1]

Oranges have excellent amounts of vitamin C, a vitamin that the body requires but is unable to store. As a result, sources of vitamin C must be consumed every day. Oranges also contain a very good amount of dietary fiber and good amounts of calcium, folate, potassium, and vitamins A and B_1.[2] In addition, oranges have the flavanones (the dominant flavonoid class in the genus citrus) hesperidin and naringin and carotenoids, such as beta-cryptoxanthin and zeaxanthin. But, what have the researchers learned?

CARDIOVASCULAR HEALTH

In a study published in 2007 in the *Journal of the Science of Food and Agriculture*, researchers from Israel, Poland, and Korea randomly assigned 60 male Wistar rats to one of six groups. The rats in one group, which were fed the normal diet, served as the control. The rats in the other five groups ate the normal diet plus supplemental hesperidin, naringin, cholesterol, hesperidin plus cholesterol, or naringin plus cholesterol. Researchers found that both hesperidin and naringin increased the antioxidant levels of the rats. But, hesperidin increased the level more than naringin. Moreover, after 30 days on the diets, the rats consuming hesperidin or naringin and high-cholesterol foods had cholesterol levels that were about in 16 percent lower than the rats consuming just the high cholesterol foods. Their LDL ("bad" cholesterol) levels were 27 percent lower. The researchers concluded that "diets supplemented with hesperidin and naringin significantly hindered the increase in plasma lipid levels caused by cholesterol feeding."[3]

In a study published in 2009 in the *British Journal of Nutrition*, researchers randomly assigned 48 people with peripheral arterial disease to one of four dietary groups: orange and blackcurrant juices and vitamin E, orange and blackcurrant juices and placebo, sugar drink and vitamin E, or sugar drink and placebo. The dose for the juice was 500 ml; for the vitamin E, it was 15 mg. The different combinations were consumed for four weeks; there were four-week washout periods between the interventions.

The researchers found that the juices lowered levels of C-reactive protein, a marker for inflammation, by 11 percent. They also reduced the amount of fibrinogen, another marker for inflammation, by three percent. On the other hand, the sugar drink raised these markers by 13 and two percent, respectively. Vitamin E did not appear to have any significant effects on these markers.[4]

In a study presented to the July 2009 American Heart Association Basic Cardiovascular Sciences Conference, French researchers supplemented the diet of 24 overall healthy men who had cardiovascular risk factors such as obesity. During three one-month periods, the men drank one of three drinks every day: 500 milliliters of orange juice which naturally contained 292 milligrams of hesperidin, 500 milliliters of an energy drink, or 500 milliliters of the energy drink enriched with hesperidin. The researchers found that the men who consumed hesperidin, in either the orange juice or in the energy drink, had improved blood pressure and better functioning of the endothelium, the inner lining of blood vessels.[5]

OSTEOPOROSIS

In a study published in 2006 in *Nutrition*, Texas researchers divided 36 rats into two groups: nine rats served as the control and 27 rats had their testes removed (orchidectomy), thereby lowering the levels of testosterone in their bodies and increasing their risk for osteoporosis. The rats were then divided into three groups: orchidectomy, orchidectomy plus supplemental orange juice, or orchidectomy plus supplemental grapefruit juice.

After 60 days, all of the rats were sacrificed. Blood was collected, and serum was studied for antioxidant status and evidence of bone formation and resorption. Researchers found that when compared to the castrated rats that received no supplementation, the hipbone (femoral) strength of the rats on orange juice increased significantly. They also had a significant reduction in hipbone fracture rate and an increase in serum antioxidant capacity. (Similar, but smaller, results were obtained with grapefruit juice.) The researchers noted that their study "supports the supposition that drinking citrus juice positively affects serum antioxidant status and bone strength."[6]

OSTEOARTHRITIS

In a study published in 2007 in *Arthritis Research & Therapy*, Australian researchers recruited 293 healthy adults, with an average age of 58. None of the adults had knee pain or knee injuries. Ten years later, the knees of the participants were assessed by magnetic resonance imaging (MRI). The researchers found that those participants who ate the most fruit and the highest amounts of vitamin C, as is available from oranges and orange juice, were less likely to have the bone degeneration that results in the development of knee osteoarthritis.[7]

In a study published in 2005 in *The American Journal of Clinical Nutrition*, English researchers analyzed data from a study of more than 25,000 participants to determine if the intake of dietary carotenoids, including beta-cryptoxanthin and zeaxanthin, was associated with the risk of an inflammatory form of arthritis, such as rheumatoid arthritis. The subjects were followed from 1993 to 2001. During that time, 88 people developed some form of inflammatory arthritis. When compared to the 176 healthy people who served as controls, the mean daily intake of zeaxanthin was found to be 20 percent lower in those who became ill. Even more notable was the finding that the mean daily intake of beta-cryptoxanthin was 40 percent lower in those who developed inflammatory arthritis. The researchers noted that their "data are consistent with previous evidence showing that a modest increase in ß-cryptoxanthin intake, equivalent to one glass of freshly squeezed orange juice per day, is associated with a reduced risk of developing inflammatory disorders such as rheumatoid arthritis."[8]

PREVENTING ALZHEIMER'S DISEASE

In a study published in 2008 in the *Journal of Food Science*, researchers exposed PC12 cells (similar to nerve cells or neurons) to apple, banana, and orange extracts, and then placed the cells under oxidative stress with hydrogen peroxide. Using ultrasound on dried fruit samples in an aqueous methanol solution, researchers extracted fruit phenolics. They found the fruits' antioxidants, specifically the phenolic phytochemicals, prevented oxidative stress. A number of studies have found that the brains of people with Alzheimer's disease are subjected to higher amounts of oxidative stress. The resulting cellular dysfunctions are thought to cause nerve degeneration. The researchers concluded that "fresh apples, banana, and orange in our daily diet along with other fruits may protect neuron cells against oxidative stress-induced neurotoxicity and may play an important role in reducing the risk of neurodegenerative disorders such as Alzheimer's disease."[9]

ONE CAVEAT

A study published in 2009 in the *Journal of Dentistry* described researchers at the University of Rochester Eastman Dental Center in Rochester, New York who were attempting to determine if whitening dental products had any negative effects on teeth. While conducting their studies on enamel in the laboratory, the researchers learned that the effects of orange juice are far more significant than the whitening products. Because of a new scanning microscope, the researchers observed that the orange juice decreased enamel hardness by 84 percent.[10] Of course, in the mouth these effects may be moderated by saliva. So what should the average person do? To reduce the amount of exposure to tooth enamel, people should not linger over a glass of orange juice. Orange juice should be consumed quickly. Whenever possible, after drinking orange juice, people should brush their teeth.

Should oranges and orange juice be included in the diet? Of course.

NOTES

1. The George Mateljan Foundation Website. www.whfoods.com.

2. The George Mateljan Foundation Website.

3. Gorinstein, Shela, Hanna Leontowicz, Maria Leontowicz, et al. 2007. "Effect of Hesperidin and Naringin on the Plasma Lipid Profile and Plasma Antioxidant Activity in Rats Fed a Cholesterol–Containing Diet." *Journal of the Science of Food and Agriculture* 87(7): 1257–1262.

4. Dalgård, Christine, Flemming Nielsen, Jason D. Morrow, et al. 2009. "Supplementation with Orange and Blackcurrant Juice, But Not Vitamin E, Improves Inflammatory Markers in Patients with Peripheral Arterial Disease." *British Journal of Nutrition* 101: 263–269.

5. "Studies Show Genetic Activity of Antioxidants: Clues Found on How They Help Arteries Stay Clear and Healthy." http://medlineplus.gov: July 21, 2009.

6. Deyhim, Farzad, Kristy Garica, Erica Lopez, et al. May 2006. "Citrus Juice Modulates Bone Strength in Male Senescent Rat Model of Osteoporosis." *Nutrition* 22(5): 559–563.

7. Wang, Yuanyuan, Allison M. Hodge, Anita E. Wluka, et al. 2007. "Effect of Antioxidants on Knee Cartilage and Bone in Health, Middle-Aged Subjects: A Cross-Sectional Study." *Arthritis Research & Therapy* 9(4): R66.

8. Pattison, Dorothy J., Deborah P. M. Symmons, Mark Lunt, et al. August 2005. "Dietary beta-Cryptoxanthin and Inflammatory Polyarthritis: Results from a Population-Based Prospective Study." *The American Journal of Clinical Nutrition* 82(2): 451–455.

9. Heo, H. J., S. J. Choi, S. -G. Choi, et al. 2008. "Effects of Banana, Orange, and Apple on Oxidative Stress-Induced Neurotoxicity in PC12 Cells." *Journal of Food Science* 73(2): H28–H32.

10. Ren, Yan-Fang, Azadeh Amin, and Hans Malmstrom. June 2009. "Effects of Tooth Whitening and Orange Juice on Surface Properties of Dental Enamel." *Journal of Dentistry* 37(6): 424–431.

REFERENCES AND RESOURCES

Magazines, Journals, and Newspapers

Dalgård, Christine, Flemming Nielsen, Jason Morrow, et al. 2009. "Supplementation with Orange and Blackcurrant Juice, But Not Vitamin E, Improves Inflammatory Markers in Patients with Peripheral Arterial Disease." *British Journal of Nutrition* 101: 263–269.

Deyhim, Farzad, Kristy Garica, Erica Lopez, et al. May 2006. "Citrus Juice Modulates Bone Strength in Male Senescent Rat Model of Osteoporosis." *Nutrition* 22(5): 559–563.

Gorinstein, Shela, Hanna Leontowicz, Maria Leontowicz, et al. 2007. "Effect of Hesperidin and Naringin on the Plasma Lipid Profiles and Plasma Antioxidant Activity in Rats Fed a Cholesterol-Containing Diet." *Journal of the Science of Food and Agriculture* 87(7): 1257–1262.

Heo, H. J., S. J. Choi, S. -G. Choi, et al. 2008. "Effects of Banana, Orange, and Apple on Oxidative Stress-Induced Neurotoxicity in PC12 Cells." *Journal of Food Science* 73(2): H28–H32.

Pattison, Dorothy J., Deborah P. M. Symmons, Mark Lunt, et al. August 2005. "Dietary beta-Cryptoxanthin and Inflammatory Polyarthritis: Results From a Population-Based Prospective Study." *The American Journal of Clinical Nutrition* 82(2): 451–455.

Ren, Yan-Fang, Azadeh Amin, and Hans Malmstrom. June 2009. "Effects of Tooth Whitening and Orange Juice on Surface Properties of Dental Enamel." *Journal of Dentistry* 37(6): 424–431.

Wang, Yuanyuan, Allison M. Hodge, Anita E. Wluka, et al. 2007. "Effect of Antioxidants on Knee Cartilage and Bone in Healthy, Middle-Aged Subjects: A Cross-Sectional Study." *Arthritis Research & Therapy* 9(4): R66.

Websites

The George Mateljan Foundation. www.whfoods.com.
MedlinePlus. http://medlineplus.gov.

PEARS

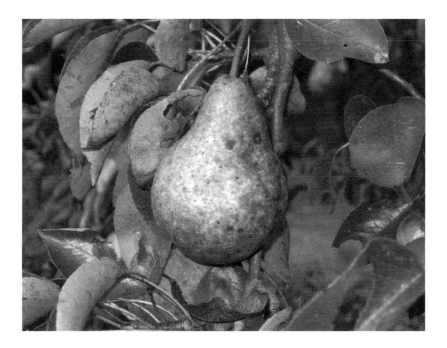

Like so many other types of fruit, pears have prehistoric roots. In those earliest of years, they grew wild. Many centuries later, pears were cultivated during the Roman Empire. By the seventeenth century, more than 300 varieties were grown in France. Pears came to America via the early colonists. They brought pear tree stock cuttings, which could easily be replanted.

Today, there are about 5,000 types of pears. But only a small number of these are available commercially. In the United States, most pears are grown in California, Oregon, and Washington. The most common varieties are Anjou, Asian, Bartlett, Bosc, and Comice.[1]

Pears are a good source of dietary fiber, vitamins C and K, and copper. But, what have the researchers learned?

WEIGHT LOSS

In a 12-week study published in 2003 in *Nutrition*, Brazilian researchers divided 411 overweight women between the ages of 30 and 50 into three groups. All of the women ate essentially the same type of diet and participated in the same amount of exercise. However, the women supplemented their diets with three daily apples, three daily pears, or three daily low-fat oat cookies.

The researchers determined that the women who ate apples or pears consumed fewer total calories than the women who ate the cookies. On average, the fruit eaters lost three pounds and the cookie eaters lost less than two—a statistically significant difference. The researchers theorized that the addition of fruit to the diet, especially apples and pears, may "contribute to weight loss."[2]

A follow-up to this study was published in 2008 in *Appetite*. This time, 49 overweight women, between the ages of 30 and 50, were randomly assigned to add three apples, three pears, or three oat cookies to their daily diets for ten weeks. The women eating apples or pears found that their daily caloric intake decreased; they also lost an average of two pounds. The women eating the cookies had increases in their daily caloric intake, but their weight remained about the same. The researchers noted that their findings, "suggest that energy densities of fruits, independent of their fiber amount, can reduce energy consumption and body weight over time."[3]

Another Brazilian study on weight loss was published in 2008 in *Nutrition Research*. This study included 80 overweight adults between the ages of 30 and 65 who attended a six-month nutrition counseling program. Half of the participants received an intervention; the other half served as the control. The members of both groups were given written information and listened to 30-minute group sessions. But, the members of the intervention group also had three individualized dietary counseling sessions in which a nutritionist recommended increasing the consumption of olive oil, fruits such as pears, and vegetables, and decreasing the consumption of saturated fat.

At the end of the six months, the researchers found that each 100-gram increase in fruit consumption was associated with a 300-gram reduction of body weight. In addition, a 100-gram increase in vegetable intake was associated with a 500-gram reduction in body weight. The researchers commented that their "findings support the relevance of increased intakes of fruits [such as pears] and vegetables that may help avoid weight gain in overweight adults."[4]

REDUCE RISK FOR ASTHMA

In a community-based, cross-sectional study published in 2003 in *The American Journal of Clinical Nutrition*, Australian researchers evaluated the food consumption and respiratory health of 1,601 young adults. In total, 25 nutrients and 47 food groups were investigated. The researchers found that the young adults who included whole milk and fruits, such as apples and pears, in their diets were less likely to develop asthma.[5]

CARDIOVASCULAR HEALTH

In a study published in 2007 in *The American Journal of Clinical Nutrition*, researchers reviewed, over a 16-year period of time, the association between the amount of dietary flavonoids contained in foods such as pears, and heart disease and death in 34,489 postmenopausal women. Pears, in addition to apples and red wine, were found to reduce the risk of both cardiovascular disease and coronary heart disease.[6]

A Japanese study published in 2008 in *Hypertension Research* examined the association between the consumption of fruits, such as pears, and the risk of hypertension, or high blood pressure. Data were obtained from 1,569 men and women (642 men and 927 women) over the age of 35 who lived in Ohasama, Japan. All of the participants measured their blood pressure at home and completed a dietary intake questionnaire. Subjects were considered to have hypertension if their home systolic/diastolic blood pressure was at or over 135/85 mm Hg and/or they were taking a medication for hypertension. Researchers found that the prevalence of home hypertension was 39.4 percent for the men and 29.3 percent for the women. They learned that the subjects who ate the most fruits, vegetables, potassium, and vitamin C were associated with "a significantly lower risk of hypertension." As for fruits, such as pears, when compared with those who ate the lowest amounts of fruits (15.6 g/day), those who ate the highest amounts of fruits (222.7 g/day) had a 45 percent lower risk for hypertension.[7]

COLORECTAL CANCER

In a study published in 2008 in *The American Journal of Clinical Nutrition*, researchers used data from the National Institutes of Health-AARP Diet and Health Study to examine the association between diet and incidence of colorectal cancer. The data included information on 293,615 men and 198,767 women. Three main dietary patterns were identified: a fruit and vegetable diet (including pears), a diet of diet foods, and a red meat and potatoes pattern diet. The researchers found that diets that included reduced amounts of meat and higher intake of fat-reduced foods and fruits and vegetables were associated with decreased risk for colorectal cancer.[8]

In another study published in 2007 in *The Journal of Nutrition*, researchers from North Carolina examined data from 725 people who had undergone colonoscopies. Within this cohort, physicians identified 203 cases of adenomas, benign tumors formed from the cells lining the inside of the large intestine (colon). In the remaining cases, a total of 522 people, no adenomas were found.

The researchers then studied the types of foods that these people ate. Three types of diets emerged: high fruit (such as pears)–low meat, high vegetable–moderate meat, and high meat. The researchers found that when compared to the people who ate a high fruit–low meat diet, the people who ate the high vegetable–moderate meat diet and the high meat diet had a significantly higher risk for adenomas. They concluded that, "a high-fruit, low-meat diet appears to be protective against colorectal adenomas compared with a dietary pattern of increased vegetable and meat consumption."[9] Why is it important to reduce the risk of the growth of benign (noncancerous) tumors? Because, these growths have the potential to increase in size and become cancerous. Over time, they may develop into colorectal cancer.

ONE CAVEAT

It is well-known that farmers tend to use a good deal of pesticides on their pear trees. People who wish to reduce their intake of pesticides should purchase pears that have been grown organically.

Should pears be included in the diet? Absolutely.

NOTES

1. Daniels-Zeller, Debra. May–June 2004. "Perfect Pears." *Vegetarian Journal* 23(3): 6–9.

2. de Oliveira, Maria Conceição, Rosely Sichieri, and Anibal Sanchez Moura. March 2003. "Weight Loss Associated with a Daily Intake of Three Apples or Three Pears Among Overweight Women." *Nutrition* 19(3): 253–256.

3. de Oliveira, Maria Conceição, Rosely Sichieri, and Renzo Venturim Mozzer. September 2008. "A Low-Energy-Dense Diet Adding Fruit Reduces Weight and Energy Intake in Women." *Appetite* 51(2): 291–295.

4. Sartorelli, Daniela Saes, Laércio Franco, and Marly Augusto Cardoso. April 2008. "High Intake of Fruits and Vegetables Predicts Weight Loss in Brazilian Overweight Adults." *Nutrition Research* 28(4): 233–238.

5. Woods, Rosalie K., E. Haydn Walters, Joan M. Raven, et al. September 2003. "Food and Nutrient Intakes and Asthma Risk in Young Adults." *The American Journal of Clinical Nutrition* 78(3): 414–421.

6. Mink, Pamela J., Carolyn G. Scrafford, Leila M. Barraj, et al. March 2007. "Flavonoid Intake and Cardiovascular Disease Mortality: A Prospective Study in Postmenopausal Women." *The American Journal of Clinical Nutrition* 85(3): 895–909.

7. Utsugi, M. T., T. Ohkubo, M. Kikuya, et al. July 2008. "Fruit and Vegetable Consumption and the Risk of Hypertension Determined by Self Measurement of Blood Pressure at Home: the Ohasama Study." *Hypertension Research* 31(7): 1435–1443.

8. Flood, Andrew, Tanuja Rastogi, Elisabet Wirfalt, et al. July 2008. "Dietary Patterns as Identified by Factor Analysis and Colorectal Cancer Among Middle-Aged Americans." *The American Journal of Clinical Nutrition* 88(1): 176–184.

9. Austin, Gregory L., Linda S. Adair, Joseph A. Galanko, et al. April 2007. "A Diet High in Fruits and Low in Meats Reduces the Risk of Colorectal Adenomas." *The Journal of Nutrition* 137: 999–1004.

REFERENCES AND RESOURCES
Magazines, Journals, and Newspapers

Austin, Gregory L., Linda S. Adair, Joseph A. Galanko, et al. April 2007. "A Diet High in Fruits and Low in Meats Reduces the Risk of Colorectal Adenomas." *The Journal of Nutrition* 137: 999–1004.

Colwyn, Kim. January 2006. "Pears: Sweet Consequences Could Come from Picking the Perfect Pear. Here's How to Ensure a Succulent Choice Year-Round." *Better Nutrition* 68(1): 28.

Daniels-Zeller, Debra. May–June 2004. "Perfect Pears." *Vegetarian Journal* 23(3): 6–9.

de Oliveira, Maria Conceição, Rosely Sichieri, and Anibal Sanchez Moura. March 2003. "Weight Loss Associated with a Daily Intake of Three Apples or Three Pears Among Overweight Women." *Nutrition* 19(3): 253–256.

de Oliveira, Maria Conceição, Rosely Sichieri, and Renzo Venturim Mozzer. September 2008. "A Low-Energy-Sense Diet Adding Fruit Reduces Weight and Energy Intake in Women." *Appetite* 51(2): 291–295.

Flood, Andrew, Tanuja Rastogi, Elisabet Wirfalt, et al. July 2008. "Dietary Patterns as Identified By Factor Analysis and Colorectal Cancer Among Middle-Aged Americans." *The American Journal of Clinical Nutrition* 88(1): 176–184.

Mink, Pamela J., Carolyn G. Scrafford, Leila M. Barraj, et al. March 2007. "Flavonoid Intake and Cardiovascular Disease Mortality: A Prospective Study in Postmenopausal Women." *The American Journal of Clinical Nutrition* 85(3): 895–909.

Sartorelli, Daniela Saes, Laércio Joel Franco, and Marly Augusto Cardoso. April 2008. "High Intake of Fruits and Vegetables Predicts Weight Loss in Brazilian Overweight Adults." *Nutrition Research* 28(4): 233–238.

Utsugi, M.T., T. Ohkubo, M. Kikuya, et al. July 2008. "Fruit and Vegetable Consumption and the Risk of Hypertension Determined by Self Measurement of Blood Pressure at Home: The Ohasama Study." *Hypertension Research* 31(7): 1435–1443.

Woods, Rosalie K., E. Haydn Walters, Joan M. Raven, et al. September 2003. "Food and Nutrient Intakes and Asthma Risk in Young Adults." *The American Journal of Clinical Nutrition* 78(3): 414–421.

Websites

The George Mateljan Foundation. www.whfoods.com.
Pear Bureau Northwest. www.usapears.com.

PINEAPPLES

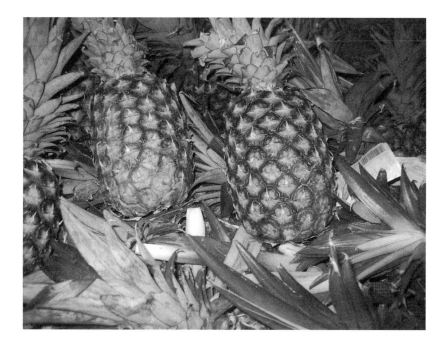

While it is generally believed that pineapples originated in Central and South America, where they were used by the indigenous peoples as both food and medicine, they were not discovered by Europeans until 1493. That was the year that Christopher Columbus, during his second voyage to the Caribbean, found them on the island that is now known as Guadalupe.[1]

Columbus, and other explorers who followed him, brought pineapples back to Europe where people attempted to grow them. Not surprisingly, since it is now known that pineapples require a tropical environment, the Europeans had little success. Still, it is known that by the 18th century, pineapples were growing in Hawaii. Today, Hawaii is the only state in which they are grown. However, pineapples are also grown in Mexico, China, Brazil, Thailand, and the Philippines.[2]

Pineapples contain huge amount of the trace element manganese and very high amounts of vitamin C. Still, pineapples are probably best known for the bromelain found in the core and stem. Bromelain, which is actually a family of enzymes, is believed to be effective for treating a wide variety of medical problems such as the inflammation and pain associated with arthritis, ulcerative colitis, sinusitis, and allergic airway disease or asthma. But are those claims supported by research?

ARTHRITIS

In a six week Pakistani study published in 2004 in *Clinical Rheumatology*, researchers treated 103 patients with osteoarthritis of the knee with either an oral enzyme combination (ERC) containing rutin, bromelain, and trypsin, or diclofenac, a non-steroidal anti-inflammatory drug available by prescription. Researchers found that 54.1 percent of the people taking ERC and 37.2 percent of the people taking diclofenac reported at least at least "good" improvement. So, in this study, people taking ERC had better results than those on prescription medication.[3]

A Mumbai, India, study published in 2001 in the *Journal of Association of Physicians of India* also investigated how the combination of the same three enzymes compared with diclofenac. The researchers randomly placed 50 patients between the ages of 40 and 75 with osteoarthritis of the knee on either two to three tablets of the enzymes twice each day, or diclofenac, 50 mg, twice each day. The treatment continued for three weeks. The researchers noted that at the end of the treatment and at a follow-up appointment at seven weeks, both groups had a reduction in pain and joint tenderness. The study group had a slight improvement in the range of motion.[4]

In a British study published in 2002 in *Phytomedicine*, researchers reviewed the effect bromelain may have on healthy adults who experience mild acute knee pain for less than three months. At the beginning of the study, the volunteers completed two questionnaires. Then, they were placed on either 200 mg or 400 mg bromelain for one month. Seventy-seven people completed the study. People in both groups reported reductions in their symptoms, such as stiffness. But, the volunteers taking the higher dose had greater improvement. The researchers concluded that, "bromelain may be effective in ameliorating physical symptoms and improving general well-being in otherwise healthy adults suffering from mild knee pain in dose-dependent manner."[5]

In another British study published in 2006 in *QJM*, 47 subjects with moderate to severe osteoarthritis of the knee were placed on 12 weeks of bromelain 800 mg/day or a placebo, with a four-week follow-up. Fourteen bromelain and 17 placebo patients completed the study. The researchers found no statistical differences in outcomes between the two groups. They concluded that, "this study suggests that bromelain is not efficacious as an adjunctive treatment of moderate to severe OA [osteoarthritis]."[6] One cannot help but wonder if bromelain tends to be more useful when the condition is relatively mild and less useful when the condition is more advanced.

Another British study, published in 2004 in the *Annals of Rheumatic Diseases*, examined the relationship between intake of fruits and vegetables high in vitamin C, such as pineapples, and the incidence of inflammatory polyarthritis or the inflammation of multiple joints as in rheumatoid arthritis. The researchers found that the people who ate the least amount of foods with vitamin C had three times the risk of developing inflammatory polyarthritis than those who ate the most foods with vitamin C.[7] Commenting on the study, one of the researchers noted that vitamin C is known to be a "scavenger of free radicals," which cause inflammatory conditions such as arthritis. Moreover, it is also possible that vitamin C is protective against infections that may cause arthritis.[8]

ULCERATIVE COLITIS

Ulcerative colitis, an inflammatory bowel disease that primarily affects the colon, may seriously impair an individual's ability to lead a normal life. Symptoms include diarrhea, joint pain, anemia, profound fatigue, abdominal pain, weight loss, and intestinal bleeding. Additionally, ulcerative colitis has also been associated with higher rates of colorectal cancer. Laura P. Hale, MD, PhD, a Duke University researcher who has been studying the use of bromelain to control the bowel inflammation in mice, reported in a study published in 2005 in *Clinical Immunology*, "Daily treatment with oral bromelain beginning at age five weeks decreased the incidence and severity of spontaneous colitis in. . . . mice. Bromelain also significantly decreased the clinical histologic severity of colonic inflammation when administered to . . . mice with established colitis."[9]

SINUSITIS

In a German study published in *In Vivo* in 2005, researchers analyzed the use of bromelain for 116 children under the age of 11 who suffered from sinusitis. Sixty-two of the children were treated with bromelain; 34 were treated with bromelain and standard therapies; and 20 were treated with standard therapies. (The standard therapies included antibiotics, pain relievers, and cortisone sprays.) The researchers found that the children who were treated only with bromelain had the fastest improvement—6.66 days. Those treated with the standard therapy improved in 7.95 days. The children who received bromelain and standard therapies required the longest time to see improvement in their symptoms—9.06 days. The researchers wrote that the children who received only bromelain "showed a statistically significant faster recovery from symptoms ($p = 0.005$) compared to the other treatment groups." Only one child, who was known to have an allergy to pineapples, had a mild allergic reaction to the bromelain. So, it is not surprising that, in Germany, bromelain is commonly used for sinusitis in children.[10]

ALLERGIC AIRWAY DISEASE OR ASTHMA

In a study published in 2005 in *Cellular Immunology*, Connecticut researchers studied three groups of mice that were induced with acute asthma. For four days, one group was treated with 2 mg of bromelain per kg twice daily, and the second group was treated with 6 mg of bromelain per kg twice daily. The third group, the control, was treated with saline. The researchers determined that the bromelain reduced the levels of white blood cells, which increases with asthma. Furthermore, bromelain lowered the inflammatory cells that occur with asthma, known as eosinophils, more than 50 percent. No such improvement was seen in the mice in the control group. The researchers noted that, "bromelain may have similar effects in the treatment of human asthma and hypersensitivity disorders."

Should pineapples be included in the diet? For the vast majority of people, absolutely.

NOTES

1. Walsh, Nancy. June 1, 2006. "Bromelain for Osteoarthritis." *Internal Medicine News* 39(11): 24.

2. The George Mateljan Foundation Website. www.whfoods.org.

3. Akhtar, Naseer M., Rizwan Naseer, Abid Z. Farooqi, et al. October 2004. "Oral Enzyme Combination Versus Diclofenac in the Treatment of Osteoarthritis of the Knee—A Double-Blind Prospective." *Clinical Rheumatology* 23(5): 410–415.

4. Tilwe, G. H., S. Beria, N. H. Turakhia, et al. June 2001. "Efficacy and Tolerability of Oral Enzyme Therapy as Compared to Diclofenac in Active Osteoarthritis of Knee Joint: An Open Randomized Controlled Clinical Trial." *Journal of Association of Physicians of India* 49(617–621).

5. Walker, A. F., R. Bundy, S. M. Hicks, and R. W. Middleton. 2002. "Bromelain Reduces Mild Acute Knee Pain and Improves Well-Being in a Dose-Dependent Fashion in an Open Study of Otherwise Healthy Adults." *Phytomedicine* 9(8): 681–686.

6. Brien, S., G. Lewith, A. F. Walker, et al. 2006. "Bromelain as an Adjunctive Treatment for Moderate-to-Severe Osteoarthritis of the Knee: A Randomized Placebo-Controlled Pilot Study." *QJM* 99(12): 841–850.

7. Pattison, D. J., A. J. Silman, N. J. Goodson, et al. 2004. "Vitamin C and the Risk of Developing Inflammatory Polyarthritis: Prospective Nested Case-Control Study." *Annals of Rheumatic Diseases* 63: 843–847.

8. "Stay Nimble with C." October 2004. *Natural Health* 34(9): 22.

9. Hale, Laura P., Paula K. Greer, Chau T. Trinh, and Marcia R. Gottfried. August 2005. "Treatment with Oral Bromelain Decreases Colonic Inflammation in the IL-10-Deficient Murine Model of Inflammatory Bowel Disease." *Clinical Immunology* 116(2): 135–142.

10. Braun, J. M., B. Schneider, and H. J. Beuth. March–April 2005. "Therapeutic Use, Efficacy and Safety of the Proteolytic Pineapple Enzyme Bromelain-POS® in Children with Acute Sinusitis in Germany." *In Vivo* 19(2): 417–421.

REFERENCES AND RESOURCES
Magazines, Journals, and Newspapers

Akhtar, Naseer M., Rizwan Naseer, Abid Z. Farooqi, et al. October 2004. "Oral Enzyme Combination Versus Diclofenac in the Treatment of Osteoarthritis of the Knee—A Double Blind Prospective Randomized Study." *Clinical Rheumatology* 23(5): 410–415.

Braun, J. M., B. Schneider, and H. J. Beuth. March-April 2005. "Therapeutic Use, Efficacy and Safety of the Proteolytic Pineapple Enzyme Bromelain-POS® in Children with Acute Sinusitis in Germany." *In Vivo* 19(2): 417–421.

Brien, S., G. Lewith, A. F. Walker, et al. 2006. "Bromelain as an Adjunctive Treatment for Moderate-to-Severe Osteoarthritis of the Knee: A Randomized Placebo-Controlled Pilot Study." *QJM* 99(12): 841–850.

Hale, Laura P., Paula K. Greer, Chau T. Trinh, and Marcia R. Gottfried. August 2005. "Treatment with Oral Bromelain Decreased Colonic Inflammation in the IL-10-Deficient Murine Model of Inflammatory Bowel Disease." *Clinical Immunology* 116(2): 135–142.

Pattison, D. J., A. J. Silman, N. J. Goodson, et al. 2004. "Vitamin C and the Risk of Developing Inflammatory Polyarthritis: Prospective Nested Case-Control Study." *Annals of Rheumatic Diseases* 63: 843–847.

Secor, Jr., Eric R., William F. Carson IV, Michelle M. Cloutier, et al. September 2005. "Bromelain Exerts Anti-Inflammatory Effects in an Ovalbumin-Induced Murine Model of Allergic Airway Disease." *Cellular Immunology* 237(1): 68–75.

"Stay Nimble with C." October 2004. *Natural Health* 34(9): 22.

Tilwe, G. H., S. Beria, N. H. Turakhia, et al. June 2001. "Efficacy and Tolerability of Oral Enzyme Therapy as Compared to Diclofenac in Active Osteoarthritis of Knee Joint: An Open Randomized Controlled Clinical Trial." *Journal of Association of Physicians of India* 49: 617–621.

Walker, A. F., R. Bundy, S. M. Hicks, and R. W. Middleton. 2002. "Bromelain Reduces Mild Acute Knee Pain and Improves Well-Being in a Dose-Dependent Fashion in an Open Study of Otherwise Healthy Adults." *Phytomedicine* 9(8): 681–686.

Walsh, Nancy. June 1, 2006. "Bromelain for Osteoarthritis." *Internal Medicine News* 39(11): 24.

Website

The George Mateljian Foundation. www.whfoods.org.

POMEGRANATES

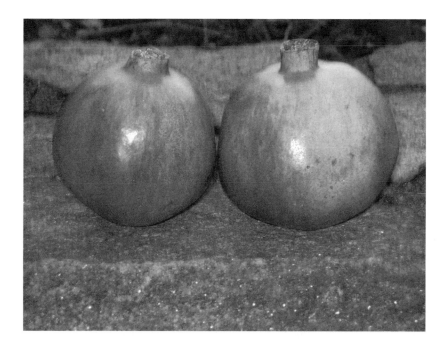

Though it is a relatively new fruit in American kitchens, the pomegranate, *Punica granatum* L., has an ancient history. In fact, it is believed that pomegranates were grown in the Garden of Eden.[1] The Bible's Old Testament praises pomegranates, and pomegranates were an integral part of the lives of the ancient Egyptians and Greeks.[2] To the Babylonians, pomegranate seeds were agents of resurrection; the Persians thought they gave soldiers invincibility during battles. To the ancient Chinese, the seeds were symbols of longevity and immortality. And, the Koran, the Moslem sacred text, envisions paradise as a place with an abundance of pomegranates.[3]

Though native to Iran, for countless generations pomegranates have been grown in many parts of the world, including the Mediterranean, China, Japan, India, Russia, and the Middle East. More recently, they have been cultivated in California and Arizona. The average pomegranate is rounded and hexagonal in shape, and the diameter is between five and twelve centimeters. The skin is thick and reddish. About 80 percent of a pomegranate is edible. Of this, 80 percent is juice and 20 percent is seed.

In a 2007 article in *Chiropractic Nutritional Wellness*, James D. Krystosik, DC, maintained that pomegranates should be considered a "superfood." According to Krystosik, pomegranates do much more than provide nutrients to the body. They fight diseases and support the immune system and youthful vigor. In addition, they offer protection from heart disease and fatigue. "Most importantly, superfoods pack a powerful, knock-out punch to free radicals—unstable and harmful molecules generated from the environment, before they can cause damage to the body cells, tissues, and organs. . . . Antioxidants mop up free radicals and render them harmless. Superfoods contain mega doses of antioxidants. . . ."[4] And, the scientific evidence currently supports such claims.

An article in *Harvard Men's Health Watch* stated that pomegranates have high amounts of vitamin C as well as polyphenols and tannins, which have powerful antioxidant activity. Moreover, the seeds are filled with fiber, estrone, genistein, daidzein, steroid estrogen, and isoflavones. These have "strong biological actions and potential medical benefits." Furthermore, the seeds have "a unique oil that contains an uncommon fatty acid, punicic acid."[5]

CARDIOVASCULAR DISEASE

An article published in 2005 in *The American Journal of Cardiology* described a study of 45 patients with a mean age of 69. All of the patients had coronary heart disease (their heart arteries have narrowed). Patients were assigned to one of two groups. One group drank 240 ml/day of pomegranate juice; the other group drank a non-pomegranate juice that looked like pomegranate juice. After three months, researchers determined that the narrowing of the arteries of the patients who drank the pomegranate juice had decreased by 17.8 percent. Meanwhile, the narrowing of the arteries of patients in the placebo group had increased by 20.3 percent. The researchers concluded that a daily consumption of pomegranate juice may well be beneficial for those dealing with coronary heart disease.[6]

In a study published in 2004 in *Clinical Nutrition*, researchers examined the effect of drinking a daily eight-ounce glass of pomegranate juice on people who already had high levels of plaque lining their arteries. Nineteen people between the ages of 65 and 75 were divided into two groups. Ten participants drank the juice and nine were given no juice. Those who drank the juice experienced a significant reduction in arterial plaque; those who did not drink the juice had increases in plaque.[7]

In 2006, the *International Journal for Vitamin and Nutrition Research* included information on an Iranian study in which researchers examined the effect of the consumption of pomegranate juice in 22 people with type 2 diabetes who also had elevated levels of cholesterol. Each day, the subjects drank 40 g of concentrated pomegranate juice for a period of eight weeks. Researchers found that the addition of pomegranate juice to the diet lowered levels of total and LDL (bad) cholesterol and improved total/HDL (good) and LDL/HDL cholesterol ratios.[8]

CANCER
Prostate Cancer

A number of different in vitro and animal studies have demonstrated that pomegranates may well play a role in inhibiting the growth of prostate cancer, the second-leading cause of cancer-related death in the United States. As a result, researchers decided to conduct clinical trials on men who had undergone surgery or radiation for prostate cancer. Even though these men had been treated, shortly after treatment, the levels of prostate-specific antigen (PSA) in their blood had risen, indicating that cancer cells had reappeared.

The goal of the research was to determine if the consumption of pomegranate juice could alter the rate of "doubling time," or the amount of time it takes for PSA levels to double. Patients with short doubling times are more likely to die from their illness. According to Allan Pantuck, MD, a UCLA associate professor of urology and the lead researcher on this study, the average doubling time is approximately 15 months. Among the 50 men who participated in the study, drinking a daily eight-ounce glass of pomegranate juice increased the doubling time to 54 months.

Commenting on the study, Dr. Pantuck said, "That's a big increase. I was surprised when I saw such an improvement in PSA numbers. In older men 65 to 70 who have been treated for prostate cancer, we can give them pomegranate juice and it may be possible for them to outlive their risk of dying from cancer. We are hoping we may be able to prevent or delay the need for other therapies usually used in this population such as hormone treatment or chemotherapy, both of which bring with them harmful side effects."[9]

Lung Cancer

Researchers at the University of Wisconsin have determined that there is now evidence that pomegranate fruit extract may alter the progression of lung disease—at least in mice. After five months of pomegranate supplementation, mice that had received a tumor-inducing agent had 62 percent fewer tumors than the mice that did not receive the supplementation.[10]

ALZHEIMER'S DISEASE

Richard Hartman, PhD, an assistant professor of psychology at the School of Science and Technology at Loma Linda University, has been studying whether mice predisposed to develop Alzheimer's disease may benefit from pomegranate-juice concentrate. Dr. Hartman and his colleagues separated a cohort of mice into two groups. One received water with pomegranate juice concentrate; the other received water with sugar. Typically, each mouse drank about five milliliters of fluid each day. That is equivalent to a human drinking one to two glasses of pomegranate juice every day. The results were more than significant. "After six months, the pomegranate juice-treated mice learned water maze tasks more quickly and swam faster, and the mice that drank the pomegranate juice had 50 percent less beta-amyloid plaques in the hippocampus of their brains [an indication of Alzheimer's disease]."[11]

GENERAL WELL-BEING

Researchers at the Institute of Hygiene and Environmental Medicine in Tianjin, China, have found that pomegranate juice is far more effective than apple juice in improving the body's antioxidant defenses. Twenty-six people, with an average age of 63.5 years, were divided into two groups. For four weeks, members of each group drank 250 ml of either pomegranate or apple juice every day. Researchers found that the people who drank the pomegranate juice had increased plasma antioxidant capacity. There was no significant change in those drinking the apple juice.[12]

BE AWARE OF A POTENTIAL CAVEAT

In a 2006 article in *Harvard's Women's Health Watch*, Celeste Robb-Nicholson, MD, responded to a reader's question about pomegranate juice. The reader wanted to know if pomegranate juice could interfere with medications, such as Lipitor. Dr. Robb-Nicholson noted that such interference is within the realm of possibility. So, "if you like the juice enough to drink a glass every day, be sure to tell your clinician so that she or he can keep it in mind when monitoring your Lipitor and other medication."[13] Should pomegranates and pomegranate juice be part of the diet? Absolutely.

NOTES

    1. "Pomegranates for the Prostate and the Heart: Seeds of Hope." April 2007. *Harvard Men's Health Watch*: NA.

    2. Jurenka, Julie. June 2008. "Therapeutic Applications of Pomegranate (*Punica granatum* L): A Review." *Alternative Medicine Review* 13(2): 128–144.

    3. Louba, Ben-Nun. September 2007. "What Are the Medical Properties of Pomegranates?" *Journal of Chinese Clinical Medicine* 2(9): 530–538.

    4. Krystosik, James D. November 2007. "Superfoods to Save the Day." *Chiropractic Nutritional Wellness* 3(4): 4–5.

    5. "Pomegranates for the Prostate and the Heart: Seeds of Hope." April 2007. *Harvard Men's Health Watch*: NA.

    6. Sumner, Michael D., Melanie Elliott-Eller, Gerdi Weidner, et al. September 15, 2005. "Effects of Pomegranate Juice Consumption on Myocardial Perfusion in Patients with Coronary Heart Disease." *The American Journal of Cardiology* 96(6): 810–814.

7. Aviram, M., M. Rosenblat, D. Gaitini, et al. 2004. "Pomegranate Juice Consumption for Three Years by Patients with Carotid Artery Stenosis Reduces Common Carotid Intima-Media Thickness, Blood Pressure and LDL Oxidation." *Clinical Nutrition* 23: 423–433.

8. Esmaillzadeh A., F. Tahbaz, I. Gaieni, et al. May 2006. "Cholesterol-Lowering Effect of Concentrated Pomegranate Juice Consumption in Type II Diabetic Patients with Hyperlipidemia." *International Journal for Vitamin and Nutrition Research* 76(3): 147–151.

9. "Pomegranate Juice Keeps PSA Levels Stable in Men Treated for Prostate Cancer." UCLA Jonsson Comprehensive Cancer Center Website, www.cancer.ucla.edu.

10. Burke, Cathy. October 2007. "Pomegranate Hinders Lung Tumors." *Life Extension*: NA.

11. Thio, Patricia, "Pomegranate Juice May Reduce Alzheimer's Disease Risk." Website of the School of Science and Technology, Loma Linda University, www.llu.edu/llu/sst/.

12. Guo, C., J. Wei, J. Wang, et al. February 2008. "Pomegranate Juice Is Potentially Better Than Apple Juice in Improving Antioxidant Function in Elderly Subjects." *Nutrition Research* 28(2): 72–77.

13. Robb-Nicholson, Celeste. July 2006. "By the Way, Doctor; Does Pomegranate Juice Interfere with Medications?" *Harvard Women's Health Watch*: NA

REFERENCES AND RESOURCES
Magazine, Journals, and Newspapers

Aviram, M., M. Rosenblat, D. Gaitini, et al. 2004. "Pomegranate Juice Consumption for Three Years by Patients with Carotid Artery Stenosis Reduces Common Carotid Intima-Media Thickness, Blood Pressure and LDL Oxidation." *Clinical Nutrition* 23: 423–433.

Burke, Cathy. May 2006. "Pomegranate Hinders Lung Tumors." *Life Extension*: NA.

Esmaillzadeh A., F. Tahbaz, I. Gaieni, et al. May 2006. "Cholesterol Lowering Effect of Concentrated Pomegranate Juice Consumption in Type II Diabetic Patients with Hyperlipidemia." *International Journal for Vitamin and Nutrition Research* 76(3): 147–151.

Guo, C., J. Wei, J. Yang, et al. February 2008. "Pomegranate Juice is Potentially Better Than Apple Juice in Improving Antioxidant Function in Elderly Subjects." *Nutrition Research* 28(2): 72–77.

Jurenka, Julie. June 2008. "Therapeutic Applications of Pomegranate (*Punica granatum* L.): A Review." *Alternative Medicine Review* 13(2): 128–144.

Khan, Naghma, Farrukh Afaq, Mee-Hyang Kweon, et al. April 1, 2007. "Oral Consumption of Pomegranate Fruit Extract Inhibits Growth and Progression of Primary Lung Tumors in Mice." *Cancer Research* 67(7): 3475–3482.

Krystosik, James D. November 2007. "Superfoods to Save the Day." *Chiropractic Nutritional Wellness* 3(4): 4–5.

Louba, Ben-Nun. September 2007. "What Are the Medical Properties of Pomegranates?" *Journal of Chinese Clinical Medicine* 2(9): 530–538.

"Pomegranate Juice Could Fight Alzheimer's." December 3, 2005. *Science News* 168(23): 366.

"Pomegranates for the Prostate and the Heart: Seeds of Hope." April 2007. *Harvard Men's Health Watch*: NA.

Robb-Nicholson, Celeste. July 2006. "By the Way, Doctor; Does Pomegranate Juice Interfere with Medications?" *Harvard's Women's Health Watch*: NA.

Sumner, Michael D., Melanie Elliott-Eller, Gerdi Weidner, et al. September 15, 2005. "Effects of Pomegranate Juice Consumption on Myocardial Perfusion in Patients with Coronary Heart Disease." *The American Journal of Cardiology* 96(6): 810–814.

Walsh, Nancy. April 1, 2006. "Pomegranate for Cardiovascular Disease." *Internal Medicine News* 39(7): 51.

Websites

Loma Linda University, School of Science and Technology. www.llu.edu/llu/sst/.

UCLA Jonsson Comprehensive Cancer Center. www.cancer.ucla.edu.

PUMPKINS

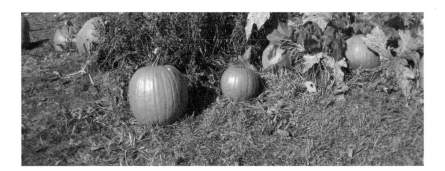

Pumpkins go hand-in-hand with Halloween. After all, pumpkins are in abundance during the fall, and, in preparation for Halloween, it is not uncommon for people to decorate their homes with pumpkins. Still, there appears to be a great deal more to pumpkins than Halloween.

Pumpkins, which belong to the gourd or Cucurbitaceae family, were consumed by Native Americans, who considered them both food and medicine. When the European explorers came to the "New World," they often returned home with pumpkins. Eventually, pumpkins spread throughout the world. Today, pumpkins are commercially cultivated primarily in the United States, Mexico, India, and China.[1]

Pumpkins contain very good amounts of dietary fiber, vitamins A and C, riboflavin, potassium, copper, and manganese; they have good amounts of vitamin E and B_6, thiamin, niacin, iron, magnesium, and phosphorus.[2] Pumpkins are filled with carotenoids, which are believed to decrease the risk of several types of cancer and other medical problems. Though all too often discarded, pumpkin seeds are a very good source of manganese, magnesium, and phosphorus; and, they are a good source of tryptophan, iron, copper, vitamin K, zinc, and protein.[3] But, what have researchers learned?

BENIGN PROSTATIC HYPERPLASIA (BPH)

As men age, it is not uncommon for their prostate glands to enlarge, a condition known as benign prostatic hyperplasia. So, researchers have searched for ways to decrease the size of the gland. One group from the West Indies decided to investigate whether pumpkin seed oil could reduce this enlargement in rats. Their findings were published in 2006 in the *Journal of Medicinal Food*.

In this study, for 20 days, testosterone was injected into rats to enlarge their prostate glands. At the same time, the diets of the rats were supplemented with two different doses of either pumpkin seed oil or corn oil. Every week, the researchers checked the weight of each of the rats. On the 21st day, the rats were sacrificed, and the prostate glands were removed, cleaned, and weighed. The researchers found that the testosterone significantly increased the prostate size. However, in the rats fed the higher dose of pumpkin seed oil, "this increase was inhibited." The researchers concluded that, "pumpkin seed oil can inhibit testosterone-induced hyperplasia of the prostate and therefore may be beneficial in the management of benign prostatic hyperplasia."[4]

DIABETES

In a study published in 2007 in the *Journal of the Science of Food and Agriculture*, researchers from East China Normal University divided a total of 12 diabetic rats and 12 normal rats into four groups, each with six rats. For 30 days, the rats were fed either a normal diet or a diet supplemented with pumpkin extract. Compared to the untreated rats, the diabetic rats fed pumpkin extract had a 36-percent increase in plasma insulin, which was only five percent less than the control group. Moreover, the percentage of insulin-positive cells in the pumpkin-fed diabetic rats was only eight percent lower than the normal rats. Though the rats used in this study modeled type 1 diabetes, the researchers noted that pumpkin extract may also help those with type 2 diabetes.[5]

BREAST CANCER

Two studies published in 2009 examined the association between consumption of carotenoids, which are found in abundance in pumpkins, and breast cancer. In one study, which was published in *Cancer Epidemiology, Biomarkers & Prevention*, researchers from the University of California, San Diego, studied a cohort of 3,043 women who had been diagnosed with early-stage breast cancer. The researchers found that the women with the highest intake of carotenoids were the least likely to experience a cancer recurrence. "Higher biological exposure to carotenoids, when assessed over the time frame of the study, was associated with greater likelihood of breast cancer-free survival."[6]

And, in a Harvard School of Public Health study published in 2009 in the *International Journal of Cancer*, researchers reviewed the intake of carotenoids in 5,707 premenopausal and postmenopausal women with incident invasive breast cancer and 6,389 premenopausal and postmenopausal controls. The researchers found that a high intake of carotenoids reduced the risk of breast cancer in premenopausal, but not postmenopausal woman.

A high carotenoid intake was particularly protective for premenopausal women who had been smokers.[7]

IRON DEFICIENCY/ANEMIA

In a study published in 2007 in *BioFactors*, Iranian researchers noted that iron deficiency "is the most prevalent nutritional problem in the world today." As a result, they decided to investigate whether the daily consumption of iron-fortified, ready-to-eat cereal and pumpkin seed kernels would improve the iron status of young adult women. Their sample size was small—only eight healthy female subjects between the ages of 20 sand 37 years. For four weeks, the women consumed 30 g of the cereal (providing 7.1 mg of iron/day) and 30 g of the pumpkin seed kernels (providing 4.0 mg of iron/day). After the four weeks, all eight women had higher levels of serum iron. The researchers wrote that, "adding another food source of iron, such as pumpkin seed kernels, improves the iron status."[8]

MANAGEMENT OF HYPERGLYCEMIA AND HYPERTENSION

In a study published in 2007 in the *Journal of Medicinal Food*, University of Massachusetts, Amherst, researchers noted that the indigenous communities in North America tend to have high rates of hyperglycemia (high concentrations of glucose in the blood) and hypertension (high blood pressure). Most likely, this is related to their high intake of high calorie foods "such as sugar, refined grain flour, and sweetened beverages." The researchers wondered if a return to the traditional foods, such as corn, beans, and pumpkins, which have a "better balance of calories and beneficial nutrients," may be helpful. In their in vitro studies, the researchers found that to be true. And, of the three foods, pumpkins "showed the best overall potential." The researchers concluded that, "this phenolic antioxidant-enriched dietary strategy using specific traditional plant food combinations can generate a whole food profile that has the potential to reduce hyperglycemia-induced pathogenesis and also associated complications linked to cellular oxidation stress and hypertension."[9]

INSOMNIA

In a double blind, placebo-controlled study published in 2005 in *Nutritional Neuroscience*, Craig Hudson, MD, a Canadian psychiatrist, and his colleagues investigated whether pumpkin seeds, a good source of tryptophan, could help people dealing with chronic insomnia. Fifty-seven subjects were randomly assigned to one of three groups: people who took a protein source of tryptophan (pumpkin seeds) in combination with carbohydrate, people who took pharmaceutical grade tryptophan in combination with carbohydrate, and people who took only a carbohydrate. Forty-nine people completed the three-week trial. The researchers found that people who took both the protein source and pharmaceutical grade tryptophan experienced, "significant improvement on subjective and objective measures of insomnia." Furthermore, "protein source tryptophan with carbohydrate alone proved effective in significantly reducing time awake during the night." As a result, the researchers concluded, "protein source of tryptophan is comparable to pharmaceutical grade tryptophan for the treatment of insomnia."[10]

SOCIAL ANXIETY DISORDER

In 2007, another study led by Dr. Hudson was published in the *Canadian Journal of Physiology and Pharmacology*. In this double blind, placebo-controlled, crossover trial, subjects were randomly placed on either a protein-source tryptophan (pumpkin seeds) in combination with carbohydrate or on carbohydrate alone for one week. There was a one-week washout period between the sessions. Though there were only seven subjects, they all completed the study. The researchers noted that, "protein-source tryptophan with carbohydrate, but not carbohydrate alone, resulted in significant improvement on an objective measure of anxiety."[11]

Should the various forms of pumpkins be part of the diet? Of course.

NOTES

1. The George Mateljan Foundation Website. www.whfoods.com.

2. Nutrition Data Website. www.nutritiondata.com.

3. The George Mateljan Foundation Website.

4. Gossell-Williams, M., A. Davis, and N. O'Connor. Summer 2006. "Inhibition of Testosterone-Induced Hyperplasia of the Prostate of Sprague-Dawley Rats by Pumpkin Seed Oil." *Journal of Medicinal Food* 9(2): 284–286.

5. Xia, Tao and Qin Wang. July 2007. "Hypoglycaemic Role of *Cucurbita ficifolia* (Cucurbitaceae) Fruit Extract in Streptozotocin-Induced Diabetic Rats." *Journal of the Science of Food and Agriculture* 87(9): 1753–1757.

6. Rock, Cheryl L., Loki Natarajan, Minya Pu, et al. 2009. "Longitudinal Biological Exposure to Carotenoids Is Associated with Breast Cancer-Free Survival in the Women's Healthy Eating and Living Study." *Cancer Epidemiology, Biomarkers & Prevention* 18(2): 486–494.

7. Mignone, L. I., E. Giovannucci, P. A. Newcomb, et al. June 15, 2009. "Dietary Carotenoids and the Risk of Invasive Breast Cancer." *International Journal of Cancer* 124(12): 2929–2937.

8. Naghii, M. R. and M. Mofid. 2007. "Impact of Daily Consumption of Iron Fortified Ready-to-Eat Cereal and Pumpkin Seed Kernels (*Cucurbita pepo*) on Serum Iron in Adult Women." *BioFactors* 30(1): 19–26.

9. Kwon, Y. I., E. Apostolidis, Y. C. Kim, and K. Shetty. June 2007. "Health Benefits of Traditional Corn, Beans, and Pumpkin: In Vitro Studies for Hyperglycemia and Hypertension Management." *Journal of Medicinal Food* 10(2): 266–275.

10. Hudson, Craig, Susan Patricia Hudson, Tracy Hecht, and Joan MacKenzie. April 2005. "Protein Source Tryptophan versus Pharmaceutical Grade Tryptophan as an Efficacious Treatment for Chronic Insomnia." *Nutritional Neuroscience* 8(2): 121–127.

11. Hudson, Craig, Susan Hudson, and Joan MacKenzie. 2007. "Protein-Source Tryptophan as an Efficacious Treatment for Social Anxiety Disorder: A Pilot Study." *Canadian Journal of Physiology and Pharmacology* 85(9): 928–932.

REFERENCES AND RESOURCES
Journals, Magazines, and Newspapers

Gossell-Williams, M., A. Davis, and N. O'Connor. Summer 2006. "Inhibition of Testosterone-Induced Hyperplasia of the Prostate of Sprague-Dawley Rats by Pumpkin Seed Oil. *Journal of Medicinal Food* 9(2): 284–296.

Hudson, Craig, Susan Hudson, and Joan MacKenzie. 2007. "Protein-Source Tryptophan as an Efficacious Treatment for Social Anxiety Disorder: A Pilot Study." *Canadian Journal of Physiology and Pharmacology* 85(9): 928–932.

Hudson, Craig, Susan Patricia Hudson, Tracy Hecht, and Joan MacKenzie. April 2005. "Protein Source Tryptophan versus Pharmaceutical Grade Tryptophan as an Efficacious Treatment for Chronic Insomnia." *Nutritional Neuroscience* 8(2): 121–127.

Kwon, Y. I., E. Apostolidis, Y. C. Kim, and K. Shetty. June 2007. "Health Benefits of Traditional Corn, Beans, and Pumpkin: In Vitro Studies for Hyperglycemia and Hypertension Management." *Journal of Medicinal Food* 10(2): 266–275.

Mignone, L. I., E. Giovannucci, P. A. Newcomb et al. June 15, 2009. "Dietary Carotenoids and the Risk of Invasive Breast Cancer." *International Journal of Cancer* 124(12): 2929–2937.

Naghii, M. R. and M. Mofid. 2007. "Impact of Daily Consumption of Iron Fortified Ready-to-Eat Cereal and Pumpkin Seed Kernels (*Cucurbita pepo*) on Serum Iron in Adult Women." *BioFactors* 30(1): 19–26.

Rock, Cheryl L., Loki Natarajan, Minya Pu, et al. 2009. "Longitudinal Biological Exposure to Carotenoids Is Associated with Breast Cancer-Free Survival in the Women's Healthy Eating and Living Study." *Cancer Epidemiology, Biomarkers & Prevention* 18(2): 486–494.

Xia, Tao and Qin Wang. July 2007. "Hypoglycemic Role of *Cucurbita ficifolia* (*Cucurbitaceae*) Fruit Extract in Streptozotocin-Induced Diabetic Rats." *Journal of the Science of Food and Agriculture* 87(9): 1753–1757.

Websites

The George Mateljan Foundation. www.whfooods.com.
Nutrition Data. www.nutritiondata.com.

SARDINES

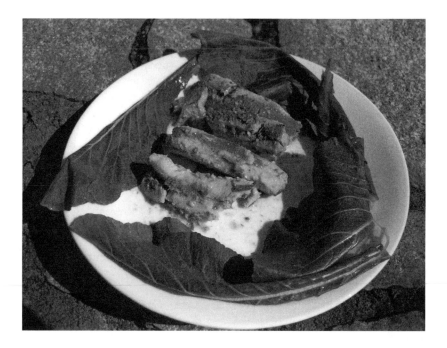

In all probability, most people do not realize that sardines are not a single species of fish. Instead, the word "sardine" is a name given to a variety of small types of fish. The name is actually derived from Sardinia, a Mediterranean island.

Sardines vary according to their point of origin. So, sardines from Maine are small herrings; sardines from Denmark and Norway are silds and brisling; and, sardines from Spain, Portugal, and France are pilchards, a type of herring.[1]

Sardines are considered to be an excellent source for vitamin B_{12} and tryptophan and a very good source for selenium, vitamin D, omega-3 fatty acids, protein, and phosphorus. They are also a good source for calcium and vitamin B_3 (niacin).[2] But, it is important to review the research.

CARDIOVASCULAR HEALTH

In a Harvard study published in 2002 in *The New England Journal of Medicine*, researchers used Physicians' Health Study data to review the blood samples of 94 men "in whom sudden death occurred as the first manifestation of cardiovascular disease" and 184 controls, who were apparently healthy. The researchers determined that the men with the highest blood levels of omega-3, which may be obtained from sardines, were far less likely to suffer a fatal heart attack during the 17 years that the data were collected. The researchers concluded that, "The n-3 fatty acids found in fish are strongly associated with a reduced risk of sudden death among men without evidence or prior cardiovascular disease."[3] Commenting on the results of this study, a 2002 article in *Environmental Nutrition* noted that omega-3 fatty acids in fish, such as sardines, prevent irregular heartbeats, also known as arrhythmias, which may cause sudden death. Furthermore, these fatty acids reduce the likelihood of blood clots, improve the elasticity of blood vessels, and lower triglycerides levels and blood pressure.[4]

In a study published in 2002 in *JAMA, The Journal of the American Medical Association*, researchers used data from the Health Professional Follow-Up Study to examine the association between consumption of long-chain omega-3 polyunsaturated fatty acid, which is found in sardines, and the incidence of stroke. The subjects included 43,671 men between the ages of 40 and 75 who did not have cardiovascular disease at baseline in 1986. During the 12-year follow-up period, the men had 608 strokes—377 ischemic, 106 hemorrhagic, and 125 unclassified. While no significant relationship was found between the consumption of long-chain omega-3 polyunsaturated fatty acid and hemorrhagic stroke, the men who ate fish one to three times per month had significantly lower rates of ischemic stroke than the men who consumed fish less than once per month.[5]

In another study published in 2002 in *JAMA, The Journal of the American Medical Association*, researchers reviewed the association between fish and long-chain omega-3 fatty acid consumption, which is found in sardines, and the risk of coronary heart disease in women. The researchers used data from 84,688 female nurses, between the ages of 34 and 59, enrolled in the Nurses' Health Study. During the 16 years of follow-up, there were 1,513 cases of coronary heart disease. The researchers found that, "among women, higher consumption of fish and omega-3 fatty acids is associated with a lower risk of CHD [coronary heart disease], particularly CHD deaths."[6]

A study published in 2008 in the *Journal of the American College of Cardiology* investigated whether marine-derived n-3 fatty acids, such as those obtained from sardines, reduced the incidence of atherosclerosis. The cohort consisted of men between the ages of 40 and 49. Two-hundred eighty-one were Japanese men from Kusatsu, Shiga, Japan; another 281 were third- or fourth-generation Japanese men from Honolulu, Hawaii; 306 were white men from Alleghany County, Pennsylvania. The researchers found that the

Japanese men who lived in Japan had the lowest levels of atherosclerosis. The Japanese-American men and the white men had about the same levels of this disorder. The researchers noted that Japanese men living in Japan ate about twice as much fish-based omega-3 fatty acids as the Japanese-American men and the white men. Moreover, the researchers determined that as the amount of omega-3 fatty acids increased in the diet of Japanese men living in Japan, the thickening of the carotid arteries in the neck decreased. This inverse relationship was found to be statistically significant. The researchers concluded that, "Very high levels of marine-derived n-3 fatty acids have antiatherogenic properties that are independent of traditional cardiovascular risk factors and may contribute to lower the burden of atherosclerosis in Japanese, a lower burden that is unlikely the result of genetic factors."[7]

CANCER

Prostate Cancer

In a California study that was published in 2009 in *Clinical Cancer Research*, researchers examined the consumption of fish high in omega-3 fatty acids, such as sardines, and the incidence of aggressive prostate cancer in men who have a predisposition for developing this disease. The study included 466 men diagnosed with aggressive prostate cancer and 478 age- and ethnically matched controls. The men in the study who ate one or more servings of fatty fish per week had a 63 percent lower risk for developing aggressive prostate cancer than the men who never ate fish.[8]

A few months earlier, in a study published in 2008 in *The American Journal of Clinical Nutrition*, researchers found similar results. Using data from the Physicians' Health Study, over 20,000 men were followed for "382,144 person-years." During this time, there were 2,161 cases of prostate cancer and 230 deaths from the disease. The researchers found that the men who consumed fish and seafood n-3 fatty acids, such as sardines, five or more times per week had a 48 percent lower risk of prostate cancer death than the men who ate fish less than once weekly.[9]

Kidney Cancer

In a Swedish study published in 2006 in JAMA, *The Journal of the American Medical Association*, researchers investigated the association between consumption of fatty fish, such as sardines, and the incidence of renal cancer in women. They used data from the Swedish Mammography Cohort, which included 61,433 women between the ages of 40 and 76. At baseline, none of the women had cancer. During the 15.3 years of follow-up, 150 cases of renal cancer were diagnosed. Researchers found an inverse relationship between the consumption of fatty fish like sardines and renal cell carcinoma. So, eating more sardines and other fatty fish appears to reduce the risk of renal cancer.[10]

COGNITIVE PERFORMANCE

In a study published in 2007 in *The American Journal of Clinical Nutrition*, researchers reviewed the relationship between the intake of seafood and cognitive performance in 2,031 Norwegian subjects between the ages of 70 and 74. Led by a researcher from the University of Oslo, the researchers found that the more fish the subjects ate, the better their performance on the battery of tests used to check cognition. The relationship appeared to level out around an average daily consumption of 75 grams of fish—about 2.5 ounces. The association appeared to be strongest among those who ate fatty fish, such as sardines, and those who ate nonprocessed lean fish, such as cod.[11]

Should sardines be included in the diet? They are clearly quite healthful. Of course, it is best to obtain fresh sardines. But, when not available, canned sardines are sold throughout the year. However, it is important to check the sodium content and avoid those products with excessive amounts.

NOTES

1. "Fishy Facts." September 2003. *Better Nutrition* 65(9): 30.

2. The George Mateljan Foundation Website. http://whfoods.com.

3. Albert, Christine M., Hannia Campos, Meir J. Stampfer, et al. April 11, 2002. "Blood Levels of Long-Chain n-3 Fatty Acids and the Risk of Sudden Death." *The New England Journal of Medicine* 346(15): 1113–1118.

4. "A Good Time for Seafood Lovers: Three New Studies Confirm Heart Benefits." June 2002. *Environmental Nutrition* 25(6): 3.

5. He, Ka, Eric B. Rimm, Anwar Merchant, et al. December 25, 2002. "Fish Consumption and Risk of Stroke in Men." *JAMA, The Journal of the American Medical Association* 288(24): 3130–3136.

6. Hu, Frank B, Leslie Bronner, Walter C. Willet, et al. April 10, 2002. "Fish and Omega-3 Fatty Acid Intake and Risk of Coronary Heart Disease in Women." *JAMA, The Journal of the American Medical Association* 287(14): 1815–1821.

7. Sekikawa, Akira, J. David Curb, Hirotsugu Ueshima, et al. 2008. "Marine-Derived n-3 Fatty Acids and Atherosclerosis in Japanese, Japanese American, and White Men." *Journal of the American College of Cardiology* 52: 417–424.

8. Fradet, Vincent, Iona Cheng, Graham Casey, and John S. Witte. April 1, 2009. "Dietary Omega-3 Fatty Acids, Cyclooxygenase-2 Genetic Variation, and Aggressive Prostate Cancer Risk." *Clinical Cancer Research* 15(7): 2559–2566.

9. Chavarro, Jorge E., Meir J. Stampfer, Megan N. Hall, et al. November 2008. "A 22-Year Prospective Study of Fish Intake in Relation to Prostate Cancer Incidence and Mortality." *The American Journal of Clinical Nutrition* 88(5): 1297–1303.

10. Walk, Alicja, Larsson, Susanna C., Jan-Erik Johansson, and Peter Ekman. September 20, 2006. "Long-Term Fatty Fish Consumption and Renal Cell Carcinoma Incidence in Women." *JAMA, The Journal of the American Medical Association* 296(11): 1371–1376.

11. Nurk, Eha, Christian A. Drevon, Helga Refsum, et al. November 2007. "Cognitive Performance Among the Elderly and Dietary Fish Intake: The Hordaland Health Study." *The American Journal of Clinical Nutrition* 86(5): 1470–1478.

REFERENCES AND RESOURCES
Magazines, Journal, and Newspapers

Albert, Christine M., Hannia Campos, Meir J. Stampfer, et al. April 11, 2002. "Blood Levels of Long-Chain n-3 Fatty Acids and the Risk of Sudden Death." *The New England Journal of Medicine* 346(15): 1113–1118.

Chavarro, Jorge E., Meir J. Stampfer, Megan N. Hall, et al. November 2008. "A 22-Year Prospective Study of Fish Intake in Relation to Prostate Cancer Incidence and Mortality." *The American Journal of Clinical Nutrition* 88(5): 1297–1303.

"Fishy Facts." September 2003. *Better Nutrition* 65(9): 30.

Fradet, Vincent, Iona Cheng, Graham Casey, and John S. Witte. April 1, 2009. "Dietary Omega-3 Fatty Acids, *Cyclooxygenase-2* Genetic Variation, and Aggressive Prostate Cancer Risk." *Clinical Cancer Research* 15(7): 2559–2566.

"A Good Time for Seafood Lovers: Three New Studies Confirm Heart Benefits." June 2002. *Environmental Nutrition* 25(6): 3.

He, Ka, Eric B. Rimm, Anwar Merchant, et al. December 25, 2002. "Fish Consumption and Risk of Stroke in Men." *JAMA, The Journal of the American Medical Association* 288(24): 3130–3136.

Hu, Frank B., Leslie Bronner, Walter C. Willett, et al. April 10, 2002. "Fish and Omega-3 Fatty Acid Intake and Risk of Coronary Heart Disease in Women." *JAMA, The Journal of the American Medical Association* 287(14): 1815–1821.

Nurk, Eha, Christian A. Drevon, Helga Refsum, et al. November 2007. "Cognitive Performance Among the Elderly and Dietary Fish Intake: The Hordaland Health Study." *The American Journal of Clinical Nutrition* 86(5): 1470–1478.

Sekikawa, Akira, J. David Curb, Hirotsugu Ueshima, et al. 2008. "Marine-Derived n-3 Fatty Acids and Atherosclerosis in Japanese, Japanese-American, and White Men." *Journal of the American College of Cardiology* 52: 417–424.

Wolk, Alicja, Susanna C. Larsson, Jan-Erik Johansson, and Peter Ekman. September 20, 2006. "Long-Term Fatty Fish Consumption and Renal Cell Carcinoma Incidence in Women." *The Journal of the American Medical Association* 296(11): 1371–1376.

Website

The George Mateljan Foundation. http://whfoods.com.

SEA VEGETABLES

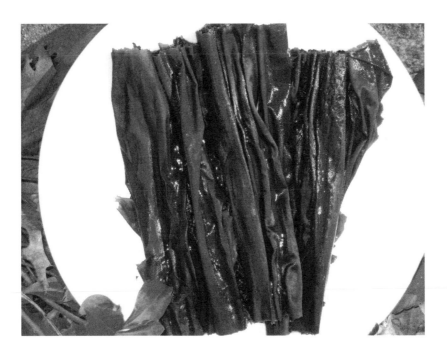

According to archeological studies, sea vegetables have been consumed by the Japanese for more than 10,000 years. In the ancient Chinese cultures, they were considered a delicacy that was served on very special occasions and to honored guests. Sea vegetables are thought to have been included in the diet of prehistoric people who lived near water in regions such as Scotland, Ireland, Norway, Iceland, New Zealand, the Pacific Islands, and coastal South American countries. Today, Japan is the largest producer and exporter of sea vegetables.[1]

Throughout the world, there are thousands of types of sea vegetables, which may also be referred to as seaweed and algae. Not all of these are suitable for human consumption; in fact, most are probably not. They tend to be classified into categories by color---brown, red, or green. The following are some of the best known sea vegetables:

- Nori: Although nori are dark purple-black, they turn green when toasted. Nori are frequently used to make sushi rolls.
- Kombu: Kombu is dark and tends to be sold in strips or sheets. It is often used to flavor soups.
- Kelp: Generally available as flakes, kelp may be light brown to dark green.
- Hijiki: This type of sea vegetable, which has a strong flavor, looks like "black wiry pasta."
- Arame: Sweeter and milder than most types of sea vegetables, arame is "wiry."
- Dulse: Reddish brown, dulse has a soft and chewy texture.
- Wakame: Wakame is like Kombu and is used to make miso soup.[2]

Sea vegetables are an excellent source of iodine and vitamin K. They are a very good source of folate and magnesium, and they are a good source of calcium, iron, and tryptophan.[3] But what have the researchers learned?

CANCER

Breast Cancer

In a study published in 2005 in *The Journal of Nutrition*, California researchers divided 24 rats into two groups. One group was fed a regular diet, and a second group was fed a diet enhanced with kelp. After four weeks, the rats that ate the diet with kelp showed a 25 to 38 percent reduction in estrogen levels in the blood. (Higher amounts of serum estrogen are associated with increased risk for breast cancer.) In addition, the kelp lengthened the rats' menstrual cycles by up to 37 percent. It is known that women who have longer menstrual cycles have fewer cycles during their lifetime. So, less of their life is spent with high amounts of estrogen in their blood.

The researchers also tested the kelp on human ovarian cells. They found that it reduced the estrogen production by 18 to 35 percent. These findings at least partially explain why people who consume Asian diets, which contain relatively high amounts of sea vegetables, "have a lower incidence of hormone-dependent cancers than populations consuming Western diets." The research indicates that, "anti-estrogenic effects of dietary kelp . . . may contribute to these reduced cancer rates."[4]

Skin Cancer

In a study published in 2006 in the *International Journal of Cancer*, researchers investigated nine groups of mice, each containing 20 hairless mice specially bred to be strongly susceptible to UVB-induced skin cancer.

The researchers applied varying amounts of brown algae polyphenols (BAPs) to the skin (3 milligrams or 6 milligrams in a mild solvent) of some of the mice and fed other mice different amounts of BAPs. Many of the mice were exposed to UVB rays. There was also a group of mice that served as controls.

The researchers determined that the mice exposed only to UVB (without treatment) developed an average of 8.5 skin tumors; the mice fed the lower and higher amounts of BAPs, respectively, had 4.7 and 3.7 tumors. But, the best results were seen in the topical application of BAPs. The lower dose mice had 3.4 tumors and the higher dose had 4.6. Furthermore, the mice that were treated with BAPs had tumor volumes that were markedly lower than in the mice that were exposed to UVB without any type of treatment.[5]

CARDIOVASCULAR HEALTH

In a randomized, double blind, placebo-controlled trial that was published in 2007 in *The Journal of Nutrition*, British researchers gave 38 healthy men and women, between the ages of 40 and 65, either daily 0.7 g of docosahexaenoic (DHA), an omega-3 fatty acid found in algae and fish oil, or a placebo. After four months, the treatments were switched. The researchers found that when the subjects took the DHA, their diastolic blood pressure dropped by 3.3 mm Hg, and their heart rate decreased by 2.1 beats per minute. So, taking a relatively modest amount of DHA has the potential to enhance cardiovascular health.[6]

In a study published in 2008 in the *Journal of the American Dietetic Association*, researchers compared the heart-protective effects of two weeks of daily 600-ml capsules of algae-derived supplementation in 32 healthy men and women, between the ages of 20 and 65, to the consumption of salmon. The results were similar. "Algal-oil DHA capsules and cooked salmon appear to be bioequivalent in providing DHA to plasma and red blood cells, and, accordingly, . . . algal-oil DHA capsules represent a safe and convenient source of non-fish-derived DHA."[7]

OSTEOARTHRITIS

In a study published in 2008 in *Nutrition Journal*, researchers randomly placed 70 subjects with mild to severe osteoarthritis in one of four parallel investigation groups. The subjects, who were between 25 and 70 years old, were then assigned to take one of the following for 12 weeks: Aquamin (a multi-mineral supplement from seaweed, 2400 mg/day), glucosamine sulfate (1500 mg/day), a combination of Aquamin (2400 mg/day) and glucosamine sulfate (1500 mg/day), or a placebo.

Only 50 subjects completed the study. Still, the subjects on either Aquamin or glucosamine sulfate had significant improvement in their osteoarthritis symptoms. The subjects who received the combined supplement or the placebo did not experience any significant changes. The researchers wrote that their study "suggested that a multi mineral supplement (Aquamin) may reduce the pain and stiffness of osteoarthritis over 12 weeks of treatment and warrants further study."[8]

WEIGHT CONTROL

A study published in 2008 in the *Asia Pacific Journal of Clinical Nutrition* may be of particular importance to the millions of people who are either overweight, obese, or simply trying to maintain a healthful weight.

Japanese researchers compared the weight of rats and mice fed regular diets or diets enhanced with fucoxanthin, brown pigment found in some types of sea vegetables. The researchers found that fucoxanthin, which stimulated a protein that increased the metabolism of abdominal fat, caused the animals to lose weight and abdominal fat. Would fucoxanthin do the same for humans? That is uncertain. Nevertheless, companies are now selling concentrated forms of fucoxanthin, and there is anecdotal evidence that these may be effective. The researchers concluded that fucoxanthin "is an important bioactive carotenoid that . . . should be beneficial for the prevention of metabolic syndrome."[9]

In a randomized, controlled, two-way crossover trial published in 2008 in *Appetite*, British researchers compared the effects of seven-day consumption of a seaweed-based drink ("strong-gelling sodium alginate formulation") against a control in 68 men and women with an average body mass index (BMI) of 23.5. The researchers found that the subjects who drank the seaweed product reduced their energy intake by about seven percent. They concluded that products like the one they used may be able to play a role "in the future management of overweight and obesity."[10]

ONE CAVEAT

Sea vegetables are known for their ability to absorb minerals from the water. Often, these are healthy minerals such as calcium, iron, magnesium, and iodine. However, when sea vegetables are located in polluted waters, they may also absorb heavy metals such as arsenic and lead. As a result, whenever possible, it is best to purchase organic sea vegetables.

Are sea vegetables a valuable part of the diet? They certainly seem to be.

NOTES

1. The George Mateljan Foundation Website. www.whfoods.com.
2. The George Mateljan Foundation Website.
3. The George Mateljan Foundation Website.
4. Skibola, Christine F., John D. Curry, Catherine VandeVoort, et al. February 2005. "Brown Kelp Modulates Endocrine Hormones in Female Sprague-Dawley Rats and in Human Luteinized Granulosa Cells." *The Journal of Nutrition* 135: 296–300.

5. Hwang, Hyejeong, Tong Chen, Ronald G. Nines, et al. December 15, 2006. "Photochemoprevention of UVB-Induced Skin Carcinogenesis in SKH-1 Mice by Brown Algae Polyphenols." *International Journal of Cancer* 119(12): 2742–2749.

6. Theobald, Hannah E., Alison H. Goodall, Naveed Sattar, et al. April 2007. "Low-Dose Docosahexaenoic Acid Lowers Diastolic Blood Pressure in Middle-Aged Men and Women." *The Journal of Nutrition* 137: 973–978.

7. Arterburn, Linda M., Harry A. Oken, Eileen Bailey Hall, et al. July 2008. "Algal-Oil Capsules and Cooked Salmon: Nutritionally Equivalent Sources of Docosahexaenoic Acid." *Journal of the American Dietetic Association* 108(7): 1204–1209.

8. Frestedt, Joy L., Melanie Walsh, Michael A. Kuskowski, and John L. Zenk. February 17, 2008. "A Natural Mineral Supplement Provides Relief from Knee Osteoarthritis Symptoms: A Randomized Controlled Pilot Trial." *Nutrition Journal* 7: 9.

9. Maeda, Hayato, Takayuki Tuskui, Tokutake Sashima, et al. 2008. "Seaweed Carotenoid, Fucoxanthin, as a Multi-Functional Nutrient." *Asia Pacific Journal of Clinical Nutrition* 17(S1): 196–199.

10. Paxman, J. R., J. C. Richardson, P. W. Dettmar, and B. M. Corfe. November 2008. "Daily Ingestion of Alginate Reduces Energy Intake in Free-Living Subjects." *Appetite* 51(3): 713–719.

REFERENCES AND RESOURCES
Magazines, Journals, and Newspapers

Arterburn, Linda M., Harry A. Oken, Eileen Bailey Hall, et al. July 2008. "Algal-Oil Capsules and Cooked Salmon: Nutritionally Equivalent Sources of Docosahexaenoic Acid." *Journal of the American Dietetic Association* 108(7): 1204–1209.

Frestedt, Joy L., Melanie Walsh, Michael A. Kuskowski, and John L. Zenk. February 17, 2008. "A Natural Mineral Supplement Provides Relief from Knee Osteoarthritis Symptoms: A Randomized Controlled Pilot Trial." *Nutrition Journal* 7: 9

Hwang, Hyejeong, Tong Chen, Ronald G. Nines, et al. December 15, 2006. "Photochemoprevention of UVB-Induced Skin Carcinogenesis in SKH-1 Mice by Brown Algae Polyphenols." *International Journal of Cancer* 119(12): 2742–2749.

Maeda, Hayato, Takayuki Tsukui, Tokutake Sashima, et al. 2008. "Seaweed Carotenoid, Fucoxanthin, as a Multi-Functional Nutrient." *Asia Pacific Journal of Clinical Nutrition* 17(S1): 196–199.

Paxman, J. R., J. C. Richardson, P. W. Dettmar, and B. M. Corfe. November 2008. "Daily Ingestion of Alginate Reduces Energy Intake in Free-Living Subjects." *Appetite* 51(3): 713–719.

Skibola, Christine F., John D. Curry, Catherine VandeVoort, et al. February 2005. "Brown Kelp Modulates Endocrine Hormones in Female Sprague-Dawley Rats and in Human Luteinized Granulosa Cells." *The Journal of Nutrition* 135: 296–300.

Theobald, Hannah E., Alison H. Goodall, Naveed Sattar, et al. April 2007. "Low-Dose Docosahexaenoic Acid Lowers Diastolic Blood Pressure in Middle-Aged Men and Women." *The Journal of Nutrition* 137: 973–978.

Website

The George Mateljan Foundation. www.whfoods.com.

SESAME SEEDS

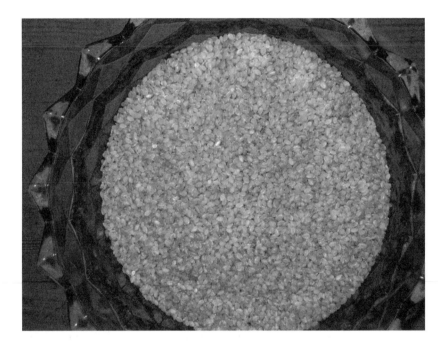

During prehistoric times, sesame seeds were grown throughout the tropical regions of the world. They were an early condiment and one of the first crops that were used to make oil. Interestingly, in Egypt, there is a tomb painting that depicts a baker adding sesame seeds to bread dough.

It was in the 17th century that sesame seeds were brought to the United States from Africa. Today, India, China, and Mexico are the largest commercial producers.[1]

Sesame seeds are considered a very good source of copper and manganese and a good source of tryptophan, calcium, magnesium, iron, phosphorus, zinc, vitamin B_1, and dietary fiber.[2] But, what have the researchers learned?

OVERALL HEALTH AND WELL-BEING

In a randomized, placebo-controlled, crossover study published in 2006 in *The Journal of Nutrition*, researchers from Taiwan investigated the association between the ingestion of sesame seeds and blood lipids, antioxidant status, and sex hormones in postmenopausal women. During the first part of the study, half of the 26 postmenopausal women consumed 50 grams of sesame seed powder per day for five weeks. After a three-week washout period, they had five weeks of 50 grams per day of rice powder, a placebo. The other half of the women received the supplements in the reverse order. Following the sesame supplementation, the 24 women who completed the study had significant improvements in blood lipids, antioxidant status, and sex hormones. The researchers concluded that the ingestion of sesame, "benefits postmenopausal women by improving blood lipids, antioxidant status, and possibly sex hormone status."[3]

In a study conducted in Honolulu, Hawaii, and published in 2001 in *Nutrition and Cancer*, researchers examined the effects of the consumption of sesame seeds on tocopherol levels in the blood. (Tocopherol is a class of compounds, many of which have vitamin E activity.) Nine subjects were fed muffins containing the same amount of gamma-tocopherol from sesame seeds, walnuts, or soy oil. The researchers found that the consumption of as little as 5 mg of sesame lignans over a three-day period significantly increased serum levels of gamma-tocopherol by 19 percent. Similar results were not obtained from the consumption of walnuts or soy oil. The researchers concluded that the "consumption of moderate amounts of sesame seeds appears to significantly increase plasma γ-tocopherol and alter plasma tocopherol ratios in humans and is consistent with the effects of dietary sesame seeds observed in rats."[4]

In a laboratory study published in 2008 in the *Journal of the Science of Food and Agriculture*, researchers from the Netherlands and Italy wanted to determine if any food-related products could offer protection against strains of *E. coli* and *Salmonella* bacteria. As a result, they exposed 18 food-related products, including sesame seed extract, to various types of bacteria. The bacteria attached themselves to the test products, and the researchers evaluated the amounts of bound bacteria. They found that sesame seed extract (and konjac gum) had the highest amount of adhered bacteria. Thus, the bacteria attached themselves to the sesame seed extract instead of gut cells, thereby reducing the severity of the symptoms that may be caused by *E. coli* or *Salmonella*. The researchers wrote that their study "highlights the potential of different food and feed components as alternative binding matrices for enteropathogens."[5]

CARDIOVASCULAR HEALTH

In a double blind, crossover, placebo-controlled study published in 2009 in *Journal of Nutritional Science and Vitaminology*, Korean researchers reviewed the association between consumption of sesamin, a lignan found in sesame, and blood pressure levels in mildly hypertensive humans. The cohort, which consisted of 25 middle-aged subjects, was divided into two groups. For four weeks, 12 subjects took capsules of 60 milligrams of sesamin per day, and 13 subjects took a placebo. After a four-week washout period, the subjects took the alternate supplements for another four weeks. Those who took sesamin experienced significant reductions in blood pressure; essentially no change was evident from the placebo. The researchers noted that their results suggested that "sesamin has an antihypertensive effect in humans." Such a reduction "may be meaningful to prevent cardiovascular disease."[6]

In a study published in 2005 in *Nutrition Research*, researchers from Taiwan attempted to determine if sesame could lower serum lipids and increase the antioxidant capacity in 21 subjects who had elevated levels of cholesterol. For two weeks, the subjects ate their usual diets. Then, for four weeks, the subjects ate an experimental diet that included 40 grams of roasted sesame. That was followed by the regular diet for another four weeks. The researchers found that "the diet with sesame significantly decreased the levels of serum total cholesterol and low-density lipoprotein (LDL) cholesterol." However, "the beneficial effects of sesame disappeared when patients returned to their regular diets."[7]

In a study published in 2005 in the *Journal of Agricultural and Food Chemistry*, Virginia researchers analyzed 27 nut and seed products. They found that sesame seed and wheat germ had the highest amounts of phytosterol content. Foods containing phytosterol help lower levels of serum cholesterol.[8]

In a study published in 2003 in *Lipids*, Japanese researchers compared the effects that sesame seeds and flaxseeds had on plasma and tissue gamma-tocopherol and TBARS (thiobarbituric acid-reactive substances assay, a measure of oxidative stress). For four weeks, rats were fed one of the following experimental diets: vitamin E-free, gamma-tocopherol, flaxseed, sesame seed, flaxseed oil, flaxseed oil with sesamin, and defatted flaxseed. The researchers found that the sesame seed diet and the flaxseed oil with sesamin diet "induced significantly higher γ-tocopherol concentrations in plasma and liver." The researchers noted that "sesame seed and its lignans induced higher γ-tocopherol and lower TBARS concentrations, whereas flaxseed lignans had no such effects."[9]

PROSTATE CANCER

In a laboratory study published in 2004 in the *Proceedings of the National Academy of Sciences*, researchers from Oakland and Berkeley, California, found that the gamma-tocopherol in sesame seeds inhibited the growth of human prostate cells. Apparently, gamma-tocopherol interfered with the synthesis of fatty molecules known as sphingolipids, which are an integral part of cell membranes. And, the gamma-tocopherol stopped the growth of human prostate cancer cells without harming any of the healthy prostate cells. The researchers said that "this study demonstrates that γT [gamma-tocopherol] induces cell death in a prostate cancer cell line by interrupting de novo [from the beginning] synthesis of sphingolipids."[10]

In a study published in 2004 in *Clinica Chimica Acta*, researchers from India examined how the consumption of three different edible oils affected people with hypertension (high blood pressure). All members of the cohort, which included 530 people, were taking a nifedipine (calcium channel blocker) medication for high blood pressure. The subjects were divided into three groups. The first group, which included 356 people, took sesame oil; the second group of 87 took sunflower oil; and, the third group of 47 took groundnut oil. The control group of 40 took no oil. The trial continued for 60 days; each day, the subjects taking the oil consumed 35 grams. Of the three oils, sesame oil appeared to have the most cardiovascular benefit. The researchers concluded that "sesame oil offers better protection over blood pressure, lipid profiles and lipid peroxidation and increases enzymatic and nonenzymatic antioxidants."[11]

Should people eat sesame seeds and use sesame oil? In most cases, sesame seeds and sesame oil are a wonderful addition to the diet. However, according to an article published in 2005 in the *Annals of Allergy, Asthma and Immunology*, the number of reports of "hypersensitivity to sesame" has been growing.[12] So, in some instances, consumers should use sesame seeds and sesame oil with caution.

NOTES

1. The George Mateljan Foundation Website. www.whfoods.com.

2. The George Mateljan Foundation Website.

3. Wu, Wen-Huey, Yu-Ping Kang, Nai-Hung Wang, et al. May 2006. "Sesame Ingestion Affects Sex Hormones, Antioxidant Status, and Blood Lipids in Postmenopausal Women." *The Journal of Nutrition* 136: 1270–1275.

4. Cooney, Robert V., Laurie J. Custer, Leila Okinaka, and Adrian A. Franke. January 2001. "Effects of Dietary Sesame Seeds on Plasma Tocopherol Levels." *Nutrition and Cancer* 39(1): 66–71.

5. Becker, Petra and Sara Galletti. August 30, 2008. "Food and Feed Components for Gut Health-Promoting Adhesion of *E. coli* and *Salmonella enterica*." *Journal of the Science of Food and Agriculture* 88(11): 2026–2035.

6. Miyawaki, Takashi, Hideshi Aono, Yoshiko Toyoda-Ono, et al. 2009. "Antihypertensive Effects of Sesamin in Humans." *Journal of Nutritional Science and Vitaminology* 55(1): 87–91.

7. Chen, Pey Rong, Kuo Liong Chien, Ta Chen Su, et al. June 2005. "Dietary Sesame Reduces Serum Cholesterol and Enhances Antioxidant Capacity in Hypercholesterolemia." *Nutrition Research* 25(6): 559–567.

8. Phillips, Katherine M., David M. Ruggio, and Mehdi Ashraf-Khorassani. November 30. 2005. "Phytosterol Composition of Nuts and Seeds Commonly

Consumed in the United States." *Journal of Agricultural and Food Chemistry* 53(24): 9436–9445.

9. Yamashita, Kanae, Saiko Okeda, and Mariko Obayashi. December 2003. "Comparative Effects of Flaxseed and Sesame Seed on Vitamin E and Cholesterol Levels in Rats." *Lipids* 38(12): 1249–1255.

10. Jiang, Qing, Jeffrey Wong, Henrik Fyrst, et al. December 21, 2004. "Gamma-Tocopherol or Combinations of Vitamin E Forms Induce Cell Death in Human Prostate Cancer Cells by Interrupting Sphingolipid Synthesis." *Proceedings of the National Academy of Sciences* 101(51): 17825–17830.

11. Sankar, D., G. Sambandam, M. Ramakrishna Rao, and K. V. Pugalendi. May 2005. "Modulation of Blood Pressure, Lipid Profiles and Redox Status in Hypertensive Patients Taking Different Edible Oils." *Clinica Chimica Acta* 355(1–2): 97–104.

12. Gangur, Venu, Caleb Kelly, and Lalitha Navuluri. 2005. "Sesame Allergy: A Growing Food Allergy of Global Proportions?" *Annals of Allergy, Asthma and Immunology* 95(1): 4–11.

REFERENCES AND RESOURCES
Magazines, Journals, and Newspapers

Becker, Petra M. and Sara Galletti. August 30, 2008. "Food and Feed Components for Gut Health-Promoting Adhesion of *E. coli* and *Salmonella enterica*." *Journal of the Science of Food and Agriculture* 88(11): 2026–2035.

Chen, Pey Rong, Kuo Liong Chien, Ta Chen Su, et al. June 2005. "Dietary Sesame Reduces Serum Cholesterol and Enhances Antioxidant Capacity in Hypercholesterolemia." *Nutrition Research* 25(6): 559–567.

Cooney, Robert V., Laurie J. Custer, Leila Okinaka, and Adrian A. Franke. January 2001. "Effects of Dietary Sesame Seeds on Plasma Tocopherol Levels." *Nutrition and Cancer* 39(1): 66–71.

Gangur, Venu, Caleb Kelly, and Lalitha Navuluri. 2005. "Sesame Allergy: A Growing Food Allergy of Global Proportions?" *Annals of Allergy, Asthma and Immunology* 95(1): 4–11.

Jiang, Qing, Jeffrey Wong, Henrik Fyrst, et al. December 21, 2004. "Gamma-Tocopherol or Combinations of Vitamin E Forms Induce Cell Death in Human Prostate Cancer Cells by Interrupting Sphingolipid Synthesis." *Proceedings of the National Academy of Sciences* 101(51): 17825–17830.

Miyawaki, Takashi, Hideshi Aono, Yoshiko Toyoda-Ono, et al. 2009. "Antihypertensive Effects of Sesamin in Humans." *Journal of Nutritional Science and Vitaminology* 55(1): 87–91.

Phillips, Katherine M., David M. Ruggio, and Mehdi Ashraf-Khorassani. November 30, 2005. "Phytosterol Composition of Nuts and Seeds Commonly Consumed in the United States." *Journal of Agricultural and Food Chemistry* 53(24): 9436–9445.

Sankar, D., G. Sambandam, M. Ramakrishna Rao, and K. V. Pugalendi. May 2005. "Modulation of Blood Pressure, Lipid Profiles and Redox Status in Hypertensive Patients Taking Different Edible Oils." *Clinica Chimica Acta* 355(1–2): 97–104.

Wu, Wen-Huey, Yu-Ping Kang, Nai-Hung Wang, et al. May 2006. "Sesame Ingestion Affects Sex Hormones, Antioxidant Status, and Blood Lipids in Postmenopausal Women." *The Journal of Nutrition* 136: 1270–1275.

Yamashita, Kanae, Saiko Ikeda, and Mariko Obayashi. December 2003. "Comparative Effects of Flaxseed and Sesame Seed on Vitamin E and Cholesterol Levels in Rats." *Lipids* 38(12): 1249–1255.

Websites

American Sesame Growers Association. www.sesamegrowers.org.
The George Mateljan Foundation. www.whfoods.com.

SOY

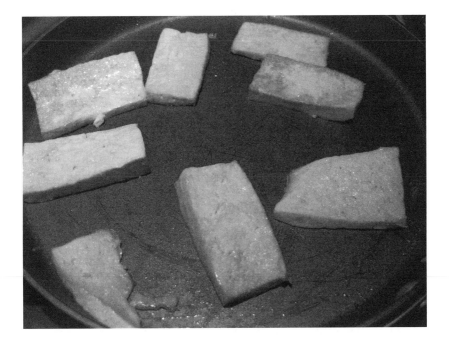

Around 3,000 years ago, soybeans originated in China. They were introduced to Japan in the eighth century, and, later, they traveled to other
parts of Asia including Thailand, Malaysia, Korea, and Vietnam.

Soybeans first appeared in the United States in the 18th century, planted
by Americans who brought them from China. Today, the United States leads
the world in the commercial production of soybeans. Soybeans are sold in a
wide variety of forms. Fresh soybeans are known as edamame. But, soybeans
may be processed into foods such as dried soybean seeds, soymilk, soynuts,
and tofu.[1]

Soybeans contain excellent amounts of molybdenum and tryptophan. They
are a very good source of manganese and protein, and a good source of iron,

omega-3 fatty acids, phosphorus, dietary fiber, vitamin K, magnesium, copper, vitamin B_2, and potassium.[2] But what have researchers learned?

CANCER
Breast Cancer

In a Korean study that was published in 2008 in *Nutrition and Cancer*, researchers compared the soy protein intake of 362 women who had been diagnosed with breast cancer to the same number of healthy women matched for age and menopausal status. The researchers found that the women with the highest intake of soy protein had a significantly lower risk of breast cancer than the women with the lowest intake of soy. The researchers noted that, "Increased regular soy food intake at a level equivalent to traditional Korean consumption levels may be associated with a reduced risk of breast cancer, and this effect is more pronounced in premenopausal women."[3]

In a study published in 2009 in *Cancer Epidemiology, Biomarkers & Prevention*, researchers investigated the consumption of soy during childhood in women of Chinese, Japanese, and Filipino decent who lived in San Francisco, Oakland, or Los Angeles, California, or in Hawaii. Of the women, 597 had a history of breast cancer, and 966 were considered healthy. They ranged in age from 20 to 55. The researchers found that high intake of soy during childhood was associated with a 58 percent reduction in rates of breast cancer. Furthermore, a high level of soy intake during adolescence and adulthood caused a 20 to 25 percent reduction.[4]

Ovarian Cancer

In a European study published in 2008 in the *International Journal of Cancer*, researchers compared the flavonoid intake (including the flavonoid known as isoflavone which is found in soy foods) of 1,031 women who were diagnosed with epithelial ovarian cancer to 2,411 women who were hospitalized for an acute, non-cancer medical problem. The researchers found that the women with a high intake of isoflavones reduced their risk of ovarian cancer by about half. "On the basis of our findings and the relevant literature," the researchers wrote, "we infer that isoflavones . . . may have favorable effects with respect to ovarian cancer risk."[5]

Colorectal Cancer

In a study published in 2009 in *The American Journal of Clinical Nutrition*, researchers prospectively examined 68,412 women between the ages of 40 and 70 who were initially free of cancer. During the mean follow-up period of 6.4 years, there were 321 cases of colorectal cancer. The researchers determined that the women who ate the highest amount of soy had 30 percent fewer cases of colorectal cancer. These benefits were primarily seen in postmenopausal women.[6]

CARDIOVASCULAR SUPPORT

In a study published in 2008 in the *European Heart Journal*, Chinese researchers reviewed the effects on blood vessel functioning of the 12-week consumption of 80 mg/day of isoflavone supplementation or a placebo by 102 patients
who had previously suffered from a stroke. When compared with the control
group, the researchers found that the subjects who took the isoflavone supplementation had significant improvement in blood vessel functioning. Even
more encouraging was the finding that the response was best for those with
the more severe cardiovascular disease. Moreover, the isoflavone supplementation reduced levels of C-reactive protein, an indicator of vascular inflammation. The researchers concluded that their findings "may have important
implication for the use of isoflavone for secondary prevention in patients
with cardiovascular disease, on top of conventional interventions."[7]

HOT FLASHES

In a randomized crossover eight-week study published in 2007 in the *Journal
of Women's Health*, Boston researchers studied the effect on hot flashes of a
diet with or without the inclusion of a daily one-half cup of soy nuts "divided
into three or four portions spaced throughout the day." During each study
period, the subjects recorded the numbers of hot flashes they experienced. At
the end of each period, they also completed a "menopausal symptom quality
of life questionnaire." The researchers found that when the women ate the
diet that included soy nuts they had a 45 percent reduction in hot flashes.
Eating the soy nuts also resulted in improvements in other menopause-
related symptoms, such as psychosocial issues, mentioned on the questionnaire. The researchers wrote that, "Substituting soy nuts for nonsoy protein . . .
and consumed three or four times throughout the day is associated with a
decrease in hot flashes and improvement in menopausal symptoms."[8]

OVERALL HEALTH OF POSTMENOPAUSAL WOMEN

In a study published in 2009 in *Menopause*, researchers randomly divided 203
healthy postmenopausal women into one of three groups. For two years, one
group took 25 g of soy protein without isoflavones; a second group took 25 g
of soy protein with 90 mg of isoflavones; and the third (control) group took
25 g of milk protein (casein and whey). At the end of two years, the women
in all three groups had significant decreases in the bone mineral density of
the lumbar spine and femoral neck. In addition, all three groups had
decreases in physical performance measurements. The researchers concluded
that, "Twenty-five grams of soy protein with 90 mg of isoflavones has no
added benefit in preventing bone loss or improving physical performance."[9]

An article published in 2009 in *Internal Medicine News* summarizes a
16-week study conducted in Brazil that divided 60 women, who were one to

13 years past menopause, into one of three groups. One group received soy supplements containing 90 mg of isoflavones; a second group received hormone replacement; and a third group took placebos. The researchers found that the woman on soy supplements and hormone replacement experienced improvement in menopause related symptoms, such as hot flashes and joint and muscle pain. However, the woman on hormone replacement saw improvements in cardiovascular factors such as total cholesterol and LDL (bad) cholesterol. The total cholesterol saw a 12 percent reduction, and the LDL cholesterol decreased 18 percent. No such improvements were seen in the women on soy supplementation.[10]

WEIGHT CONTROL

A study published in 2008 in the *European Journal of Nutrition* examined whether soy products may play a role in controlling weight gain. Researchers in Seattle and Honolulu reviewed the association between lifetime intake of soy foods and body mass index (BMI) of 1,418 women who lived in Hawaii. The researchers found that the women with a higher soy consumption in adulthood had lower levels of BMI. However, this association was only significant for Caucasian and postmenopausal women. "The women in the highest category also experienced a smaller annual weight change since age 21 (by 0.05 kg/year) than the low soy intake group. . . ."[11]

ONE CAVEAT

Much of the world's soybean crop is genetically modified. People who wish to avoid genetically modified foods should eat organic soy products.

Should soy products be part of the diet? For most people, there is no reason to exclude them. And, they may well have some benefits.

NOTES

1. The George Mateljan Foundation Website. www.whfoods.com.

2. The George Mateljan Foundation Website.

3. Kim, Mi Kyung, Jin Hee Kim, Seok Jin Nam, et al. September 5, 2008. "Dietary Intake of Soy Protein and Tofu in Association with Breast Cancer Risk Based on a Case-Control Study." *Nutrition and Cancer* 60: 568–576.

4. Korde, Larissa A., Anna H. Wu, Thomas Fears, et al. April 1, 2009. "Childhood Soy Intake and Breast Cancer Risk in Asian American Women." *Cancer Epidemiology, Biomarkers & Prevention* 18(4): 1050–1059.

5. Rossi, Marta, Eva Negri, Pagona Lagiou, et al. 2008. "Flavonoids and Ovarian Cancer Risk: A Case-Control Study in Italy." *International Journal of Cancer* 123(4): 895–898.

6. Yang, Gong, Xiao-Ou Shu, Honglan Li, et al. February 2009. "Prospective Cohort Study of Soy Food Intake and Colorectal Cancer Risk in Women." *The American Journal of Clinical Nutrition* 89(2): 577–583.

7. Chan, Yap-Hang, Kui-Kai Lau, Kai-Hang Yiu, et al. 2008. "Reduction of C-Reactive Protein with Isoflavone Supplement Reverses Endothelial Dysfunction in Patients with Ischaemic Stroke." *European Heart Journal* 29(22): 2800–2807.

8. Welty, Francine K., Karen S. Lee, Natalie S. Lew, et al. April 2007. "The Association Between Soy Nut Consumption and Decreased Menopausal Symptoms." *Journal of Women's Health* 16(3): 361–369.

9. Vupadhyayula, Phanni M., J. C. Gallagher, Thomas Templin, et al. March–April 2009. "Effects of Soy Protein Isolate on Bone Mineral Density and Physical Performance Indices in Postmenopausal Women—A 2-Year Randomized, Double-Blind, Placebo-Controlled Trial." *Menopause* 16(2): 320–328.

10. McNamara, Damien. January 15, 2009. "Soy Matches HT for Menopause Symptoms." *Internal Medicine News* 42(2): 17.

11. Maskarinec, Gertraud, Alison G. Aylward, Eva Erber, et al. April 2008. "Soy Intake Is Related to a Lower Body Mass Index in Adult Women." *European Journal of Nutrition* 47(3): 138–144.

REFERENCES AND RESOURCES
Magazines, Journals, and Newspapers

Chan, Yap-Hang, Kui-Kai Lau, Kai-Hang Yiu, et al. 2008. "Reduction of C-Reactive Protein with Isoflavone Supplement Reverses Endothelial Dysfunction in Patients with Ischaemic Stroke." *European Heart Journal* 29(22): 2800–2807.

Kim, Mi Kyung, Jin Hee Kim, Seok Jin Nam, et al. September 5, 2008. "Dietary Intake of Soy Protein and Tofu in Association with Breast Cancer Risk Based on a Case-Control Study." *Nutrition and Cancer* 60: 568–576.

Korde, Larissa A., Anna H. Wu, Thomas Fears, et al. April 1, 2009. "Childhood Soy Intake and Breast Cancer Risk in Asian American Women." *Cancer Epidemiology, Biomarkers & Prevention* 18(4): 1050–1059.

Maskarinec, Gertraud, Alison G. Aylward, Eva Erber, et al. April 2008. "Soy Intake Is Related to a Lower Body Mass Index in Adult Women." *European Journal of Nutrition* 47(3): 138–144.

McNamara, Damien. January 15, 2009. "Soy Matches HT for Menopause Symptoms." *Internal Medicine News* 42(2): 17.

Rossi, Marta, Eva Negri, Pagona Lagiou, et al. 2008. "Flavonoids and Ovarian Cancer Risk: A Case-Control Study in Italy." *International Journal of Cancer* 123(4): 895–898.

Vupadhyayula, Phanni M., J. C. Gallagher, Thomas Templin, et al. March–April 2009. "Effects of Soy Protein on Bone Mineral Density and Physical Performance Indices in Postmenopausal Women—A 2-Year Randomized, Double-Blind, Placebo-Controlled Trial." *Menopause* 16(2): 320–328.

Welty, Francine K., Karen S. Lee, Natalie S. Lew, et al. April 2007. "The Association Between Soy Nut Consumption and Decreased Menopausal Symptoms." *Journal of Women's Health* 16(3):361–369.

Yang, Gong, Xiao-Ou Shu, Honglan Li, et al. February 2009. "Prospective Cohort Study of Soy Food Intake and Colorectal Cancer Risk in Women." *The American Journal of Clinical Nutrition* 89(2): 577–583.

Website

The George Mateljan Foundation. www.whfoods.com.

SPINACH

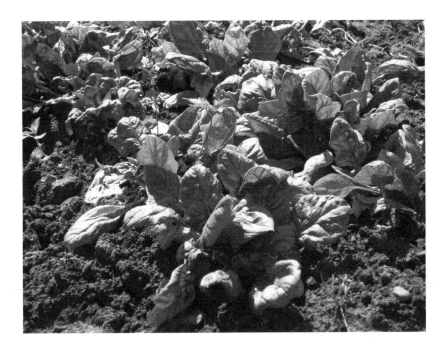

Remember Popeye, the cartoon figure? Whenever he needed to recharge his superhuman strength, he would swallow canned spinach. Thanks in part to Popeye, spinach has become a popular food. Today, with its many nutrients, such as magnesium, iron, folic acid, potassium, vitamin K, alpha-lipoic acid (ALA), vitamins C and A, lutein, and zeaxanthin, spinach is viewed as an exceedingly healthful food choice. But what does the research say?

EYE HEALTH

In short-term and long-term studies that were published in 2002 in two separate journals, Harvard researchers determined that dietary zeaxanthin, a carotenoid that is found in spinach, serves a vital role in shielding eyes from damaging light. As a result, spinach may help protect against age-related macular degeneration and the formation of cataracts.

In the first study, which was published in *Investigative Ophthalmology & Visual Science,* quails, whose eyes are similar to human eyes, were raised on a carotenoid-deficient diet. Then, the quails were divided into two groups. Before exposure to light damage, one group was fed a zeaxanthin-supplemented diet for a week. The quails whose eyes had low concentrations of zeaxanthin experienced severe light damage; the quails with higher concentrations of zeaxanthin had only minor damage.[1]

In the second study, published in *Experimental Eye Research,* quails were raised for six months on one of three types of diets: normal, carotenoid-deficient, or carotenoid-deficient diet supplemented with high doses of zeaxanthin. All the quails were exposed to bright light. The healthiest eyes were found in the quails who received zeaxanthin; the worst eyes were in those quails that had a carotenoid-deficient diet.[2]

In a study that was published in 2004 in *The Journal of Nutrition,* Ohio State University researchers treated human eye lens cells with lutein (another carotenoid), zeaxanthin, or vitamin E. Then, these cells, as well as a group of untreated cells, were exposed to ultraviolet-beta radiation. Researchers found that lutein and zeaxanthin were almost ten times more protective than vitamin E. And, this protection was obtained using far less lutein and zeaxanthin than vitamin E.[3]

CANCER

Evidence has emerged suggesting that the consumption of spinach helps prevent and/or treat several types of cancers. For example, a study published in *The Journal of Nutrition* in 2004 described research conducted at the National Food Research Institute in Japan. The researchers examined the effect that neoxanthin, a carotenoid found in green leafy vegetables such as spinach, had on human prostate cancer cells. They studied the "gastrointestinal metabolism of neoxanthin in mice and the in vitro digestion of spinach." During digestion, a good deal of the neoxanthin was converted to neochrome. In turn, neoxanthin "induced evident apoptotic cell death," while "neochrome inhibited the cell proliferation." Thus, the ingestion of spinach hampered "the proliferation of human prostate cancer cells."[4]

Another study of the association between prostate cancer and fruits and vegetables, including spinach, was published in 2007 in the *Journal of the National Cancer Institute.* Researchers investigated the intake of fruits and vegetables in 1,338 patients with prostate cancer. While the researchers did not find a relationship between the overall risk of prostate cancer and vegetable and fruit consumption, the risk of extraprostatic prostate cancer, or prostate cancer that had spread outside the prostate gland, did decrease with increased vegetable intake. In addition, there was "some evidence that risk of aggressive prostate cancer decreased with increasing spinach consumption."[5]

A Harvard study on the consumption of foods high in the flavonoid kaempferol, such as spinach, and ovarian cancer was published in 2007 in the *International Journal of Cancer*. Using a cohort of 66,940 women from the Nurses' Health Study, the researchers found that women with the higher intake of kaempferol developed 40 percent fewer cases of ovarian cancer than those with the lowest intake of kaempferol. The researchers concluded that "dietary intake of certain flavonoids may reduce ovarian cancer risk."[6]

A 2005 article in *JAMA, The Journal of the American Medical Association*, reviewed the association between lung cancer and phytoestrogens, cancer-fighting agents in foods such as spinach. People who ate more phytoestrogens tended to have lower rates of lung cancer. This was most apparent in current smokers and people who had never smoked, and less evident in former smokers. The researchers noted that their "data provide further support for the limited but growing epidemiologic evidence that phytoestrogens are associated with a decrease in the risk of lung cancer."[7]

Spinach is even proving to be effective in preventing pancreatic cancer. A study reported in the October 2007 in the *American Journal of Epidemiology* noted that people with higher levels of flavonol consumption have rates of pancreatic cancer that are about half those who eat lower levels of flavonols. Of the three flavonols studies, kaempferol, found in spinach, provided the largest risk reduction.[8]

CARDIOVASCULAR HEALTH

An American Heart Association study published in 2002 in *Stroke* reviewed the association between dietary intake of the B vitamin folate, found in spinach, and the risk of stroke and cardiovascular disease. In the almost 20-year study that included more than 9,700 men and women aged 25 to 74, researchers determined that those people who consumed at least 300 micrograms of folate per day had a 20 percent lower risk of stroke than those who ate less.[9]

Moreover, in a 2005 study published in *Experimental Neurology*, researchers fed rats a diet with blueberries, spinach, or spirulina for one month. Other rats received regular diets. After inducing strokes, researchers determined that the rats who had received the added supplements experienced half the brain damage of the control rats.[10]

In November 2007, the *Proceedings of the National Academy of Sciences* describes a study of dietary nitrite, found in leafy vegetables like spinach, conducted at the Albert Einstein College of Medicine in New York. Researchers added nitrite to the drinking water of mice for seven days. A control group of mice received the standard diet. All the mice had a simulated heart attack that was followed by 24 hours of restoring blood to the heart and tissues. The hearts of the mice that received nitrite had 48 percent less heart damage.[11]

METABOLIC SYNDROME

In order to study the relationship between the intake of foods high in magnesium, such as spinach, and the development of metabolic syndrome, researchers reviewed the dietary intake of 4,637 people between the ages of 18 and 30. The cohort was divided into four groups, according to the amount of magnesium in the diet. At the beginning of the study, none of the participants had metabolic syndrome. The study continued for 15 years. During that time, 608 cases of metabolic syndrome were identified. Those who had the highest intake of magnesium were least likely to develop metabolic syndrome.[12]

BONE MINERAL DENSITY

A study published in 2003 in *The American Journal of Clinical Nutrition* reviewed the association between vitamin K consumption and bone mineral density of the hip and spine. (Spinach contains lots of vitamin K.) Bone mineral density was measured in over 1,100 men and almost 1,500 women. Low dietary intake of vitamin K was consistently related to low bone mineral density in women; no association was found in men.[13] People with lower bone mineral density are at increased risk for osteoporosis and fractures.

ONE CAVEAT

Though clearly spinach is a truly healthful food, people who are on the drug warfarin (Coumadin), a medication used to prevent blood clots, should use foods with large amounts of vitamin K with care. Vitamin K plays an integral role in clotting. But, warfarin reduces the amount of vitamin K and "interferes with the cascade of events that clots blood." So, people on warfarin should be sure to discuss vitamin K with their medical providers. And, it is important not to make significant changes in vitamin K consumption. "Suddenly eating a lot of spinach or kale, for example, might decrease Coumadin's effectiveness."[14]

NOTES

        1. Thomson, Lauren R., Yoko Toyoda, Andrea Langner, et al. November 2002. "Elevated Retinal Zeaxanthin and Prevention of Light-Induced Photoreceptor Cell Death in Quail." *Investigative Ophthalmology & Visual Science* 43: 3538–3549.

        2. Thomson, L. R., Y. Toyoda, and F. C. Delori. November 2002. "Long-Term Dietary Supplementation with Zeaxanthin Reduces Photoreceptor Death in Light-Damaged Japanese Quail." *Experimental Eye Research* 75(5): 529–542.

        3. Chitchumroonchokchai, Chureeporn, Joshua A. Bomser, Jayme E. Glamm, and Mark L. Failla. December 2004. "Xanthophylls and Alpha-Tocopherol Decrease UVB-Induced Lipid Peroxidation and Stress Signaling in Human Lens Epithelial Cells." *The Journal of Nutrition* 134: 3225–3232.

        4. Asai, Akira, Masaru Terasaki, and Akihiko Nagao. September 2004. "An Epoxide-Furanoid Rearrangement of Spinach Neoxanthin Occurs in the Gastrointestinal

Tract of Mice and In Vitro: Formation and Cytostatic Activity of Neochrome Steroisomers." *The Journal of Nutrition* 134: 2237–2243.

5. Kirsh, Victoria A., Ulrike Peters, Susan T. Mayne, et al. August 1, 2007. "Prospective Study of Fruit and Vegetable Intake and Risk of Prostate Cancer." *Journal of the National Cancer Institute* 99(15): 1200–1209.

6. Gates, Margaret A., Shelley S. Tworoger, Jonathan L. Hecht, et al. April 2007. "A Prospective Study of Dietary Flavonoid Intake and Incidence of Epithelial Ovarian Cancer." *International Journal of Cancer* 121(10): 2225–2232.

7. Schabath, Matthew B., Ladia M. Hernandez, Xifeng Wu, et al. September 28, 2005. "Dietary Phytoestrogens and Lung Cancer Risk." *JAMA: The Journal of the American Medical Association* 294(12): 1493–1504.

8. Nöthlings, Ute, Suzanne P. Murphy, Lynne R. Wilkens, et al. October 15, 2007. "Flavonols and Pancreatic Cancer Risk." *American Journal of Epidemiology* 166(8): 924–931.

9. Bazzano, Lydia A., Jiang He, Lorraine G. Ogden, et al. May 1, 2002. "Dietary Intake of Folate and Risk of Stroke in US Men and Women." *Stroke* 33(5): 1183–1189.

10. Wang, Yun, Chen-Fu Chang, Jenny Chou, et al. May 2005. "Dietary Supplementation with Blueberries, Spinach, or Spirulina Reduces Ischemic Brain Damage." *Experimental Neurology* 193(1): 75–84.

11. Bryan, Nathan S., John W. Calvert, John W. Elrod, et al. November 27, 2007. "Dietary Nitrite Supplementation Protects Against Myocardial Ischemia-Reperfusion Injury." *Proceedings of the National Academy of Sciences* 104(48): 19144–19149.

12. He, Ka, Kiang Liu, Martha L. Daviglus, et al. April 4, 2006. "Magnesium Intake and Incidence of Metabolic Syndrome Among Young People." *Circulation* 113: 1675–1682.

13. Booth, Sarah L., Kerry E. Broe, David R. Gagnon, et al. February 2003. "Vitamin K Intake and Bone Mineral Density in Women and Men." *The American Journal of Clinical Nutrition* 77(2): 512–516.

14. "On Coumadin? Tell Your Doctor if You Love Spinach or Take Fish Oils." October 2005. *Environmental Nutrition* 28(10): 7

REFERENCES AND RESOURCES
Magazines, Journals, and Newspapers

Asai, Akira, Masaru Terasaki, and Akihiko Nagao. September 2004. "An Epoxide-Furanoid Rearrangement of Spinach Neoxanthin Occurs in the Gastrointestinal Tract of Mice and In Vitro: Formation and Cytostatic Activity of Neochrome Stereoisomers." *The Journal of Nutrition* 134: 2237–2243.

Bazzano, Lydia A., Jiang He, Lorraine G. Ogden, et al. May 1, 2002. "Dietary Intake of Folate and Risk of Stroke in US Men and Women." *Stroke* 33(5): 1183–1189.

Booth, Sarah L, Kerry E. Broe, David R. Gagnon, et al. February 2003. "Vitamin K Intake and Bone Mineral Density in Women and Men." *The American Journal of Clinical Nutrition* 77(2): 512–516.

Bryan, Nathan S., John W. Calvert, John W. Elrod, et al. November 27, 2007. "Dietary Nitrite Supplementation Protects Against Myocardial Ischemia-Reperfusion Injury." *Proceedings of the National Academy of Sciences* 104(48): 19144–19149.

Chitchumroonchokchai, Chureeporn, Joshua A. Bomser, Jayme E. Glamm, and Mark L. Failla. December 2004. "Xanthophyll and Alpha-Tocopherol Decrease UVB-Induced Lipid Peroxidation and Stress Signaling in Human Lens Epithelial Cells." *The Journal of Nutrition* 134: 3225–3232.

Gates, Margaret A., Shelley S. Tworoger, Jonathan L. Hecht, et al. April 2007. "A Prospective Study of Dietary Flavonoid Intake and Incidence of Epithelial Ovarian Cancer." *International Journal of Cancer* 121(10): 2225–2232.

He, Ka, Kiang Liu, Martha L. Daviglus, et al. April 4, 2006. "Magnesium Intake and Incidence of Metabolic Syndrome among Young Adults." *Circulation* 113: 1675–1682.

Kirsh, Victoria A., Ulrike Peters, Susan T. Mayne, et al. August 1, 2007. "Prospective Study of Fruit and Vegetable Intake and Risk of Prostate Cancer." *Journal of the National Cancer Institute* 99(15): 1200–1209.

Moeller, Suzen M., Niyati Parekh, Lesley Tinker, et al. August 2006. "Associations Between Intermediate Age-Related Macular Degeneration and Lutein and Zeaxanthin in the Carotenoids in Age-Related Eye Disease Study (CAREDS)." *Archives of Ophthalmology* 124(8): 1151–1162.

Nöthlings, Ute, Suzanne P. Murphy, Lynne R. Wilkens, et al. October 15, 2007. "Flavonols and Pancreatic Cancer Risk." *American Journal of Epidemiology* 166(8): 924–931.

"On Coumadin? Tell Your Doctor if You Love Spinach or Take Fish Oils." October 2005. *Environmental Nutrition* 28(10): 7.

Schabath, Matthew B., Ladia M. Hernandez, Xifeng Wu, et al. September 28, 2005. "Dietary Phytoestrogens and Lung Cancer Risk." JAMA, *The Journal of the American Medical Association* 294(12): 1493–1504.

Thomson, L. R., Y. Toyoda, and F. C. Delori. November 2002. "Long-Term Supplementation with Zeaxanthin Reduces Photoreceptor Death in Light-Damaged Japanese Quail." *Experimental Eye Research* 75(5): 529–542.

Thomson, Lauren R., Yoko Toyoda, Andrea Langner, et al. November 2002. "Elevated Retinal Zeaxanthin and Prevention of Light-Induced Photoreceptor Cell Death in Quail." *Investigative Ophthalmology & Visual Science* 43: 3538–3549.

Wang, Yun, Chen-Fu Chang, Jenny Chou, et al. May 2005. "Dietary Supplementation with Blueberries, Spinach, or Spirulina Reduces Ischemic Brain Damage." *Experimental Neurology* 193(1): 75–84.

Website

The George Mateljan Foundation. http://www.whfoods.com.

SUNFLOWER SEEDS

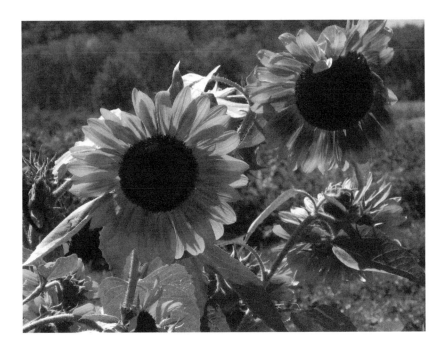

Sunflower plants, the source of sunflower seeds, are believed to have originated in Peru and Mexico. They were one of the first plants cultivated in the United States, where Native Americans have used them for over 5,000 years.

It was the Spanish explorers who carried sunflowers from the "New World" to Spain, and from Spain, they made their way to other European countries. Today, sunflower seeds are ubiquitous, and sunflower oil, derived from the seeds, is one of the most popular oils in the world. Leading commercial producers of sunflower seeds include Russia, Peru, Argentina, Spain, France, and China.[1]

Sunflower seeds are an excellent source of vitamin E and a very good source of vitamin B_1. Additionally, sunflower seeds are considered a good source of manganese, magnesium, copper, tryptophan, selenium, phosphorus, vitamin B_5, and folate.[2] Sunflower seeds are filled with phytosterol, a plant-based compound that lowers levels of cholesterol in the blood. The amount of research on sunflower seeds appears to be somewhat limited. Yet, it is still interesting to review some of the relevant studies.

CARDIOVASCULAR HEALTH

In a study published in the 2005 in *Journal of Agricultural and Food Chemistry*, Virginia researchers analyzed the phytosterol content of 27 varieties of nuts and seeds. Although wheat germ and sesame seeds were found to have the highest amount of phytosterol, they are not commonly eaten in the United States. Of the nuts and seeds frequently consumed, sunflower seeds (and pistachios) were on the top of the list (270–289 mg/100 g).[3]

In a crossover study published in 2005 in *Journal of the American Dietetic Association*, researchers from Pennsylvania and Massachusetts recruited 31 men and women, between the ages of 25 and 64 years, with moderate hypercholesterolemia (elevated levels of cholesterol). The women's LDL ("bad") cholesterol was between 140 and 188; the men's was between 129 and 177. The subjects consumed one of the following three diets for four weeks, with two-week washout periods between each diet: a typical American high-fat diet, an olive oil-based diet, or a diet that replaced the saturated fat in foods with NuSun sunflower oil. (Named by the National Sunflower Association, NuSun is a class of sunflower seeds and oil. It has higher amounts of the healthful oleic oil and lower amounts of the less healthful linoleic oil than traditional sunflower oil.) The typical American diet contained 34 percent fat calories; the two oil-based diets limited fat to 30 percent of calories. When compared to the average American diet and the olive oil-based diet, the subjects who ate the NuSun diet experienced a 4.7 drop in the total cholesterol levels and a 5.8 percent drops in their LDL cholesterol levels.[4]

KNEE OSTEOARTHRITIS

In 2005, Joanne M. Jordan, MD, of the University of North Carolina School of Medicine, and her fellow researchers presented findings on the association between the intake of selenium, which is found in abundance in sunflower seeds, and knee osteoarthritis to the annual meeting of the American College of Rheumatology. The study, which included 940 subjects enrolled in the Johnston County [North Carolina] Osteoarthritis Project, determined that for every extra tenth of a part per million of selenium in the body, there is a 15 to 20 percent reduction in the risk of knee osteoarthritis. Moreover, in a striking finding, the severity of knee osteoarthritis appeared to be directly related to the amount of selenium in the body. Commenting on their findings, Dr. Jordan said, "Our results suggest that we might be able to prevent or delay osteoarthritis of the knees and possibly other joints in some people if they are not getting enough selenium. That's important because the condition, which makes walking painful, is the leading cause of activity limitation among adults in developed countries."[5]

METABOLIC SYNDROME

In a study published in 2006 in *Circulation*, researchers prospectively examined the association between magnesium intake and metabolic syndrome in 4,637 Americans between the ages of 18 and 30. (As has previously been noted, sunflower seeds contain good amounts of magnesium.) When the study began, all the subjects were free of diabetes and metabolic syndrome, a disorder that is characterized by excess waist circumference, high blood pressure, elevated triglycerides, low levels of HDL ("good") cholesterol, and increased fasting glucose levels. The symptoms associated with metabolic syndrome place people at increased risk for heart disease and diabetes.

During the 15-year follow-up period, the researchers identified 608 cases of metabolic syndrome. They found that magnesium intake was inversely associated with the incidence of metabolic syndrome. So, the people who consumed the most magnesium were the least likely to develop this disorder. The researchers commented that their "findings suggest that young adults with higher magnesium intake have lower risk of development of metabolic syndrome."[6]

PHYSICAL DECLINE IN OLDER PEOPLE

In a study published in 2008 in *JAMA, The Journal of the American Medical Association*, researchers recruited 698 people, with an average age of 73.7, who lived independently in Tuscany, Italy. The subjects were followed for three years. During that time, the researchers obtained measurements of several micronutrients that the people consumed, including folate, and vitamins B_6, B_{12}, D, and E. Only vitamin E was found to be associated with physical decline. So, older people who did not take in adequate amounts of vitamin E had increased risk for physical decline. As has been noted, sunflower seeds are an excellent source of vitamin E. The researchers wrote that their results "provide empirical evidence that a low serum concentration of vitamin E is associated with subsequent decline in physical function among community-living older adults."[7]

BLADDER CANCER

A 2004 article in the *Oakland Tribune* described research on the eating habits of about 1,000 residents of Houston, Texas, which was presented to a meeting of the American Association for Cancer Research. The researchers found that those residents with the highest intake of alpha-tocopherol vitamin E, which is found in sunflower seeds, had a risk of bladder cancer that was 50 percent lower than the residents with the least intake of vitamin E.[8]

Meanwhile, in a study published in 2009 in *Cancer Prevention Research*, researchers found that selenium, such as the selenium found in sunflower seeds, may help prevent bladder cancer. The researchers compared the selenium levels in the toenails of 767 people with newly diagnosed bladder cancer to the selenium levels in the toenails of 1,108 people from the general population. Although no association was found between the selenium levels and the entire cohort, there were significant reductions found for women, moderate smokers, and those with p53-positive cancer, a type of bladder cancer.[9]

CHILDHOOD ASTHMA

In a longitudinal study published in 2006 in the *American Journal of Respiratory and Critical Care Medicine*, English researchers reviewed 1,861 children who were recruited during their mother's pregnancy and followed for five years. Data on the symptoms associated with asthma and dietary intakes from food questionnaires were available for 1,253 and 1,120 children, respectively. The researchers found that the children who were born to mothers with the lowest intake of vitamin E, such as the vitamin E found in sunflower seeds and sunflower oil, were five times more likely to have asthma than the children who were born to women with the highest intake of vitamin E. Moreover, the researchers also determined that the pregnant women with the highest amounts of alpha-tocopherol in their blood were more likely to have children with better lung function. The researchers noted that, "the results of this present study suggest that dietary modification or supplementation during pregnancy to reduce the likelihood of childhood asthma warrants further investigation."[10]

Should sunflower seeds be included in the diet? They certainly appear to be a good addition.

NOTES

1. The George Mateljan Foundation Website. www.whfoods.com.

2. The George Mateljan Foundation Website.

3. Phillips, Katherine M., David M. Ruggio, and Mehdi Ashraf-Khorassani. 2005. "Phytosterol Composition of Nuts and Seeds Commonly Consumed in the United States." *Journal of Agricultural and Food Chemistry* 53(24): 9436–9445.

4. Binkoski, Amy E., Penny M. Kris-Etherton, Thomas A. Wilson, et al. July 2005. "Balance of Unsaturated Fatty Acids Is Important to a Cholesterol-Lowering Diet: Comparison of Mild-Oleic Sunflower Oil and Olive Oil on Cardiovascular Disease Risk Factors." *Journal of the American Dietetic Association* 105(7): 1080–1086.

5. The Medical News Website. www.news-medical.net.

6. He, Ka, Kiang Liu, Martha L. Daviglus, et al. 2006. "Magnesium Intake and Incidence of Metabolic Syndrome Among Young Adults." *Circulation* 113: 1675–1682.

7. Bartali, Benedetta, Edward A. Frongillo, Jack M. Guralnik, et al. January 23, 2008. "Serum Micronutrient Concentrations and Decline in Physical Function

Among Older Persons." *JAMA, The Journal of the American Medical Association* 299(3): 308–315.

    8. Haney, Daniel Q. March 29, 2004. "Vitamin E May Fight Bladder Cancer." *Oakland Tribune*: NA.

    9. Wallace, Kristin, Karl T. Kelsey, Alan Schned, et al. 2009. "Selenium and Risk of Bladder Cancer: A Population-Based Case-Control Study." *Cancer Prevention Research* 2: 70–73.

    10. Devereux, Graham, Stephen W. Turner, Leone C. A. Craig, et al. 2006. "Low Maternal Vitamin E Intake During Pregnancy Is Associated with Asthma in 5-Year-Old Children." *American Journal of Respiratory and Critical Care Medicine* 174: 499–507.

REFERENCES AND RESOURCES
Magazines, Journals, and Newspaper

Bartali, Benedetta, Edward A. Frongillo, Jack M. Guralnik, et al. January 23, 2008. "Serum Micronutrient Concentrations and Decline in Physical Function Among Older Persons." *JAMA, The Journal of the American Medical Association* 299(3): 308–315.

Binkoski, Amy E., Penny M. Kris-Etherton, Thomas A. Wilson, et al. July 2005. "Balance of Unsaturated Fatty Acids Is Important to a Cholesterol-Lowering Diet: Comparison of Mid-Oleic Sunflower Oil and Olive Oil on Cardiovascular Disease Risk Factors." *Journal of the American Dietetic Association* 105(7): 1080–1086.

Devereux, Graham, Stephen W. Turner, Leone C. A. Craig, et al. 2006. "Low Maternal Vitamin E Intake During Pregnancy Is Associated with Asthma in 5-Year-Old Children." *American Journal of Respiratory and Critical Care Medicine* 174: 499–507.

Haney, Daniel Q. March 29, 2004. "Vitamin E May Fight Bladder Cancer." *Oakland Tribune*: NA.

He, Ka, Kiang Liu, Martha L. Daviglus, et al. 2006. "Magnesium Intake and Incidence of Metabolic Syndrome Among Young Adults." *Circulation* 113: 1675–1682.

Phillips, Katherine M., David M. Ruggio, and Mehdi Ashraf-Khorassani. 2005. "Phytosterol Composition of Nuts and Seeds Commonly Consumed in the United States." *Journal of Agriculture and Food Chemistry* 53(24): 9436–9445.

Wallace, Kristin, Karl T. Kelsey, Alan Schned, et al. 2009. "Selenium and Risk of Bladder Cancer: A Population-Based Case-Control Study." *Cancer Prevention Research* 2: 70–73.

Websites

The George Mateljan Foundation. www.whfoods.com.
The Medical News. www.news-medical.net.
National Sunflower Association. www.sunflowernsa.com.

TEA

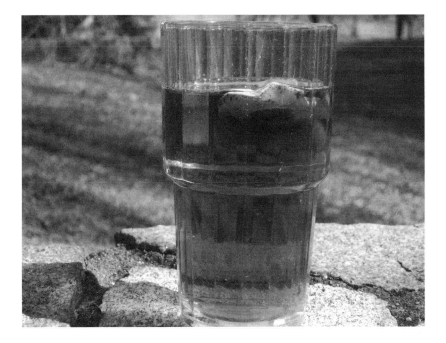

Tea. When it's hot, it's the perfect drink for a cold winter morning. When it's iced, it's ideal for an after-exercise pick-me-up or to help cope with a sweltering hot day.

Throughout the world, tea is loved. In fact, after water, it is the second most popular drink. In the United States, every day, about half the population drinks tea. Most tea drinkers live in the Northeast or South.

At present, there are four main types of tea—black, green, oolong, and white. They are all derived from the same plant—*Camellia sinensis*. The differences among teas are a direct result of varying types of processing and levels of oxidation.[1] Teas contain a variety of different biologically active chemicals such as flavonoids, caffeine, and fluoride. When green tea is fermented to become black or oolong tea, theaflavins are produced. And, theanine is found in green tea. But is tea a healthful drink? Should people be drinking as much as they do?

CARDIOVASCULAR HEALTH

A number of studies have found solid evidence that drinking tea is good for the cardiovascular system. For example, a study of healthy non-smoking men between the ages of 18 and 55 appeared in 2007 in *Atherosclerosis*. During a four-week period, half of the men drank black tea and the other half drank a placebo. The tea drinkers were found to have reductions in platelet activation and C-reactive protein, both signs of improved cardiovascular health. The researchers noted that the "effects cannot be attributed to observer bias or lifestyle cofounders." The tea clearly "contributes to sustained cardiovascular health."[2]

Another study published in *Circulation* in 2001 asked 66 people with coronary artery disease to consume both black tea and water. The study had a "crossover design"–subjects drank both black tea and water at different times. The researchers examined both the short-term effects—two hours after drinking 450 ml tea or water—and long-term effects—900 ml of tea or water daily for four weeks. In the 50 subjects who completed the study, the results were rather dramatic. As detected by ultrasound, the short- and long-term consumption of tea improved the flow of blood in the arteries.[3]

Similar results were obtained in a Greek study published in 2008 in the *European Journal of Cardiovascular Prevention & Rehabilitation*. Researchers studied 14 healthy people around the age 30. The consumption of green tea relaxed the arteries and improved the flow of blood. Researchers believe that drinking green tea may well benefit cardiovascular health.[4]

A study published in 2003 in the *Archives of Internal Medicine* included a total of 240 Chinese men and women with mild to moderately elevated cholesterol. For 12 weeks, the subjects received either a placebo or theaflavin- (black tea extract)-enriched green tea extract. By the end of the study, those receiving enriched green tea had an average cholesterol decrease of 11 percent. Their LDL (bad cholesterol) levels dropped an average of 16 percent. The researchers noted that, "The theaflavin-enriched green tea extract we studied is an effective adjunct to a low-saturated-fat diet to reduce LDL-C in hypercholesterolemic adults [adults with high levels of cholesterol] and is well tolerated."[5]

POTENTIAL ANTI-CANCER BENEFIT

Research published in 2008 in *Cancer Epidemiology, Biomarkers & Prevention* reported that green tea may be useful in the prevention of ovarian cancer. In 781 women diagnosed with ovarian cancer and 1,263 without the disease, researchers evaluated the association between the consumption of caffeine-containing drinks and ovarian cancer. The researchers found that the women who drank one or more cups of green tea per day had a 54 percent reduction in risk. The researchers commented that green tea is commonly consumed in countries with low ovarian cancer incidence.[6]

In a study presented to the 121st Annual Meeting of the American Physiological Society in 2008, researchers from the University of Mississippi Medical Center added the green tea antioxidant epigallocatechin-3-gallate (EGCG) to the water of seven-week-old female mice for five weeks. A control group of mice received regular water. During the second week of the study, all the mice were injected with breast cancer cells. Compared to the control mice, the mice that drank EGCG had a reduction in tumor weight of 68 percent and tumor size of 66 percent. The researchers believed that the consumption of EGCG "significantly inhibits breast tumor growth in female mice." Dr. Jian-Wei Gu, the senior researcher, noted that their findings "will help lead to new therapies for the prevention and treatment of breast cancer in women."[7]

ALTER COURSE OF DIABETES TYPE 1

In a study that was published in 2008 in *Life Sciences*, researchers, who were studying Sjögren's syndrome, an autoimmune disorder, realized that the EGCG found in green tea helped the symptoms of Sjögren's syndrome, but it could also prevent or delay insulin-dependent type 1 diabetes. During the research, mice were given EGCG in drinking water, while a control group was given regular water. At the age of 16 weeks, the EGCG-fed mice were 6.1 times more likely to be free of diabetes than the regular water-fed group. At 22 weeks, they were 4.2 times more likely.[8]

IMPROVED MENTAL ALERTNESS AND COGNITION

In a study conducted in Israel and published in 2008 in *The Journal of Nutrition*, researchers determined that green tea prevented brain cell death of laboratory animals. Moreover, in sharp contrast to the past belief that damaged brain cells were unable to be repaired, the EGCG in green tea was able to mend brain cells, as well as reduce the prevalence of compounds that trigger lesions in the brain. So, it is possible that green tea may be useful in preventing and treating the destruction to the brain caused by illnesses such as Alzheimer's and Parkinson's disease.[9] However, it is important to remember that what happens in laboratory animals is not, necessarily, repeated in humans. Still, it is certainly worthy of further study.

A study published in *The Journal of Nutrition* in 2008 noted that New York researchers found that only 20 minutes after the intake of theanine, subjects experienced improvement in attention and they had increased activity in the sections of the brain responsible for attention. When the consumption of theanine was combined with caffeine, the improvement in attention was even greater.[10]

Surely, tea sounds like a simply wonderful drink. But, there are at least two areas of concern. Researchers at the University of Southern California have observed that green tea renders a cancer drug used to treat multiple myeloma and mantle cell lymphoma ineffective.[11] Since it is possible that green tea may affect other cancer drugs, people dealing with cancer should discuss tea consumption with their oncologists. And, since tea is naturally high in fluoride levels, people who drink fluoridated water should drink green tea with some care. The intake of too much fluoride places people at risk for damage to bones and soft tissue as well as discolored teeth.[12]

NOTES

1. Tea Association of the U.S.A. Inc. Website. www.teaUSA.org.

2. Steptoe, Andrew, E. Leigh Gibson, Raisa Vuononvirta, et al. August 2007. "The Effects of Chronic Tea Intake on Platelet Activation and Inflammation: A Double-Blind Placebo Controlled Trial." *Atherosclerosis* 193(2): 277–282.

3. Duffy, Stephen J., John F. Keaney Jr., Monika Holbrook, et al. 2001. "Short- and Long-Term Black Tea Consumption Reverses Endothelial Dysfunction in Patients with Coronary Artery Disease." *Circulation* 104: 151–156.

4. Alexopoulos, Nikolaos, Charalambos Vlachopoulos, Konstantinos Aznaouridis, et al. June 2008. "The Acute Effect of Green Tea Consumption on Endothelial Function in Healthy Individuals." *European Journal of Cardiovascular Prevention & Rehabilitation* 15(3): 300–305.

5. Maron, David J., Guo Ping Lu, Nai Sheng Cai, et al. June 23, 2003. "Cholesterol-Lowering Effect of a Theaflavin-Enriched Green Tea Extract." *Archives of Internal Medicine* 163(12): 1448–1453.

6. Song, Yoon Ju, Alan R. Kristal, Kristine G. Wicklund, et al. March 1, 2008. "Coffee, Tea, Colas, and Risk of Epithelial Ovarian Cancer." *Cancer Epidemiology, Biomarkers & Prevention* 17: 712–716.

7. The American Physiological Society. Website, www.the-aps.org/press/journal/08/8.htm.

8. Gillespie, Kevin, Isamu Kodani, Douglas P. Dickinson, et al. October 2008. "Effects of Oral Consumption of the Green Tea Polyphenol EGCG in a Murine Model for Human Sjögren's Syndrome, an Autoimmune Disease." *Life Sciences* 83(17–18): 581–588.

9. Mandel, Silvia A., Tamar Amit, Limor Kalfon, et al. August 2008. "Targeting Multiple Neurodegenerative Disease Etiologies with Multimodal-Acting Green Tea Catechins." *The Journal of Nutrition* 138: 1578S–1583S.

10. Kelly, Simon P., Manuel Gomez-Ramirez, Jennifer L. Montesi, and John J. Foxe. August 2008. "L-Theanine and Caffeine in Combination Affect Human Cognition as Evidenced by Oscillatory Alpha-Band Activity and Attention Task Performance." *The Journal of Nutrition* 138: 1572S–1577S.

11. "USC Study Finds That Green Tea Blocks Benefits of Cancer Drug." February 22, 2009. *NewsRx Health:* 109.

12. "Fluoridation and Tea Don't Mix, Studies Continue to Show." October 9, 2008. *Women's Health Weekly:* 456.

REFERENCES AND RESOURCES
Magazines, Journals, and Newspapers

Alexopoulos, Nikolaos, Charalambos Vlachopoulos, Konstantinos Aznaouridis, et al. June 2008. "The Acute Effect of Green Tea Consumption on Endothelial

Function in Healthy Individuals." *European Journal of Cardiovascular Prevention & Rehabilitation* 15(3): 300–305.

Duffy, Stephen J., John F. Kearney, Jr., Monika Holbrook, et al. 2001. "Short- and Long-Term Black Tea Consumption Reverses Endothelial Dysfunction in Patients with Coronary Artery Disease." *Circulation* 104: 151–156.

"Fluoridation and Tea Don't Mix, Studies Continue to Show." October 9, 2008. *Women's Health Weekly*: 456.

Gillespie, Kevin, Isamu Kodani, Douglas P. Dickinson, et al. October 2008. "Effects of Oral Consumption of the Green Tea Polyphenol EGCG in a Murine Model for Human Sjögren's Syndrome, an Autoimmune Disease." *Life Sciences* 83(17–18): 581–588.

Kelly, Simon P., Manuel Gomez-Ramirez, Jennifer L. Montesi, and John J. Foxe. August 2008. "L-Theanine and Caffeine in Combination Affect Human Cognition as Evidenced by Oscillatory Alpha-Band Activity and Attention Task Performance." *The Journal of Nutrition* 138: 1572S–1577S.

Mandel, Silvia, Tamar Amit, Limor Kalfon, et al. August 2008. "Targeting Multiple Neurodegenerative Disease Etiologies with Multimodal-Acting Green Tea Catechins." *The Journal of Nutrition* 138: 1578S–1583S.

Maron, David J., Guo Ping Lu, Nai Sheng Cai, et al. June 23, 2003. "Cholesterol-Lowering Effect of a Theaflavin-Enriched Green Tea Extract." *Archives of Internal Medicine* 163(12): 1448–1453.

Song, Yoon Ju, Alan R. Kristal, Kristine G. Wicklund, et al. March 1, 2008. "Coffee, Tea, Colas, and Risk of Epithelial Ovarian Cancer." *Cancer Epidemiology, Biomarkers & Prevention* 17: 712–716.

Steptoe, Andrew, E. Leigh Gibson, Raisa Vuononvirta, et al. August 2007. "The Effects of Chronic Tea Intake on Platelet Activation and Inflammation: A Double-Blind Placebo Controlled Trial." *Atherosclerosis* 193(2): 277–282.

"USC Study Finds that Green Tea Blocks Benefits of Cancer Drug." February 22, 2009. *NewsRX Health*: 109.

Websites

The American Physiological Society. www.the-aps.org.
Tea Association of the U.S.A. Inc. www.teaUSA.org.

TOMATOES

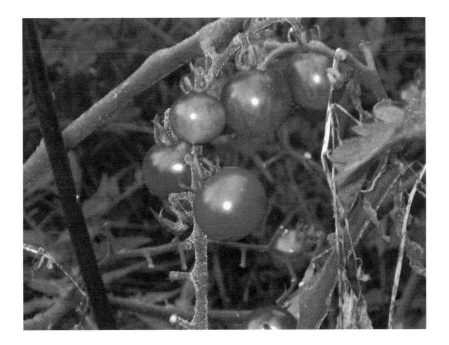

During prehistoric times, tomatoes grew wild in the western portions of South America. Over time, they migrated north to the Aztecs, where they were cultivated. Apparently, the Aztecs were intrigued with this fruit that closely resembled the tomatillo, a fruit that is a staple of their diet. Spanish conquistadors found tomatoes and brought them back to Spain. From Spain, they quickly spread to other European countries.

Tomatoes came to America with the colonists. Still, tomatoes were relatively unpopular until the late 19th century. Today, tomatoes, which are available in many varieties, are top sellers. In addition to the United States, tomatoes are commercially produced in countries such as Russia, Italy, Spain, China, and Turkey.[1]

Tomatoes are remarkably nutritious. They contain excellent amounts of vitamins C, A, and K. They have very good amounts of molybdenum, potassium, manganese, dietary fiber, chromium, and vitamin B_1. And, tomatoes are considered to have good amounts of the following: vitamins B_1, B_2, B_5, B_6, and E, folate, copper, magnesium, iron, phosphorus, tryptophan, and protein. Nevertheless, tomatoes are probably best known for containing lycopene, a carotenoid that is believed to protect the body from oxidative damage.[2]

Many researchers have studied tomatoes. It is interesting to review some of what they have learned.

CARDIOVASCULAR HEALTH

In a Finnish study published in 2007 in the *British Journal of Nutrition*, 21 healthy volunteers followed a tomato-free diet for three weeks. Then, they were placed on a three-week diet that was high in tomato consumption—a daily intake of 13.5 ounces of tomato juice and one ounce of tomato ketchup. When the study ended, the researchers found that the total cholesterol levels of the subjects had dropped an average of 5.9 percent. In addition, the LDL ("bad" cholesterol) levels had dropped by 12.9 percent. Blood tests also showed a 13-percent increase in the ability of the circulating LDL cholesterol to resist oxidation.[3]

In a study published in 2003 in *The Journal of Nutrition*, Boston researchers, led by Howard D. Sesso, ScD, examined the diets of almost 40,000 subjects from the Women's Health Study. The researchers found that when compared to the women who ate the least amount of tomato products (including tomatoes, tomato juice, and tomato sauce), the women who ate the most tomato products had almost a 30-percent reduction in risk for cardiovascular disease. The women who ate more than two servings per week of oil-based tomato products, such as tomato sauce, had a 34-percent lower risk of cardiovascular disease.[4]

Using the same data, another research study led by Dr. Sesso was published in 2004 in *The American Journal of Clinical Nutrition*. When the data were originally collected, the participating women were free of cardiovascular disease. After almost five years of follow-up, researchers found that 483 of the women had developed some type of cardiac problem. Again, the researchers determined that the women who ate the most tomato products had the lowest risk for cardiovascular disease. "Higher plasma lycopene concentrations are associated with a lower risk of CVD [cardiovascular disease] in women."[5]

In a study published in 2006 in *The American Journal of Clinical Nutrition*, researchers learned that tomato extracts lowered the activation of platelets, a situation that has the potential to cause blood clots, heart attacks, and strokes. In the double blind, placebo-controlled crossover trial, researchers selected 90 healthy people who had normal platelet functioning. Three hours after they were all given a tomato extract-enriched or control supplement, platelet function measurements were taken. While the control caused no changes in the platelets, the tomato extract resulted in a significant reduction in platelet activation. The researchers noted that "as a functional food or dietary supplement, tomato extract may have a role in primary prevention of cardiovascular disease by reducing platelet activation, which could contribute to a reduction in thrombotic events."[6]

CANCER
Colorectal Cancer

In a randomized, placebo-controlled, double blind crossover study published in 2007 in the *American Journal of Clinical Nutrition*, Dutch researchers recruited 40 men and 31 women with a family history of colorectal cancer and/or a personal history of colorectal adenoma (benign tumor). For eight weeks, they took either a daily tomato lycopene supplement or a placebo. The researchers found that lycopene supplementation was associated with an increase in levels of proteins that bind to insulin-like growth factors. In so doing, the lycopene supplementation reduced the availability of the insulin-like growth factors. Since insulin-like growth factors have been linked to cancer, the tomato supplementation appeared to lower the risk of colorectal cancer.[7]

Prostate Cancer

In a study published in 2007 in *Cancer Research*, researchers from Illinois and Ohio placed 206 male rats on one of several diets containing varying amounts of tomato powder, broccoli powder, and/or lycopene. One month later, all of the rats were implanted with prostate cancer. The researchers then compared the effects of diet to surgical castration or finasteride (a drug for prostate enlargement). At the end of 22 weeks, the rats were sacrificed, and their tumors were weighed. The diet that included 10 percent tomato powder and 10 percent broccoli powder was the most effective in shrinking prostate tumors. It shrank the tumors 52 percent. Tomato alone shrank the tumor by 34 percent; and, broccoli alone shrank the tumor by 42 percent.[8]

Meanwhile, a meta-analysis of 21 studies on the use of tomatoes, tomato products, and lycopene that was published in 2004 in *Cancer Epidemiology, Biomarkers & Prevention* determined that the men who ate the most raw tomatoes had an 11-percent reduction in risk for prostate cancer. The rate was even higher for those who ate the most cooked tomato products. Those men had a reduced risk of 19 percent. The researchers noted that "tomato products may play a role in the prevention of prostate cancer," but "this effect is modest and restricted to high amounts of tomato intake."[9]

On the other hand, a study published in 2006 also in *Cancer Epidemiology, Biomarkers & Prevention* evaluated the association between the intake of lycopene and certain tomato products in the Prostate, Lung, Colorectal, and Ovarian Cancer Screening Trial. Over an average of 4.2 years, a total of 1,338 cases of prostate cancer were found in 26,361 men. The researchers did not find any association between intake of lycopene and risk for prostate cancer. Additionally, "reduced risks were also not found for total tomato servings or for most tomato-based foods." However, "among men with a family history of prostate cancer, risks were decreased in relation to increased consumption of lycopene . . . and specific tomato-based foods commonly eaten with fat."[10]

Pancreatic Cancer

In a case-control three-year study published in 2005 in *The Journal of Nutrition*, Canadian researchers examined the dietary intake of 462 people with histologically confirmed cases of pancreatic cancer and a control group of 4,721. The researchers found that the men who consumed the most lycopene, provided primarily by tomatoes, reduced their risk of pancreatic cancer by 31 percent. Furthermore, among those who never smoked, people whose diets contained the most beta-carotene and total carotenoids lowered their risk for pancreatic cancer, respectively, by 43 percent and 42 percent.[11]

Should tomatoes be included in the diet? They certainly appear to be a healthful addition.

NOTES

1. The George Mateljan Foundation Website. www.whfoods.com.

2. The George Mateljan Foundation Website.

3. Silaste, Marja-Leena, Georg Alfthan, Antti Aro, et al. 2007. "Tomato Juice Decreases LDL Cholesterol Levels and Increases LDL Resistance to Oxidation." *British Journal of Nutrition* 98: 1251–1258.

4. Sesso, Howard D., Simin Liu, J. Michael Gaziano, and Julie E. Buring. July 2003. "Dietary Lycopene Tomato-Based Food Products and Cardiovascular Disease in Women." *The Journal of Nutrition* 133: 2336 –2341.

5. Sesso, Howard D., Julie E. Buring, Edward P. Norkus, and J. Michael Gaziano. January 2004. "Plasma Lycopene, Other Carotenoids, and Retinol and the Risk of Cardiovascular Disease in Women." *The American Journal of Clinical Nutrition* 79(1): 47–53.

6. O'Kennedy, Niamh, Lynn Crosbie, Stuart Whelan, et al. September 2006. "Effects of Tomato Extract on Platelet Function: A Double-Blinded Crossover Study in Healthy Humans." *The American Journal of Clinical Nutrition* 84(3): 561–569.

7. Vrieling, Alina, Dorien W. Voskuil, Johannes M. Bonfrer, et al. November 2007. "Lycopene Supplementation Elevates Circulating Insulin-Like Growth Factor-Binding Protein-1 and -2 Concentrations in Persons at Greater Risk of Colorectal Cancer." *American Journal of Clinical Nutrition* 86(5): 1456–1462.

8. Canene-Adams, Kirstie, Brian L. Lindshield, Shihua Wang, et al. January 15, 2007. "Combinations of Tomato and Broccoli Enhance Antitumor Activity in Dunning R3327-H Prostate Adenocarcinomas." *Cancer Research* 67(2): 836–843.

9. Etminan, Mahyar, Bahi Takkouche, and Francisco Caamaño-Isorna. March 2004. "The Role of Tomato Products and Lycopene in the Prevention of Prostate

Cancer: A Meta-Analysis of Observational Studies." *Cancer Epidemiology, Biomarkers & Prevention* 13: 340–345.

10. Kirsh, Victoria A., Susan T. Mayne, Ulrike Peters, et al. January 2006. "A Prospective Study of Lycopene and Tomato Product Intake and Risk of Prostate Cancer." *Cancer Epidemiology, Biomarkers & Prevention* 15: 92–98.

11. Nkondjock, André, Parviz, Kenneth C. Johnson, et al. March 2005. "Dietary Intake of Lycopene Is Associated with Reduced Pancreatic Cancer Risk." *The Journal of Nutrition* 135: 592–597.

REFERENCES AND RESOURCES
Magazines, Journals, and Newspapers

Canene-Adams, Kirstie, Brian L. Lindshield, Shihua Wang, et al. January 15, 2007. "Combinations of Tomato and Broccoli Enhance Antitumor Activity in Dunning R3327-H Prostate Adenocarcinomas." *Cancer Research* 67(2): 836–843.

Etminan, Mahyar, Bahi Takkouche, and Francisco Caamaño-Isorna. March 2004. "The Role of Tomato Products and Lycopene in the Prevention of Prostate Cancer: A Meta-Analysis of Observational Studies." *Cancer Epidemiology, Biomarkers & Prevention* 13: 340–345.

Kirsh, Victoria A., Susan T. Mayne, Ulrike Peters, et al. January 2006. "A Prospective Study of Lycopene and Tomato Product Intake and Risk of Prostate Cancer." *Cancer Epidemiology, Biomarkers & Prevention* 15: 92–98.

Nkondjock, André, Parviz Ghadirian, Kenneth C. Johnson, et al. March 2005. "Dietary Intake of Lycopene Is Associated with Reduced Pancreatic Cancer Risk." *The Journal of Nutrition* 135: 592–597.

O'Kennedy, Niamh, Lynn Crosbie, Stuart Whelan, et al. September 2006. "Effects of Tomato Extract on Platelet Function: A Double-Blinded Crossover Study in Healthy Humans." *The American Journal of Clinical Nutrition* 84(3): 561–569.

Sesso, Howard D., Julie E. Buring, Edward P. Norkus, and J. Michael Gaziano. January 2004. "Plasma Lycopene, Other Carotenoids, and Retinol and the Risk of Cardiovascular Disease in Women." *The American Journal of Clinical Nutrition* 79(1): 47–53.

Sesso, Howard D., Simin Liu, J. Michael Gaziano, and Julie E. Buring. July 2003. "Dietary Lycopene, Tomato-Based Food Products and Cardiovascular Disease in Women." *The Journal of Nutrition* 133: 2336–2341.

Silaste, Marja-Leena, Georg Alfthan, Antti Aro, et al. 2007. "Tomato Juice Decreases LDL Cholesterol Levels and Increases LDL Resistance to Oxidation." *British Journal of Nutrition* 98: 1251–1258.

Vrieling, Alina, Dorien W. Voskuil, Johannes M. Bonfrer, et al. November 2007. "Lycopene Supplementation Elevates Circulating Insulin-Like Growth Factor-Binding Protein-1 and -2 Concentrations in Persons at Greater Risk of Colorectal Cancer." *American Journal of Clinical Nutrition* 86(5): 1456–1462.

Website

The George Mateljan Foundation. www.whfoods.com.

TURNIPS

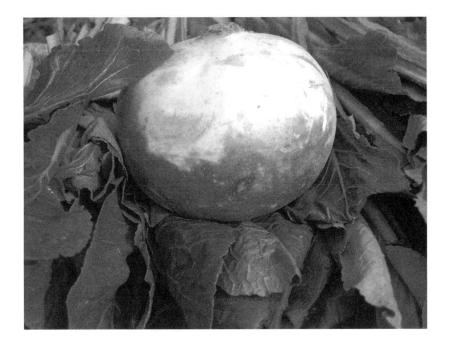

Turnips have prehistoric roots. They are believed to have been grown in the Near East almost 4,000 years ago. And, it is known that the ancient Greeks and Romans cultivated several different varieties.

Early European settlers and colonists brought turnips with them to the "New World." They grew particularly well in the southern areas, where they became a staple of the diet. It is said that slave owners ate turnip roots; the supposedly less desirable greens were reserved for the slaves.[1] Ironically, the slave owners unwittingly did themselves a disservice. Though turnips are healthful, turnip greens have an extraordinary amount of vitamins and nutrients.

Turnips contain very good amounts of vitamin C and smaller amounts of calcium, zinc, vitamin B_6, magnesium, iron, thiamin, niacin, folate, and phosphorus.[2] Meanwhile, turnip greens have excellent amounts of vitamins

A, B_6, C, and K, folate, manganese, dietary fiber, calcium, and copper. They have very good amounts of tryptophan, potassium, magnesium, and iron, and good amounts of phosphorus; vitamin, B_1, B_3, and B_5; omega-3 fatty acids; and protein.[3] They also contain lutein and zeaxanthin. But, what have the researchers learned?

CANCER

In an in vitro study published in 2009 in *Food Chemistry*, Canadian researchers evaluated the extent to which extracts from 34 vegetables inhibited the growth of stomach, lung, breast, kidney, skin, pancreas, prostate, and brain tumor cells. The extracts from cruciferous vegetables, such as turnips and turnip greens, had some of the most powerful anti-cancer properties. On the other hand, common vegetables, such as potatoes, carrots, tomatoes, and lettuce, appeared to provide essentially no cancer protection. The researchers concluded that "vegetables have very different inhibitory activities toward cancer cells and that the inclusion of cruciferous and *Allium* vegetables [such as garlic and onions] in the diet is essential for effective dietary-based chemopreventive strategies."[4]

Breast Cancer

In a study published in 2007 in the *American Journal of Clinical Nutrition*, Swedish researchers examined the association between intake of folate and risk of invasive breast cancer in 11,699 postmenopausal women over the age of 50. (As has been noted, turnips have some folate; turnip greens contain excellent amounts of folate.) During 9.5 years of follow-up, health providers diagnosed 392 cases of breast cancer. The researchers found that the women with the highest intake of folate—456 micrograms per day—had a 44-percent lower risk of invasive breast cancer than the women in the lowest intake group—160 micrograms per day. The researchers concluded that, "a high folate intake was associated with a lower incidence of postmenopausal breast cancer in this cohort."[5]

In a study published in 2008 in the *American Journal of Clinical Nutrition*, researchers from Nashville, Tennessee, and China investigated the association between intake of white turnips and Chinese cabbage, cruciferous vegetables common in the Chinese diet, and incidence of breast cancer in more than 6,000 women. The researchers found that women who had a higher consumption of white turnips and Chinese cabbage had "a significantly lower postmenopausal breast cancer risk." The benefit was most apparent in women who had two copies of a variant of a gene called GSTP1. Those with the highest intake had about half the risk of those with the lowest intake. The researchers noted that cruciferous vegetables have high amounts of compounds that the body converts into isothiocyanates, which have anti-cancer properties.[6]

Bladder Cancer

In a study published in 2007 in the *International Journal of Cancer*, researchers from the University of Texas M.D. Anderson Cancer Center in Houston, Texas, investigated 697 patients with newly diagnosed bladder cancer and 708 healthy controls. The researchers compared their intake of isothiocyanates and bladder cancer. They found that the patients with bladder cancer had a significantly lower intake of isothiocyanates than the healthy controls. The people who ate high amounts of isothiocyanates reduced their risk of bladder cancer by 29 percent. This anti-cancer response was most evident in smokers, men, and patients who were at least 64 years old. The researchers wrote that, "this is the first epidemiological report that ITCs [isothiocyanates] from cruciferous vegetable consumption protect against bladder cancer."[7]

Lung Cancer

In a study published in 2008 in *Nutrition*, Spanish researchers reviewed the food intake of 617 people—295 had lung cancer and 322 were healthy controls. The subjects who consumed at least one portion of green leafy vegetables, such as turnip greens, every day had 50 percent fewer cases of lung cancer than those who ate green leafy vegetables less than five times per week.[8]

Prostate Cancer

In a prospective study published in 2007 in the *Journal of the National Cancer Institute*, researchers reviewed the association between intake of cruciferous vegetables and incidence of prostate cancer in 1,338 men. On average, the men were followed for 4.2 years. The researchers found that the men who ate the most cruciferous vegetables had a 40 percent reduction in prostate cancer risk. They noted that "high intake of cruciferous vegetables . . . may be associated with reduced risk of aggressive prostate cancer, particularly extraprostatic disease."[9]

CARDIOVASCULAR HEALTH

In a cross-sectional study published in 2006 in *The American Journal of Clinical Nutrition*, researchers from the United Kingdom reviewed the vitamin C intake of 3,258 men between the ages of 60 and 69. None of the men had any history of diabetes or cardiovascular disease. After assessing C-reactive protein levels, the researchers determined that high blood concentrations of vitamin C, as is found in both turnips and turnip greens, was associated with a 45-percent reduction in the risk of inflammation.[10]

HEALTHIER AGING

In a study published in 2009 in *The American Journal of Clinical Nutrition*, two researchers from Children's Hospital Oakland Research Institute in

Oakland, California, poured through hundreds of published vitamin K studies conducted since the 1970s. They found that the current recommendations for vitamin K were not based on optimum long-term health. Rather, the recommendations were designed to ensure adequate blood coagulation (formation of clots). From their work with mice, these researchers learned that without adequate amounts of vitamin K, which is found in abundance in turnip greens, medical problems associated with aging, such as bone fragility, kidney calcification, cardiovascular disease, and possibly cancer, may be exacerbated. The researchers noted that they hope their work "will stimulate further efforts to redefine micronutrient adequacy on the basis of long-term effects. Methods to determine optimal micronutrient intakes on the basis of long-term needs should allow recommended intakes to be set more accurately and with less reliance on uncertain safety factors."[11]

NUCLEAR CATARACTS

In a study published in 2008 in the *Archives of Ophthalmology*, researchers reviewed the association between intake of lutein and zeaxanthin, such as found in turnip greens, and nuclear cataracts in 1,802 women, aged 50 to 79, from Iowa, Wisconsin, and Oregon. (Nuclear cataracts are the clouding of the center of the natural lens of the eyes.) The researchers found that the women with the highest intake of lutein and zeaxanthin were 32 percent less likely to have nuclear cataracts than the women with the lowest intake.[12]

Should turnips and turnip greens be part of the diet? Certainly.

NOTES

1. The George Mateljan Foundation Website. www.whfoods.com.

2. Nutrient Facts Website. www.nutrientfacts.com.

3. The George Mateljan Website.

4. Boivin, Dominique, Sylvie Lamy, Simon Lord-Dufour, et al. January 15, 2009. "Antiproliferative and Antioxidant Activities of Common Vegetables: A Comparative Study." *Food Chemistry* 112(2): 374–380.

5. Ericson, U., E. Sonestedt, B. Gullberg, et al. August 2007. "High Folate Intake Is Associated with Lower Breast Cancer Incidence in Postmenopausal Women in the Malmö Diet and Cancer Cohort." *American Journal of Clinical Nutrition* 86(2): 434–443.

6. Lee, Sang-Ah, Jay H. Fowke, Wei Lu, et al. March 2008. "Cruciferous Vegetables, the GSTP1 Ile[105] Val Genetic Polymorphism, and Breast Cancer Risk." *American Journal of Clinical Nutrition* 87(3): 753–760.

7. Zhao, Hua, Jie Lin, H. Barton Grossman, et al. May 15, 2007. "Dietary Isothiocyanates, GSTM1, GSTT1, NAT2 Polymorphisms and Bladder Cancer Risk." *International Journal of Cancer* 120(10): 2208–2213.

8. Dosil-Diaz, Olga, Alberto Ruano-Ravina, J. Gestal-Otero, and Juan M. Barros-Dios. May 2008. "Consumption of Fruit and Vegetables and Risk of Lung Cancer: A Case-Control Study in Galicia, Spain." *Nutrition* 24(5): 407–413.

9. Kirsh, V. A., U. Peters, S. T. Mayne, et al. August 1, 2007. "Prospective Study of Fruit and Vegetable Intake and Risk of Prostate Cancer." *Journal of the National Cancer Institute* 99(15): 1200–1209.

10. Wannamethee, S. Goya, Gordon D. O. Lowe, Ann Rumley, et al. March 2006. "Associations of Vitamin C Status, Fruit and Vegetable Intakes, and Markers of Inflammation and Hemostasis." *The American Journal of Clinical Nutrition* 83(3): 567–574.

11. McCann, Joyce C. and Bruce N. Ames. October 2009. "Vitamin K, An Example of Triage Theory: Is Micronutrient Inadequacy Linked to Diseases of Aging?" *The American Journal of Clinical Nutrition* 90(4): 889–907.

12. Moeller, Suzen M., Rick Voland, Lesley Tinker, et al. March 2008. "Associations Between Age-Related Nuclear Cataract and Lutein and Zeaxanthin in the Diet and Serum in the Carotenoids in the Age-Related Eye Disease Study (CAREDS), an Ancillary Study of the Women's Health Initiative." *Archives of Ophthalmology* 126(3): 354–364.

REFERENCES AND RESOURCES
Magazines, Journals, and Newspapers

Boivin, Dominique, Sylvie Lamy, Simon Lord-Dufour, et al. January 15, 2009. "Antiproliferative and Antioxidant Activities of Common Vegetables: A Comparative Study." *Food Chemistry* 112(2): 374–380.

Dosil-Diaz, Olga, Alberto Ruano-Ravina, J. Gestal-Otero, and Juan M. Barros-Dios. May 2008. "Consumption of Fruit and Vegetables and Risk of Lung Cancer: A Case Control Study in Galicia, Spain." *Nutrition* 24(5): 407–413.

Ericson, U., E. Sonestedt, B. Gullberg, et al. August 2007. "High Folate Intake is Associated with Lower Breast Cancer Incidence in Postmenopausal Women in the Malmö Diet and Cancer Cohort." *American Journal of Clinical Nutrition* 86(2): 434–443.

Kirsh, V. A., U. Peters, S. T. Mayne, et al. August 1, 2007. "Prospective Study of Fruit and Vegetable Intake and Risk and Risk of Prostate Cancer." *Journal of the National Cancer Institute* 99(15): 1200–1209.

Lee, Sang-Ah, Jay H. Fowke, Wei Lu, et al. March 2008. "Cruciferous Vegetables, the GSTP1 Ile[105] Val Genetic Polymorphism, and Breast Cancer Risk." *American Journal of Clinical Nutrition* 87(3): 753–760.

McCann, Joyce C. and Bruce N. Ames. October 2009. "Vitamin K, An Example of Triage Theory: Is Micronutrient Inadequacy Linked to Diseases of Aging." *The American Journal of Clinical Nutrition* 90(4): 889–907.

Moeller, Suzen M., Rick Voland, Lesley Tinker, et al. March 2008. "Associations Between Age-Related Nuclear Cataract and Lutein and Zeaxanthin in the Diet and Serum in the Carotenoids in the Age-Related Eye Disease Study (CAREDS), an Ancillary Study of the Women's Health Initiative." *Archives of Ophthalmology* 126(3): 354–364.

Wannamethee, S. Goya, Gordon D.O. Lowe, Ann Rumley, et al. March 2006. "Associations of Vitamin C Status, Fruit and Vegetable Intakes, and Markers of Inflammation and Hemostasis." *The American Journal of Clinical Nutrition* 83(3): 567–574.

Zhao, Hua, Jie Lin, H. Barton Grossman, et al. May 15, 2007. "Dietary Isothiocya-
    nates, *GSTM1*, *GSTT1*, *NAT2* Polymorphisms and Bladder Cancer Risk."
    International Journal of Cancer 120(10): 2208–2213.

Websites

The George Mateljan Foundation. www.whfoods.com.
Nutrient Facts. nutrientfacts.com.

WALNUTS

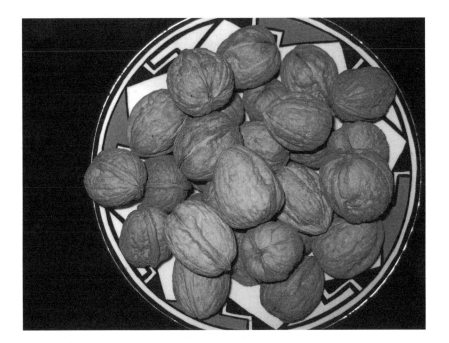

Walnuts are a truly ancient food. In fact, excavations in southwest France have found petrified walnut shells that are more than 8,000 years old.

By the 16th and 17th century, walnuts were viewed as a medicinal food. Because walnuts resembled human hearts and brains, they were believed to quell emotions and boost intelligence.[1] Today, the United States is one of the leading commercial producers of walnuts. Other producers include Turkey, China, Iran, France, and Romania.[2]

Walnuts are an excellent source of omega-3 fatty acids. In addition, they are a very good source of manganese and a good source of tryptophan.[3] But, what have researchers learned about them?

CARDIOVASCULAR HEALTH

In a study published in 2006 in the *Journal of the American College of Cardiology*, 12 healthy people and 12 people with high levels of cholesterol were randomly assigned to eat a high-fat meal (80 g of fat, 35 percent saturated fat) that included 40 g of walnuts or 30 g of olive oil. At the end of a week, the subjects repeated the study. This time, the subjects who ate walnuts consumed olive oil and the ones who consumed olive oil ate walnuts. The researchers found that after the people with high levels of cholesterol ate the meal with walnuts, the blood flow in the brachial arteries of their arms increased 24 percent. However, after they ate the meal with olive oil, there was a 36 percent decrease in blood flow. What does this mean? Apparently, walnuts were able to neutralize some of the detrimental aspects of a high-fat diet, which was not the case with olive oil. Still, the walnut and olive oil meals resulted in decreases in levels of cholesterol and triglycerides.[4] And, olive oil should be considered a food that supports cardiovascular health.

In a study published in 2007 in *Hypertension*, researchers calculated the amount of omega-3 polyunsaturated fatty acids (PFAs) in the diet of 4,680 men and women, between the ages of 40 and 59, living in Japan, China, the United Kingdom, and the United States. Of the four countries studied, people in Japan consumed the highest amounts of omega-3 PFAs, which are found in abundance in walnuts. And, people who consumed the most omega-3 PFAs had lower levels of systolic and diastolic blood pressure. The researchers concluded that "food omega-3 PFA intake related inversely to blood pressure, including in nonhypertensive persons, with small estimated effect size. Food omega-3 PFA may contribute to prevention and control of adverse blood pressure levels."[5]

In a study published in 2009 in *The American Journal of Clinical Nutrition*, Loma Linda University researchers compared the cholesterol-lowering abilities of walnuts and fatty fish. During a randomized crossover feeding trial, 25 subjects with normal to mild hyperlipidemia (elevated levels of cholesterol) consumed one of three diets, each for four weeks: a control diet containing no nuts or fish; a diet that included about 42.5 g of walnuts/day (about a handful); and, a diet in which subjects consumed 113 g of salmon twice/week.

The researchers found that, when compared to the control diet, the walnut diet lowered total cholesterol levels by more than five percent and LDL ("bad") cholesterol levels by more than nine percent. In addition to these findings, the researchers determined that the fatty fish diet decreased levels of triglyceride by 11.4 percent and HDL ("good") cholesterol by 4 percent. However, the fatty fish diet slightly increased levels of LDL cholesterol. Still, the researchers noted that it is a good idea to include both walnuts and fatty fish in the diet. Both foods support cardiovascular health.[6]

Two months later, in another study published in *The American Journal of Clinical Nutrition*, Harvard researchers analyzed 13 studies on the association between the consumption of walnuts and cardiovascular health. In total, there were 365 participants, and the diets lasted between 4 and 24 weeks; walnuts provided between 10 and 24 percent of total calories. The researchers found that, "high-walnut-enriched diets significantly decreased total and LDL cholesterol for the duration of the short-term trials." Yet, the researchers acknowledged that, "Larger and longer-term trials are needed to address the effects of walnut consumption on cardiovascular risk and body weight."[7]

Because people with diabetes are at increased risk for cardiovascular problems, researchers in Australia investigated whether walnuts could be a useful addition to their diets. In the study, published in 2004 in *Diabetes Care*, 58 men and women with type 2 diabetes, who had an average age of 59 years, ate one of three diets in which 30 percent of calories were obtained from fat: a low fat diet, a modified low-fat diet, and a modified low-fat diet that included daily consumption of one ounce of walnuts. At the end of six months, the subjects eating the diet that contained walnuts had a significantly higher increase in their HDL-to-total cholesterol ratio than the other groups. The walnut eaters also had a 10 percent reduction in their LDL cholesterol levels. So, simply by including a small amount of walnuts in their daily diets, these subjects saw improvements in their cardiovascular health.[8]

BREAST CANCER PREVENTION

In a study published in 2008 in *Nutrition and Cancer*, researchers at the Marshall University School of Medicine in West Virginia divided 22 mice with human breast cancer tumors into two groups. The diet of one group was supplemented with walnuts—the human equivalent of about two ounces a day; the diet of the other group was fed the control diet. After 35 days, the researchers noted that the breast tumors in the walnut supplemented group were only about half the size of the mice in the control group.[9] In a 2009 article in *Women's Health Weekly*, Elaine Hardman, PhD, the coresearcher of the study, noted, "It is clear that walnuts contribute to a healthy diet that can reduce breast cancer."[10]

WEIGHT CONTROL

In a randomized crossover trial published in 2005 in the *British Journal of Nutrition*, researchers placed 90 men and women, between the ages of 30 and 72, on two six-month diets. During one six-month period, the participants ate 1 to 1.5 ounces of walnuts every day; the other six-month period served as the control. The researchers found that during the six-month walnut phase, the average weight gain was less than a pound, an insignificant amount. The researchers noted that the regular consumption of walnuts "resulted in weight gain much lower than expected and which became non-significant after controlling for differences in energy intake."[11]

MEMORY

In a study published in 2009 in the *British Journal of Nutrition*, researchers at the USDA-ARS Human Nutrition Research Center on Aging at Tufts University in Boston randomly assigned aging weight-matched rats to one of four diet groups. For eight weeks, the rats were fed food that contained two percent, six percent, or nine percent walnuts or a walnut-free diet. After the feeding, they had a number of motor and memory tests. The researchers found that the rats that ate the two- and six-percent diets experienced improvements in age-related motor and cognitive difficulties. On the other hand, the nine-percent diet was associated with memory problems. The researchers commented that their findings "show for the first time that moderate dietary walnut supplementation can improve cognitive and motor performance in aged rats."[12]

Should walnuts be included in the diet? It certainly seems that a moderate intake of walnuts is beneficial.

NOTES

1. California Walnut Board Website. www.walnuts.org.

2. The George Mateljan Foundation Website. www.whfiids.com.

3. The George Mateljan Foundation Website.

4. Cortés, Berenice, Isabel Núñez, Montserrat Cofán, et al. October 17, 2006. "Acute Effects of High-Fat Meals Enriched with Walnuts or Olive Oil on Postprandial Endothelial Function." *Journal of the American College of Cardiology* 48(8): 1666–1671.

5. Ueshima, Hirotsugu, Jeremiah Stamler, Paul Elliott, et al. 2007. "Food Omega-3 Fatty Acid Intake of Individuals (Total, Linolenic Acid, Long-Chain) and Their Blood Pressure." *Hypertension* 50: 313–319.

6. Rajaram, Sujatha, Ella Hasso Haddad, Alfredo Majia, and Joan Sabaté. May 2009. "Walnuts and Fatty Fish Influence Different Serum Lipid Fractions in Normal to Mildly Hyperlipidemic Individuals: A Randomized Controlled Study." *The American Journal of Clinical Nutrition* 89(5): 1657S–1663S.

7. Banel, Deirdre K. and Frank B. Hu. July 2009. "Effects of Walnut Consumption on Blood Lipids and Other Cardiovascular Risk Factors: A Meta-Analysis and Systematic Review." *The American Journal of Clinical Nutrition* 90(1): 56–63.

8. Tapsell, Linda C., Lynda J. Gillen, Craig S. Patch, et al. December 2004. "Including Walnuts in a Low-Fat/Modified-Fat Diet Improves HDL Cholesterol-to-Total Cholesterol Ratios in Patients with Type 2 Diabetes." *Diabetes Care* 27(12): 2777–2783.

9. Hardman, W. Elaine and Gabriela Ion. September 5, 2008. "Suppression of Implanted MDA-MB 231 Human Breast Cancer Growth in Nude Mice by Dietary Walnut." *Nutrition and Cancer* 60: 666–674.

10. "Walnuts May Prevent Breast Cancer." May 7, 2009. *Women's Health Weekly*: 311.

11. Sabaté, Joan, Zaida Cordero-MacIntyre, Gina Siapco, et al. 2005. "Does Regular Walnut Consumption Lead to Weight Gain?" *British Journal of Nutrition* 94: 859–864.

12. Willis, Lauren M., Barbara Shukitt-Hale, Vivian Cheng, and James A. Joseph. 2009. "Dose-Dependent Effects of Walnuts on Motor and Cognitive Function in Aged Rats." *British Journal of Nutrition* 101: 1140–1144.

REFERENCES AND RESOURCES
Magazines, Journals, and Newspapers

Banel, Deirdre K. and Frank B. Hu. July 2009. "Effects of Walnut Consumption on Blood Lipids and Other Cardiovascular Risk Factors: A Meta-Analysis and Systematic Review." *The American Journal of Clinical Nutrition* 90(1): 56–63.

Cortés, Berenice, Isabel Núñez, Montserrat Cofán, et al. October 17, 2006. "Acute Effects of High-Fat Meals Enriched with Walnuts or Olive Oil on Postprandial Endothelial Function." *Journal of the American College of Cardiology* 48(8): 1666–1671.

Hardman, W. Elaine and Gabriela Ion. September 5, 2008. "Suppression of Implanted MDA-MB 231 Human Breast Cancer Growth in Nude Mice by Dietary Walnut." *Nutrition and Cancer* 60: 666–674.

Rajaram, Sujatha, Ella Hasso Haddad, Alfredo Mejia, and Joan Sabaté. May 2009. "Walnuts and Fatty Fish Influence Different Serum Lipid Fractions in Normal to Mildly Hyperlipidemic Individuals: A Randomized Controlled Study." *The American Journal of Clinical Nutrition* 89(5): 1657S–1663S.

Sabaté, Joan, Zaida Cordero-MacIntyre, Gina Siapco, et al. 2005. "Does Regular Walnut Consumption Lead to Weight Gain?" *British Journal of Nutrition* 94: 859–864.

Tapsell, Linda C., Lynda J. Gillen, Craig S. Patch, et al. December 2004. "Including Walnuts in a Low-Fat/Modified-Fat Diet Improves HDL Cholesterol-to-Total Cholesterol Ratios in Patients with Type 2 Diabetes." *Diabetes Care* 27(12): 2777–2783.

Ueshima, Hirotsugu, Jeremiah Stamler, Paul Elliott, et al. 2007. "Food Omega-3 Fatty Acid Intake of Individuals (Total, Linolenic Acid, Long-Chain) and Their Blood Pressure." *Hypertension* 50: 313–319.

"Walnuts May Prevent Breast Cancer." May 7, 2009. *Women's Health Weekly*: 311.

Willis, Lauren M., Barbara Shukitt-Hale, Vivian Cheng, and James A. Joseph. 2009. "Dose-Dependent Effects of Walnuts on Motor and Cognitive Function in Aged Rats." *British Journal of Nutrition* 101: 1140–1144.

Websites

California Walnut Board. www.walnuts.org.
The George Mateljan Foundation. www.whfoods.com.

GLOSSARY

Adenomas—a benign tumor formed from cells lining the inside of a surface or organ

Amino acids—building blocks of protein

Anthocyanins—antioxidant flavonoids that protect many systems of the body

Antihypertensive drug—medication to lower elevated blood pressure

Antioxidants—substances that protect cells against the actions of free radicals

Antiproliferative—pertaining to the use of a substance or substances to inhibit the growth of malignant cells

Apigenin—a class of flavonoid, a phytonutrient (plant compound) with high antioxidant activity

Apoptosis—cell death

Atherosclerosis—hardening of the arteries

Atopy—genetic tendency to develop classic allergic diseases

Benign prostatic hyperplasia—enlargement of the prostate gland (only in men)

Beta-carotene—a type of carotenoid

Beta-glucans—naturally occurring polysaccharides found in foods such as cereal and mushrooms

Body mass index (BMI)—measure of body fat based on height and weight

Brassica—any plant of the genus *Brassica* of the mustard family, including broccoli and cabbage

Carotenoids—highly pigmented fat-soluble compounds naturally present in many foods

Cataract—the clouding of the natural lens of the eye (lens is located behind the iris and pupil)

Catechins—flavonoid phytochemical compounds that are primarily found in green tea

Cholecystectomy—surgical removal of the gallbladder

Coagulation—process in which the blood forms clots

Colonoscopy—a medical procedure in which a long, flexible instrument, a colonoscope, is used to view the entire inner lining of the large intestine (colon) and rectum

Coronary artery disease—narrowing of the heart arteries

C-reactive protein—a measure of inflammation; higher amounts may be seen in individuals at increased risk for cardiovascular disease

Cruciferous vegetables—also called brassica vegetables, a family of vegetables that includes broccoli, Brussels sprouts, cabbage, cauliflower, collard greens, kale, and turnips

Cytoplasm—all the contents of a cell outside of the nucleus and enclosed within the cell membrane

De novo—a Latin expression meaning "from the beginning"

Diurnal animal—an animal that is active during the day and sleeps at night

DNA adduct—a piece of DNA covalently bonded to a cancer-causing chemical; the start of a cancer cell

Docosahexaenoic (DNA)—an omega-3 fatty acid found in algae and fish oil

Dyslipidemia—abnormal fats in the blood

Eccentric exercise—exercise in which the contracting muscle is forcibly lengthened

Endothelium—inner lining of blood vessels

Fatty acids—acids produced when fats are broken down; may be saturated, polyunsaturated, or monounsaturated

Flavanones—the dominant flavonoid class in the genus citrus

Flavonoids—also known as bioflavonoids; flavonoids are polyphenol antioxidants found in plants

Free radicals—highly reactive oxygen molecules that are a by-product of normal metabolism

Gastric dysrhythmia—abnormal electrical activity of the stomach

Gastrocnemius muscle—muscle in the back part of the leg that makes up the greater part of the calf

Glucosinolates—a group of secondary plants occurring especially in brassica vegetables such as cabbage

Hemostasis—the stoppage of bleeding

High-density lipoprotein (HDL)—good cholesterol

High-glycemic foods or high glycemic index—carbohydrates that release energy quickly and result in fluctuations in blood glucose and insulin levels

Hemorrhagic stroke—stroke cause by the bursting of a blood vessel inside the brain

Homocysteine—an amino acid; higher amounts of it in the blood have been associated with increased risk for cardiovascular disease

Hydrolysis—chemical reaction of compounds with water

Hypercholesterolemia or hypercholesterol—elevated levels of cholesterol

Hyperglycemia—high concentrations of glucose in the blood, usually associated with diabetes

Hyperlipidemia—elevated levels of cholesterol

Hypertension—high blood pressure

Hyperuricemia—abnormally high levels of uric acid in the blood

Hypocitraturia—low amount of citrate in the urine, a risk factor for kidney stone formation

Immunoglobulin E (IgE)—the primary antibody associated with an allergic response

Indole-3-carbinol—phytochemical derived from cruciferous vegetables, such as broccoli and cabbage

Inflammatory polyarthritis—rheumatoid arthritis

Insulin sensitivity—the body's ability to use glucose, a sugar

Ischemic heart disease—when the heart is receiving insufficient amounts of blood and oxygen

Ischemic stroke—stroke caused by blockage of artery in the brain

Isocaloric—having similar caloric value

Isoflavones—a type of phytoestrogen (plant estrogen) found primarily in soybeans

Isothiocyanate—compound found in cruciferous vegetables that is believed to have anti-cancer properties

Lignans—phytoestrogens that have estrogenic and anti-cancer properties

Low-density liproprotein (LDL)—bad cholesterol

Low-glycemic foods or low glycemic index—foods that release energy slowly

Luteolin—a flavonoid found in high concentrations in celery and green pepper

Metabolic syndrome—a cluster of health problems that include insulin resistance, abnormal blood fats, and borderline or elevated blood pressure; associated with chronic diseases such as cardiovascular disease and diabetes

Metabolite—any substance produced or used during metabolism (digestion)

Methionine—a sulfur-containing essential amino acid

Monosaccharide—a sugar that may no longer be broken down into simpler sugars by hydrolysis

Myocardial infarction—heart attack

Neovascular age-related macular degeneration—also called wet age-related macular degeneration; it is the more serious form of the disease that causes a loss of central vision

Neurons—nerve cells

Nifedipine—a class of drugs called calcium channel blockers that lower blood pressure by relaxing (widening) blood vessels

Obesogenic diet—a diet that fosters obesity

Orchidectomy—removal of the testes

Osteopenia—bones that have a bone marrow density that is lower than normal but not low enough to be classified as osteoporosis

Osteoporosis—a disease in which bones become more fragile and are at increased risk of breaking

Ovariectomy—surgical removal of one or both ovaries

Oxalate—naturally occurring organic acids found in humans, plants, and animals

Periodontitis—a serious gum infection that kills soft tissue and bones that support teeth

Peripheral artery disease—a build-up of fatty tissues in leg arteries resulting in the impairment of blood flow

Phytochemicals—plants compounds found in dark fruits and vegetables that are believed to have health-protecting qualities

Phytoestrogens—naturally occurring plant compounds that are thought to have a number of different health benefits

Phytosterol—a plant-based compound that lowers levels of cholesterol in the blood

Polyphenols—phytochemicals that give fruits and vegetables their colors and appear to have strong health benefits

Polysaccharide—a carbohydrate that may be broken down by hydrolysis into two or more molecules of monosaccharides

Prostatectomy—surgical removal or all or part of the prostate

Pterostilbene—a naturally occurring antioxidant in blueberries

Reperfusion—restoration of blood flow to an organ or tissue

Sham operation—a placebo surgical procedure

TBARS—thiobarbituric acid-reactive substances assay; a measure of oxidative stress

Tocopherol—a class of compounds, many of which have vitamin E activity

Trabecular bone—tissue inside bones that resembles a sponge

Tryptophan—an amino acid well-known to foster drowsiness

Tumoricidal—destructive to tumor cells

Ultraviolet light—radiation lying in the ultraviolet range: the wave lengths are shorter than light but longer than x-rays

Uric acid (urate)—a chemical created when the body breaks down purines, which are found in foods such as wine, beer, dried beans, and peas

INDEX

About the Authors

MYRNA CHANDLER GOLDSTEIN has been a freelance writer and independent scholar for two decades. Her website is "Doing Good, While Doing Business: Support Socially Responsible Companies" (www.changethemold .com). Her published works include Greenwood's *Boys into Men*, *Controversies in the Practice of Medicine*, and *Food and Nutrition Controversies Today*.

MARK A. GOLDSTEIN, MD, is Chief, Division of Adolescent and Young Adult Medicine at Massachusetts General Hospital, and assistant Professor of Pediatrics at Harvard Medical School.